Volume 1

The School Nurse's Source Book of Individualized Healthcare Plans

A Compendium of I.H.P.s Covering the Most Frequently Encountered Chronic and Acute Health Issues

Foreword by
Judith B. Igoe

Marykay B. Haas, Editor

Mary J. Villars Gerber
Kathleen M. Kalb
Ruth Ellen Luehr

Wanda R. Miller
Cynthia K. Silkworth
Susan I.S. Will

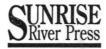

x

The publisher and authors have made a conscientious effort to ensure any recommendations or procedures outlined in this book are proper, accurate and in accordance with accepted school nursing practices at the time of publication. As is the case with health care in general and school nursing in particular, each specific health issue and each individual in question combine to form a unique situation, not easily addressed at a distance nor from the pages of a book designed to provide generic information on a wide range of subjects. While this work provides recognized structures, processes and procedures, it is mandatory for the reader to realize that recommendations found within this book are not a substitute for professional on-site assessments and recommendations. The publisher and authors make no representations or warranties of any kind regarding the materials in this work nor shall they be liable for any damages resulting, in whole or in part, from the use of or reliance upon this material.

Haas, Marykay B., 1947–
    The school nurse's source book of individualized healthcare plans
    Marykay B. Haas.
        p.   cm.
    Includes bibliographical references and index.
    ISBN 0-9624814-1-6 (softbound): $39.95
    1. School nursing.   2. Nursing care plans.   I. Title.
    [DNLM: 1. Nursing Assessment—in infancy & childhood.   2. Nursing Care—in infancy & childhood.   3. School Nursing—methods.   WY 113   H112s]
    RJ247.H32   1993
    610.73'62—dc20
    DNLM/DLC
    for Library of Congress   92-48666
                                                                                                CIP

For additional copies of this work, contact:
Sunrise River Press, 11481 Kost Dam Rd.
North Branch, MN 55056, 612-583-3239

Contributors

Marykay B. Haas, R.N.C., M.P.H.

Marykay Haas is currently employed by the Minnesota Department of Education. She holds a dual master's degree in both Public Health Nursing and Maternal-Child Health. She is currently adjunct faculty at the University of Minnesota and the University of Colorado. She was a school nurse with the St. Paul, MN school district and a faculty member of the University of Minnesota, School of Nursing, before joining the Department of Education staff.

Mary J. Villars Gerber, R.N., B.S.N.

Formerly Lead School Nurse, District 916, North East Metro Technical Institute, White Bear Lake, Minnesota

Kathleen M. Kalb, R.N.C., M.S., C.P.N.P.

Child/Adolescent Health Consultant, Minnesota Department of Health, Minneapolis, Minnesota

Ruth Ellen Luehr, M.S., R.N.

Prevention/Risk Reduction Specialist, Minnesota Department of Education, St. Paul, Minnesota. Adjunct faculty, School of Public Health and School of Nursing, University of Minnesota, Minneapolis, Minnesota

Wanda R. Miller, R.N., S.N.P., M.A.

Administrator, Student Wellness, St. Paul Public Schools, St. Paul, Minnesota. National Association of School Nurses, Past President

Cynthia K. Silkworth, M.P.H., R.N., C.S.N.P.

School Nurse, White Bear Lake Public Schools, White Bear Lake, Minnesota. Community Faculty, Metropolitan State University, St. Paul, Minnesota

Susan I. Simandl Will, R.N., M.P.H.

School Nurse, St. Paul Schools, St. Paul Minnesota. Community Faculty, Metropolitan State University, St. Paul, Minnesota

Acknowledgements

First and most importantly thanks to our families and friends who gave us uninterrupted time, space and encouragement to pursue this project.

Thanks to all of our school nursing colleagues in Minnesota, your questions and feedback have been invaluable.

A special thanks to members of our study group, Kay Williams, Betty Nowicki, Patty Rezabek and Jean Brown for their input into the planning of this project and encouraging support.

Thanks to our publishers Dave, and school nursing colleague, Martha Arnold who believed that this book was worth the extra effort of having to deal with seven authors.

Thanks to the staff of the Minnesota Department of Health library for helping all Minnesota school nurses with literature searches and document retrieval for many years. This backup was invaluable as none of us are professional researchers.

Finally we thank and dedicate this book to the thousands of children and families that we have had the opportunity to serve. You have taught us much and it is your trust in us that makes school nursing more than just a job.

December 1992

Contents

Foreword

The health needs of school children have dramatically changed in recent years. More and more students now come to schools acutely and chronically ill, with serious emotional troubles and with special healthcare needs. School administrators are also noting that many students come from such severely fractured families, that any type of healthcare is viewed as low priority. Consequently, school nurses struggle daily to provide diagnosis and treatment services and/or referral to scarce community agencies. At the same time, busy professionals who are also parents, are urging school officials to offer school-based, one-stop shopping for a wide range of health and social services for their children as well as themselves.

National commissions; federal, state, and local agencies; professional associations; and advocacy organizations for children and parents are unanimous in their recommendations that school health programs must improve. More resources must be found or existing resources must be better utilized.

The impact of the school health reform movement will be enormous for school nurses. Opportunities and challenges will abound in the decades to come. Among the first priorities will be the design of more integrated school health systems that will closely connect with community health agencies so all students will have ready access to primary healthcare. Equally important will be the further development and refinement of the school nurse role. As the future calls on all of us to become more accountable for our school nursing practice, practical, sound reference materials must be available.

The School Nurse's Source Book of Individualized Healthcare Plans is the first text to come to my attention which contains the clinical information that school nurses must have to fully function as health professionals in the school setting. This comprehensive reference contains:

- A review of pathophysiology related to the health problem and/or a description of current knowledge about the condition in children.
- A comprehensive list of history questions and assessment areas.
- A selection of pertinent NANDA approved nursing diagnoses.
- A selection of appropriate nursing and/or student goals.
- A full range of applicable nursing interventions.
- A list of expected student outcomes.

This text provides a systematic organized way to use the nursing process in the formulation of unique individualized healthcare plans (IHPs). At the same time specific assessment tools, checklists, and questions have been designed to ensure the development of comprehensive, first-rate IHPs covering forty of the most commonly encountered health issues. As school nurses begin to routinely use this reference, we will, for the first time in the history of school nursing, have a framework for documenting the impact of this type of practice in a standardized fashion.

The authors of this text represent, as a team, the best in school nursing. They understand precisely what school nurses face on a day-to-day basis because of their own experiences in the field. With this background, the authors have compiled an easy-to-use, scholarly guide that will assist school nurses in the preparation of written documents required for improved student health care, special education regulations, third party reimbursement and performance audits for quality assurance.

The goal of this reference work is to provide specific and detailed "how-to" directions concerning the formulation of IHPs designed to fit unique student health issues. I commend the authors for this achievement and for the contribution they have made to the advanced practice of school nursing.

Judith B. Igoe, R.N., M.S., F.A.A.N.
Associate Professor/Director

School Health Programs
School of Nursing

University of Colorado Health Sciences Center

Denver

Preface

As school nurses across the country look for ways to plan, describe, document, and evaluate the nursing care delivered to children in schools, tools such as Individualized Healthcare Plans (IHPs) are gaining in popularity. The primary factor influencing school nurses to look for tools such as the IHP is the increase in medically fragile and chronically ill children who are being mainstreamed into regular education settings. In the past many children with special healthcare needs would have been institutionalized, hospitalized in intensive care units or sent to special schools.

The passage of P.L. 94-142 and Section 504 of the Rehabilitation Act over ten years ago and the more recent passage of P.L. 99-457 and P.L. 101-476, the Individuals with Disabilities Education Act (IDEA) 1990, have provided access to school for children with chronic and handicapping conditions. The case has been made and demonstrated that every child has the ability to learn and to benefit from school. The challenge for the present is to integrate children with special healthcare needs into the regular school setting. This means schools have to modify and adapt the environment and program to safely and effectively accommodate children with chronic and handicapping conditions.

The challenges facing today's schools are enormous. The "new morbidity" means that the old communicable disease control problems that have challenged schools in the past have turned into today's challenges which encompass mental health and lifestyle issues, new communicable diseases, and chronic disease.

From wheelchair accessible classrooms to skilled gastrostomy feedings to complex medical regimens, the school nurse will be challenged to interpret the child's needs, recommend safe procedures, provide direct skilled nursing care such as treatments, and document the planning, interventions, and outcomes to be attained from the nursing care. For some school nurses this will represent a need to develop not only a more efficient means to plan and deliver care, but also stronger case management skills. The school nurse is in an ideal position to *coordinate* the care that a child with a chronic health condition is receiving from many different providers.

Legal Factors

While some educators have been involved in providing nursing care to students with or without appropriate nursing supervision, there is growing reticence among teachers to do nursing care as the complexity of that care increases and education funding tightens. Some teachers' organizations have also started to consider the legal liabilty issues when teachers are allowed to carry out healthcare functions for which they have little or no formal training.[1] Teachers' organizations frequently offer liability coverage for teachers, but most policies were not designed to cover the medical and nursing care that some teachers are now being asked to provide to students.

Most state nurse practice acts regulate the practice of nursing by requiring a license to sell certain nursing services to the public. School nurses are advised to obtain and read their state's nurse practice act. School nurses should become familiar with how their state nurse practice act covers the following points.

- Defines nursing practice
- Describes what nursing care can be delegated and/or the conditions under which nursing care can be delegated
- Defines the qualifications for persons providing nursing care
- Specifies the means and/or responsibility to report the unlicensed practice of nursing to the state board of nursing or other agency.
- Defines inappropriate delegation as a cause for disciplinary action

School nurses must become increasingly aware of how state nurse practice acts regulate school nursing. Failure to do this may result in litigation and/or loss of one's nursing license.

Other guides to practice include documents developed by specialty organizations. For example, The Standards of School Nursing Practice (1983) jointly published by the National Association of School Nurses, American Public Health Association, American School Health Association, American Nurses Association, National Association of Pediatric Nurse Associates and Practitioners, and National Association of State School Nurse Consultants.[2]

History

The term "Individualized Healthcare Plan" (IHP) comes from The Standards of School Nursing Practice (1983). Traditionally, hospital care plans provided a summary of the patient's history, diagnosis, doctor's orders, patient needs, and directions to the nursing staff describing the nursing care to be provided. The development of nursing as a profession has encouraged nurses to use the nursing process to expand the "nursing care" portion of the care plan to include: nursing assessment, nursing diagnosis, nursing interventions, and nursing outcomes. IHPs are the application and formalization of the nursing process in the school setting. An IHP should include information about client needs, nursing interventions designed to meet those needs, and a description of how this care supports the educational process of the school.

School nurses have been somewhat reluctant to carry the technical nursing language into the school setting. For some nurses this has meant a decreased ability to think about students as needing "nursing care." While it is probably not a good idea to use technical nursing jargon with educators, it is essential that school nurses continue to "think" nursing care as they work with students, especially those with complex healthcare needs. The school nurse's license as a nurse demands that the nurses continue to use and upgrade their nursing knowledge. In addition, school administrators hire school nurses because of their specialized knowledge and skill. Finally, school nurses are accountable to the public and the client for the adequacy of the care provided.

Nursing Care Plans as Guides

While most nurses have the education and experience to provide safe care in a supervised setting such as a doctor's office, clinic, or hospital, the provision of nursing care in school settings requires a different level of knowledge and skill. Nurses in independent settings such as schools must formulate nursing care plans without the formal structure of a healthcare institution's policies and procedures. In addition, the nurse is frequently the only healthcare professional in the school setting and must therefore make independent assessments about student needs and services.

Because of the daily contact school nurses have with children they are frequently the best case managers for these students as well. School nurses see the day-to-day variations in student needs and are often the first to notice important changes in the student's condition.

Resources like this book can provide assistance in formulating healthcare plans. However, they cannot substitute for the nursing judgement required to assess, plan, and implement nursing interventions for a particular student with a unique set of needs. The healthcare plans found in this book must be individualized based on an assessment of student information and needs. These standardized care plans are intended only as a **guide** to assist in planning for students with similar conditions.

Only the professional nurse working with a particular student can make a determination as to whether the suggested interventions are appropriate for a particular student.

REFERENCES

1. *The Medically Fragile Child in the School Setting: A Resource Guide for the Educational Team*, 1992. Available from the American Federation of Teachers, 555 Jersey Ave NW Washington, DC 20001.

2. American Nurses Association, American Public Health Association, American School Health Association, National Association of Pediatric Nurse Associates and Practitioners, National Association of School Nurses and National Association of State School Nurse Consultants. *Standards of School Nursing Practice.*. 1983. Available from the American Nurses Association, 2420 Pershing Rd, Kansas City, MO 64208.

Using the Nursing Process in the School Setting

Ruth Ellen Luehr

The nursing process is a way to describe nurses' systematic approach to understanding and dealing with the health needs of their clients—individuals, families, or communities. The nursing process organizes the work and practice of nursing into sequential steps. It outlines a knowledgeable, purposeful series of thoughts and actions that are carried out with and/or for the client.

Nursing process steps are assessment (collection of data and nursing diagnosis), planning, intervention/implementation, and evaluation. Similar to other systematic problem-solving approaches, these nursing process steps parallel the phases used in basic scientific research, teaching, medicine, and counseling and other physical and behavioral sciences.

"The public most clearly sees the intervention or treatment step of the nursing process during which the nurse is either giving direct care to the client or providing health teaching to the client. The public therefore, often mistakenly assumes that the performance of specific tasks is the essence of the practice of nursing."[1]

The steps of assessment, planning, intervention/implementation, and evaluation are discrete and sequential. Yet in actual practice these approaches are used concurrently and recurrently to meet the variety of needs of an individual student and the community of students in a school.[2]

Application of the Nursing Process in School Nursing

The nursing process is the framework that guides nursing practice in all settings. The nursing process is the cornerstone of standards of the profession (*Standards of Nursing Practice*, ANA, 1973; *Standards of Clinical Nursing Practice*, ANA, 1991 [See Supplement 1 at the end of this chapter]; *Implementation Guide for the Standards of School Nursing Practice*, ASHA, 1991). "Regardless of the setting, a professional nurse goes through a systematic process of assessing a situation, deciding what is occurring, deciding what to do, doing it, and mentally reviewing the success of the entire undertaking" writes Proctor in *Guidelines for a Model School Nursing Services Program*.[3] Adhering to the standards of practice—including the nursing process—is considered an ethical responsibility of all nurses. (See Supplement 2 at the end of this chapter for the Code for Nurses [ANA, 1985] and Code of School Nursing Practice [NASN, 1990].) For the specialty practice of school nursing, the *Standards of School Nursing Practice* present the guiding principles. Standard III describes how the nursing process applies in the school setting (see Table 1). (See Supplement 3 for all eight School Nursing Standards statements).

School nurses apply the nursing process when working with students, families, and school faculty in a variety of situations and environments. In any given day, a school nurse manages dozens of encounters with students whose problems are increasingly complex and diverse, providing direct specialized health procedures in school in more and more cases. During the same day a school nurse may participate in individual planning sessions for one or more students, draft health policies for the district, teach staff or students, and conduct home-based interviews.

School nurses' interventions are systematic. Due to the hectic pace of typical school health offices, school nurses' interactions with individuals or groups seem to be spontaneous, routine, or second-nature. With experience and continuous upgrading of knowledge and skills, school nurses are very efficient, methodical, and precise in their practice. But the school nurse's interventions are not simply automatic responses. Given time to describe each interaction with students, even brief encounters, school nurses articulate the nursing process steps—including the comprehensive assessments made, the theoretical basis for conclusions, the rationale for plans, and the effect of each interaction.

School nurses' interventions are individualized for each student. Here are some issues school nurses take into account when individualizing the assessment, planning, and intervention steps: student's and family's perceptions of the problem, capacity to deal with a given issue at the time, experiences with solving similar problems, developmental stage, resources he/she has in terms of skills and knowledge, family situation and its positive or negative impact on the problem, resources in the school, and expectations for the future. If all nursing plans and interventions are unique to each student, what is the purpose of having model Individualized

Healthcare Plans (IHPs)? There are common issues that can be outlined and used as a checklist to ensure that a plan is complete, that all variables are considered. But each plan needs to be modified—individualized—for each student. The model IHPs are not prescriptions but are to be used as a draft or template in assessment and planning for a student with special needs.

School nurses view each student holistically. The primary responsibility of the public school system is to provide students with an education. "Students in the school system often have needs to be met, in addition to their normal learning needs. The student enters the school system as a whole being, not just a mind to be educated."[1] A school nurse's skill is in identifying the meaning or impact of a given problem in the context of other life variables—crises or successes for the family, school or community events, friendships and pressures of school or work. This concept of viewing the student holistically is embedded in how school nurses develop their nursing diagnoses. As discussed in the next chapter, an element of the nursing diagnosis statement is the "life response"—the "so what"—the impact of the condition of the whole child.

The student is a partner in implementing the nursing process—an active, not passive, participant in the assessment, problem solving, planning, and evaluation phases in school nursing practice. This participation ensures that the goals meet the student's needs, supports him/her taking increasing responsibility, and increases the student's investment, thereby increasing the likelihood of success in meeting the goals. By being integrally involved, the student not only experiences the success of problem resolution, but also learns the skills of problem solving.

The focus of school nursing practice is enhancement of students' capacity for learning, growing, and developing. Therefore, the first phase of the nursing process

Table 1. Standards of School Nursing Practice, 1983

STANDARD III. Nursing Process

The nursing process includes individualized health plans which are developed by the school nurse.

A. Collection of Data

The school nurse collects information about the health and developmental status of students in a systematic and continuous manner.

B. Nursing Diagnosis

The nurse uses data collected about the health and educational status of the student to determine a nursing diagnosis.

C. Planning

The nurse develops a nursing care plan with specific goals and interventions delineating school nursing actions unique to student needs.

D. Intervention

The nurse intervenes as guided by the nursing care plan to implement actions that promote, maintain, or restore health, prevent illness, and effect rehabilitation.

E. Evaluation

The nurse assesses student responses to nursing actions in order to revise the data base, nursing diagnosis, and nursing care plan and to determine progress made toward goal achievement.

The Standards I, II and IV—VIII address theory, program management, interdisciplinary collaboration, health education, professional development, community health systems and research. (See Supplement 3)

Authored by American Nurses Association, American Public Health Association, American School Health Association, National Association of Pediatric Nurse Associates and Practitioners, National Association of School Nurses, National Association of State School Nurse Consultants.

Reprinted, with permission, from *Standards of School Nursing Practice*,[7] pp. 5-11.

addresses these goals: 1) Gain a better understanding of the nature of a student's health problem and the impact on learning; 2) Remedy the effects of the problem on learning by adjustment in the medical plan, nutrition, or activity; 3) Increase a student's self-care skills; 4) Identify ways to alter teaching/learning strategies to increase the effectiveness of learning; 5) Identify ways to alter the educational environment—physical or psychosocial—to resolve problems that would interfere, distract, or disturb the learner; and 6) Create and sustain a supportive environment for the student/family. Often several of these goals are considered when addressing a given problem, leading to an integrated and comprehensive plan of services and education.[4]

Some situations in which school nurses apply the nursing process include: 1) All individual encounters with students episodes of acute illness or injury, health education, addressing problems related to the learning process and/or the learning environment; 2) Focusing on any aspect of health—physical, developmental, emotional, and interpersonal; 3) When carrying out a variety of nursing functions—diagnostic, therapeutic, educative, and supportive; 4) When working with groups or with individuals; 5) Planning and evaluating school building or district-wide health services and educational programs; 6) Evaluation and development of one's professional practice.[5]

Another way to describe school nursing practice is to define the roles of school nurses. In each of the roles, the nursing process is the organizing framework for determining what to do when. The roles of school nurses, according to Proctor, are provider of client care, communicator, planner and coordinator of client care, health teacher, and investigator.[3] For a chart that shows the relationship between these roles and the Standards of School Nursing Practice, see Table 2.

Nursing Process Steps

The preceding section lists a number of school nursing scenarios, roles, and settings where the nursing process is applied. In this section, the steps in the nursing process are described and the role of the school nurse as coordinator and planner of client care is emphasized. Documentation of the nursing process is explained in references to the problem/progress-oriented pupil health record.

The nursing process steps are assessment (collection of data and nursing diagnosis), planning, intervention/implementation, and evaluation. Each step relates to codes in the problem/progress-oriented documentation format called SOAPIER (see Tables 3 and 4). The first three letters refer to the assessment step and organize the data collected into subjective (S) and objective (O) information. Conclusions from the data analysis, the nursing diagnoses, are recorded by (A) assessment. The second step is recorded under (P) for plan. Interventions (I) and evaluation (E) conclude the recording of the nursing process.

For each phase of the nursing process pertinent questions guide assessment, intervention, and evaluation as illustrated in Table 4. The chart also includes the steps in the development of the Individualized Education Plan (IEP) for comparison.[6]

Assessment: Data Collection and Nursing Diagnosis

The first phase, assessment, includes collecting and analyzing pertinent information. The school nurse then makes a professional judgement about the information and formulates nursing diagnoses.

Data collection and interviewing are an art and a science. Key skills include selecting questions, measurement instruments, and observations that are relevant and provide an accurate description of the presenting situation or issue.[5] When col-

Table 2. School Nurse Roles, Standards and Goals

ROLES [capitalized] and related STANDARDS [numerals]	GOALS
COORDINATOR and Planner/Manager • Program Management (V) • Interdisciplinary Collaboration (VI) • Community Health Systems (VII)	Participate in the planning, implementation, and evaluation of a school health program.
PROVIDER of Client Care/Counselor • Theory (I) • Nursing Process (III) • Program Management (II)	Deliver needed health services to the client system utilizing systematic processes to assess needs, plan interventions, and evaluate outcomes so that high-level wellness can be achieved. Provide health counseling and guidance for the client system on an individual basis or within a group setting
COMMUNICATOR/Advocate • Interdisciplinary Collaboration (IV) • Community Health Systems (VII)	Act as an advocate for the health rights of children and their families both within the school setting and between the school and the community at large
HEALTH TEACHER/Educator • Health Education (V)	Participate in health education program activities for children, youth, school personnel, and the community.
INVESTIGATOR • Research (VIII)	
ROLE WITHIN THE DISCIPLINE OF NURSING • Professional Development (VI)	

Adapted with permission, from following sources:
ROLES: Proctor.[3]
STANDARDS: ANA et al.[7]
GOALS: Wold SJ., Dagg, NV. Philosophy, roles and goals of school nursing. In: Wold, SJ.,[2] p22.

Table 3. Problem/Progress-Oriented Method of Documentation

Documentation	Nursing Process Step
S: Subjective data	
O: Objective data	ASSESSMENT
A: Assessment/Nursing diagnosis	
P: Plan	PLAN
I: Implementation	INTERVENTION/IMPLEMENTATION
E: Evaluation	EVALUATION

lecting data, school nurses identify a range of data sources so a complete picture of the situation can be assessed and so information from one source can be confirmed or complemented by a second source. It is also critical for school nurses to use discretion in choosing the data sources for the issue at hand. This conserves resources in terms of time and energy, but, more importantly, respects the privacy of the student and family by not asking them to divulge information not pertinent to the current problem. Many times the school nurse learns facts or gains insight that is useful in problem solving with the student and/or family members, but may not be necessary for the education of the student so should not be shared with other educators. In fact, the school nurse is restricted by legal and ethical guidelines from divulging information without parental permission, and even with consent, the school nurse is called upon to use discretion.

The primary source of data is the student—even young children. The first order of business is discussing with the student the nature of the problems and the relevance of that problem to his/her school experience. The family is then asked the same questions.

Some questions include: perception of the problem; attitudes toward personal health problem; attitudes toward school and learning; perception of academic progress; schedule of daily activities including classes, transportation, and work; the environment at school, home, and neighborhood; attendance; relationships with peers; and extracurricular activities. A second valuable data source is the Pupil/Student Health Record or other school sources of previous developmental, psychological, and special learning and behavior problem assessments. Relevant data should also be obtained with permission of the student/family from the physician or other healthcare providers.

Given this foundation of student/family perceptions and past records, the next step is to collect new information through pertinent, focused questions about health and developmental history, current health status, and current health practices. Next are physical assessment/measurements including sensory functions (vision and hearing), physical assessment, neurologic assessment, and growth (height and weight—graphed). Developmental assessment is also an important measure. Family circumstances that may positively or nega-

Table 4. The Nursing Practice as Applied to School Nursing Practice

| Steps | NURSING PROCESS | | SPECIAL EDUCATION PROCESS |
	Documentation Format	Pertinent Questions	
ASSESSMENT	S: Subjective data	For individuals, what does the client and family think and say? For groups and communities, what do the members think and say?	Student's and family's perception of the problem at staffings
Data Collection	O: Objective data	What is observed, measured and reported? What are the pertinent norms and standards?	Teacher referrals Child study team assessment activities
Diagnosis	A: Assessment	According to the nurse's perception and judgement, what is happening? What are the concerns? What is the resulting impact? Diagnosis = problem + etiology + response	Child study team's identification of the problems and goals Statement of the student's level of educational functioning
INTERVENTION Plan	P: Plan	What are the desired outcomes? What action will be taken? (educational, therapeutic, diagnostic, supportive) by whom? when? how? What behaviors will be measured?	Individualized Education Plan IEP Goals Objectives
Implementation	I: Implementation	Who is carrying out the plan? What agencies and others are involved?	Instructional Implementation Plan IIP
EVALUATION	E: Evaluation	Have the desired outcomes been achieved according to the set criteria?	Evaluation according to measurements and review dates incorporated into objectives
	R: Reassessment	Is more information needed? Have changes or adaptations occurred?	Review staffing
	Plan	Have priorities changed? Does the plan or implementation method need revision?	
	Reevaluation	What are the new strategies? next steps?	

Reprinted, with permission, from *Goals of School Nursing, An Interpretive Tool,*[6] *Appendix II*

tively affect the situation are essential, too, and include family structure, family function, and family health. A very important element is teacher observation; relevant information ranges from a student's academic performance to his/her attitude toward learning. Teachers are valuable historians, recalling changes in a student's behavior over time, and providing a normative perspective—how this student is alike or different in comparison with his/her peers. Finally, the school nurse and/or other child study team members' observations are valuable when completing the data collection phase. As a reminder, parental permission for health assessment activities is required, as is permission to gain information from the student's/family's healthcare providers. See Table 5 for an outline of essential baseline information.

Data analysis and nursing diagnoses are only as accurate as the data base. Data collection must be "comprehensive, accurate, systematic and continuous to allow the school nurse to reach sound conclusions and plan appropriate interventions."[7]

In the problem-oriented method of record-keeping, data are recorded as follows: S: Subjective Data—Statements by the client and family; O: Objective data—Information that the school nurse observes directly or obtains from valid sources.[5]

Data analysis is the process of interpreting the findings of the data collection process. Information is compared to norms and standards (e.g., developmental milestones, nursing theories and concepts, references from clinical experiences, and so on). The student's and family's strengths and weaknesses are also reviewed from the perception of the parent/student and from the perception of the nurse. A comprehensive approach is taken, integrating each finding with all others to reach conclusions about the student's educational, developmental, and health needs.[5]

What are some potential results of the data collection and analysis? How do the results guide or determine the next steps? Igoe[8] proposes the following range of conclusions: 1) No problem exists. The child/adolescent is well. Nursing diagnosis would focus on wellness and could propose health promotion measures. Nursing interventions could focus on anticipatory guidance—predicting and planning for changes in the child/adolescent or family; building knowledge and skills to sustain and enhance health; guaranteeing continued health maintenance visits to healthcare providers; ensuring access to resources when needed, and so on. 2) The data indicate a problem could exist in the future; this situation would require further assessment, anticipatory guidance, and/or health education. 3) An existing problem is being managed successfully by the student and/or his/her family. Nursing interventions could focus on sustaining support systems and anticipatory guidance. 4) A problem exists that requires intervention. 5) A problem exists that calls for further study and diagnosis to be resolved or managed successfully. 6) A problem exists and the client requires extensive services putting him/her in a dependent role, at least temporarily. 7) A problem exists which is taxing the client's coping ability. 8) Problems exist that are long-term and permanent.

The result of data analysis is the nursing diagnosis, the nurse's judgement of the primary issues of actual or potential health or developmental problems and, for school nurses, the relationship of the health issues and the student's ability to learn.[7]

Standardized nursing diagnoses have been in development through the North American Nursing Diagnosis Association (NANDA) since 1975. These standardized categories provide a more precise, concise method of delineating conditions ame-

Table 5. Essential Data Base for Students with Identified Needs

Sources of essential baseline information for determining whether or not health is a factor contributing to a student's educational or developmental problem, and determining the extent and nature of the interference:

- Discussion with the student and family: school experience
  - perception of the problem
  - attitudes towards personal health problem, school and learning
  - perception of academic progress
  - schedule of daily activities
  - environment: school, home and neighborhood
  - attendance
  - peers
  - extracurricular activities

- Pupil Health Record review and other sources of previous developmental, psychological and special learning and behavior problem assessments
- Health information from physician or other healthcare providers.
- Health history (if not present in the Pupil Health Record), current health status, current health practices

- Physical assessment/measurements
  - sensory functions: vision and hearing
  - physical assessment
  - neurological assessment
  - growth (height and weight graphed)

- Developmental assessment

- Family assessment
  - family structure
  - family function
  - family health

- Teacher observations

- School nurse and/or other child study team members' observations

As for other educational assessments, is it necessary to obtain written parental permission for health assessment activities.

Reprinted from *Student Health Information*. [4]

nable to nursing intervention. Also, communication among nursing professionals in different settings is improved with the standardized diagnoses.

The phrases of the standardized nursing diagnoses include the PROBLEM statement, the ETIOLOGY or source, SIGNS/SYMPTOMS that are substantiating evidence for the identified problem, and RESPONSE from the client. (See Chapter 2 for additional discussion of nursing diagnosis.)

In the problem-oriented method of record-keeping, the nursing diagnoses are recorded by A: Assessment (see Table 4).

Plan

The school nurse manages or intervenes regarding health concerns by planning and implementing strategies to resolve the concerns identified in the nursing diagnosis with the student and family. The plan is the basis of the nurse-client contract. Concepts from nursing theories and theories of other disciplines and sciences offer guidance in identifying reasonable goals, suitable nursing activities and expected student outcomes.[5] For example, Maslow's hierarchy of needs dictates that a student's safety needs should be dealt with first, then the psychosocial needs of self-esteem and empowerment through increased skills in decision-making could be addressed.

School nurses may begin the planning phase of the nursing process by articulating goals—student goals and/or nursing goals. The goals are positive and future-oriented. Diagnosis statements are often negative or problem-oriented, whereas goal statements are positive. Diagnosis defines the current state, and goals point to a future state. Goals are segmented into objectives, specific action steps that are sequential and lead collectively to a goal. These objectives are the steps of a plan.

Student goals and objectives define what the student will do. Goals and objectives on an IEP are often written in this format. Some educators also use student outcomes to clarify and more precisely describe what the state will be when goals are achieved—how do you know that you have gotten where you wanted to go. In contrast, nursing goals outline the the school nurse's actions to facilitate the student reaching his/her goals. Most plans require joint action on the part of students and the nurse to resolve the identified problems and attain goals.

What variables should be considered in a plan? How are priorities set? Basic needs for health and safety should to be addressed first, as suggested above. Next is review of the capacity to manage the plan—the resources available in the family, school, and community; these could include access to care, experience in solving similar problems, funds, support from family or friends, and the like. Another point is determining who is accountable for each plan of action. The timing and pace of the action steps can also affect the success of the plan. For example, having steps that are readily achievable early in the implementation phase can influence the belief that other elements of the plan are achievable. Finally, there needs to be evaluation criteria and a timeline for periodic and final review.

One way to prioritize which actions are to be taken first is to focus on the safety of the client (and others) and urgency the problem presents (current or future). Here are three decision-action guides: 1) For conditions that may result in an emergency or safety for self or others, a health planning conference is scheduled immediately and includes the student, parent, primary teacher, the school nurse, and perhaps an administrator. 2) Conditions that may interfere with learning are referred to the child study team (special education team). 3) Other health concerns may be addressed by scheduling a health planning conference, a child study meeting, or both.[4]

The above components of the nursing process are the elements of the Individualized Healthcare Plan (IHP)—Assessment (Data Collection and Nursing Diagnosis) and Plan. In the problem-oriented method of record-keeping, the plan is recorded by P: Plan—goals, priorities, action steps and timelines.[5]

Intervention/Implementation

The school nurse implements the plan during the intervention phase by carrying out his/her responsibilities and by assisting the student to utilize his/her own resources to do likewise. This is the most visible part of school nursing practice, the "doing" part in which nursing knowledge and skills are applied to practice, grounded in science that gives credence to nursing actions.

School nurses implement the plan with the client by assuming various roles. Those roles include providing skilled nursing care, counseling, educating, assisting the student and family in coping, and providing an interface with the community and other resources by acting as advocate, liaison, or monitor. Throughout the interventions the school nurse functions primarily as a communicator.[3]

Nursing intervention is planned and systematic. But, as discussed in the opening paragraphs of this chapter, the nursing process is cyclical and concurrent. "Nursing care is a dynamic process that implies alterations in data, diagnosis or plans previously made."[7] Adaptations are made based on whether or not certain interventions are working. Many times the plans need to be adjusted to accommodate everything else happening in the lives of a student and family—dynamic, unpredictable life events.

In the problem-oriented method of record-keeping, the implementation portion is recorded by I: Intervention/Implementation—time and date of nursing actions and response of the client or results. While the assessment and planning steps are recorded as portions of the IHP, the intervention/implementation step may be recorded as a daily log or as progress notes on actions and implications. The achievement of goals as stated in the IHP are reviewed periodically based on data in the implementation log.[5]

Evaluation

The evaluation phase allows the school nurse to make judgements about the student's progress toward goals, the appropriateness of the goals, and the effectiveness of the nursing interventions. Evaluation is seeing if the goals are met. It means scrutinizing activities to see if they were a help or a hindrance. The nurse's, student's, and family's accountability is measured according to preset criteria, by reviewing the responsibilities delineated in the plan.[5]

Besides measuring achievement of goals, evaluation can be skill-building. This is an opportunity to review the steps taken in the problem-solving process discussing with the student and family the purpose of each, and how to use the steps in other situations. In another way, evaluation identifies where a student lacks knowledge or skill in problem solving or in choosing and using resources. Evaluation enhances the capacity or self-care skills of the student and family so they can act independently in the future when identifying problems and accessing resources.[2]

In the problem-oriented method of record-keeping, the evaluation portion is recorded by E: Evaluation—record of whether desired outcomes were achieved and why or why not.[5]

Summary of Nursing Process Steps

The nursing process is continuous and cyclical. Evaluation triggers an assessment of related or new actual or potential health conditions. For school nursing, the question to be asked consistently is, how does this health issue affect the student's learning, growing, and developing?

Nursing Process as Product: Document and Communicate

The nursing process provides a structure or framework for nursing practice. The nursing process also shapes how evidence of the nursing practice being implemented is documented—the "writing about what the nurse has done and why [or] translating the experience of caring into words."[9] Although often viewed as time-consuming paperwork, recording of nursing care is essential thinking, documenting, and communicating time (see Table 6). The record is the evidence or product of the nursing process in practice.

A product that captures, in part, nursing practice in the school setting is the pupil health record. This cumulative record follows the student throughout his/her school career. In other healthcare settings this record is the patient/client chart. The focus of this book is the IHP, a product that focuses on a specific health need or problem of a student at a given time in his/her development and educational career. An IHP is one part of the pupil health record. A student with a chronic healthcare problem may have several different or sequential IHPs in his/her student career.

The IHP provides a format to record each step in the nursing process—the school nurse summarizes key information from the assessment phase, synthesizes

Table 6. Rationale for Recording the Nursing Process

TO DOCUMENT

Identify and seek remedies for health problems that may interfere with learning.

Organize material and the approach to children's health into a systematic and retrievable format.

Establish a legal record of problems identified and services provided; record the practice of health professionals and educators.

Provide a vehicle for continuity of care and service.

TO COMMUNICATE

Inform the educational team members of

student strengths and limitations

actual and potential areas of need

special services required

areas where adaptation of education is required

areas where adaptation of the environment is required

successful and unsuccessful management strategies.

Assist the student in gaining knowledge and skills about a specific problem or concern and about the decision-making process.

Relate to parents the school's response to the child and his/her special needs.

Report progress of treatment/management plans to the primary healthcare provider and others meeting a student's complex needs.

Provide a data base in the event of an emergency.

Reprinted from *Student Health Information*. [4]

problem statement(s), formulates goals and plans of action, and documents interventions and the evaluation of outcomes.

School nurses practice according to the nursing process instinctively. Reflecting on their decisions and actions using the steps of the nursing process, school nurses engage in a cognitive system of checks and balances. The written record also offers checks and balances to ensure that school nurses and their clients have done complete assessments, made logical conclusions, developed reasonable plans, and judged the effectiveness of the results.

Nursing process can be called the *why* of the profession. Documentation, the product, can be called the *what* of the profession.

The nursing process documentation or record is the vehicle to communicate what has occurred in a nurse-client partnership. In this way the record is the therapeutic language of the relationship. Second, the record is the legal language that describes the relationship. An old adage—if it is not documented, it was not done—emphasizes how important documentation is when legal questions arise. Third, the record is the fiscal language of the nurse-client relationship. In times of scarce resources, the record is reviewed for the judgements/decisions that were made and the services provided. With proper evidence of student need and nursing practice, dollars may be accessed from an increasing number of sources—regular education dollars, special education funds, private insurance, and public assistance revenues.

A pupil health record in the format of a Problem-Oriented Health Record, sometimes called the Positive-Oriented Health Record, (POHR) organizes material and the approach to a student's health in a more systematic, easily retrievable format than block charting (progress notes). Components of the record include: 1) An accurate and complete data base, 2) Problem/

concern list to which all plans are addressed and consists of medical diagnoses, nursing diagnoses, educational assessments (as appropriate), 3) Incorporation or cross references to a longer IHP for specific problems that have been the focus of a more intensive planning process, 4) Sequential narrative notes that are referenced to the problem list in the SOAP or SOAPIER formats (as described in the preceding section on nursing process), 5) Other methods for logging or documenting specific regular procedures or educational interventions (e.g., medication/procedure log, teaching checklist of knowledge and skill attainment), 6) Discharge plan—at the time a student leaves a school setting (sixth grade, eighth grade, twelfth grade, transfer). [2, 10]

Other characteristics of POHR that apply in school and other settings are outlined by Wold.[2] For example, the record should be confidential, cumulative, accurate, specific, objective, and goal-oriented and have a uniform format.

The POHR establishes a consistent format for documenting and communicating the whole picture of positive health status as well as health concerns of a student over time. How can the IHP—a time-limited and specific problem-focused plan—be incorporated as a part of the POHR? First, cite the problem or nursing diagnoses on the problem list. In the narrative notes section record a brief summary of the assessment and goals. Maintain the record by periodically summarizing (every three months) on the pupil health record whereas lengthier observations and daily/regular activity logs are kept as part of the IHP. Label the IHP as a permanent part of the pupil health record. If a student is being served through special education and the IHP is attached to or incorporated in the IEP, a summary of essential concerns and a reference to the student's special education file may be sufficient. Note these recent publications on documentation issues: *Guidelines for School Nursing Documentation: Standards, Issues and Models* [10] by Schwab for the National Association of School Nurses, 1991; and *Implementation Guide for the Standards of School Nursing Practice*,[11] ASHA, 1991.

With an increase in the number and complexity of health problems in children, an accurate, comprehensive, and current document is essential. Problems are interrelated—such as a chronic health problem complicated by depression, a student with special needs being more vulnerable to abusive situations, the complex causes and effects of chemical use/abuse, or sexual orientation/identity issues correlated with high rates of depression and suicide. Good documentation may help the school nurse predict and prevent problems for students by highlighting clusters of risk factors. Increasingly, schools and families are involved with a widening circle of agencies and specialty practices, so a record of goals and what works is necessary for coordination and to reduce duplication of services. Families are more mobile so a complete written record could improve continuity of care.

Summary

There are several unanswered questions regarding documentation—standards for amount and content of the records, confidentiality, and the ethical issues regarding recording vulnerable experiences (pregnancy, chemical use, AIDS/HIV). And there are plenty of excuses for why school nurses don't pay attention to documentation—lack of time, lack of skill, undervaluing paperwork. Nevertheless, the therapeutic, legal, and fiscal benefits of documentation outweigh the drawbacks. The challenge is for school nurses to increase their attention to and skill in documentation. School nurses must define the criteria and methods that will facilitate the translation of nursing caring into words, the development of a product that describes the nursing process.

REFERENCES

1. Oregon State Board of Nursing. *Oregon State Board of Nursing Declaratory Ruling: Petition Requested for Hillsboro Union High School (#3) employees and Carol Mitts*, Feb 16, 1989. (Oregon State Bd. of Nursing 10445 SW Canyon Rd., Suite 200, Beaverton, OR 97005).
2. Wold, S. *School Nursing: A Framework for Practice*. North Branch, MN: Sunrise River Press, 1981.
3. Proctor, S. *Guidelines for a Model School Nursing Services Program*. Scarborough, ME: National Association of School Nurses, 1990.
4. Luehr, RE. *Student Health Information*. St. Paul, MN: Minnesota Department of Education, Feb 1985, rev Dec 1986.
5. Luehr, RE. Nursing process as applied to school nursing practice. In: Iverson, C, ed. *HADHAS—Health and Developmental History Assessment Skills-Implementation Manual*. Scarborough, ME: National Association of School Nurses, 1983.
6. Minnesota Nurses Association and School Nurse Organization of Minnesota. *Goals of School Nursing, An Interpretive Tool*. St. Paul, MN: MNA and SNOM, 1983: Appendix II.
7. American Nurses Association. Authored jointly by ANA, APHA, ASHA, NAPNAP, NASN, NASSNC. *Standards of School Nursing Practice*. Washington, DC: American Nurses Association, 1983 (publication No. NP-66).
8. Igoe, JB. *School Nurse Achievement Program: Self Instructional Module #2, The Nursing Process*. Denver, CO: University of Colorado Health Sciences Center, School of Nursing Programs, 1983.
9. Hays, J. Voices in the record. *Image: J. Nursing Scholarship*, 1989; 21 (4): 200-204.
10. Schwab, N. *Guidelines for School Nursing Documentation: Standards, Issues and Models*. Scarborough, ME: National Association of School Nurses, 1991.
11. American School Health Association. *Implementation Guide for the Standards of School Nursing Practice*. Kent, OH: American School Health Association, 1991.
12. American Nurses Association. *Standards of Clinical Nursing Practice*. Washington, DC: American Nurses Association, December 1991 (publication No. NP-79).

13. American Nurses Association. *Code for Nurses with Interpretive Statements.* Washington, DC: American Nurses Association, 1985.
14. National Association of School Nurses. *Code of Ethics with Interpretive Statements for the School Nurse.* Scarborough, ME: NASN, 1990.

BIBLIOGRAPHY

American Nurses Association. Standards of Nursing Practice. Washington, DC: American Nurses Association, 1973.

American School Health Association. (authored by ANA, APHA, ASHA, NAPNAP, NASN, NASSNC). *An Evaluation Guide for School Nursing Practice Designed for Self and Peer Review.* Kent, OH: American School Health Association, 1985.

Iyer, PW, Taptich, BJ, Bernocchi-Losey, D. *Nursing Process and Nursing Diagnosis.* Philadelphia: WB Saunders, 1986.

Luehr, RE. Planning for a student with a chronic health condition. In: Larson G, ed. *Managing the School Age Child with a Chronic Health Condition: A Practical Guide for Schools, Families and Organizations.* Wayazata, MN: DCI Publishing, 1988 (Available from: Sunrise River Press, 11481 Kost Dam Rd., North Branch, MN 55056, 612-583-3239): Chap 2.

National Association of School Nurses. (authored by ANA, APHA, ASHA, NAPNAP, NASN, NASSNC). *Administrative Evaluation of School Nursing Practice.* Scarborough, ME: National Association of School Nurses, 1987.

Supplement 1. Standards of Clinical Nursing Practice, 1991
American Nurses Association

"Standards of Care" describe a competent level of nursing care as demonstrated by the nursing process... The nursing process encompasses all significant actions taken by nurses in providing care to clients and forms the foundation of clinical decision making.

STANDARDS OF CARE

Standard   I.   Assessment. The nurse collects client health data.

Standard   II.   Diagnosis. The nurse analyzes the assessment data in determining diagnosis.

Standard   III. Outcome Identification. The nurse identifies expected outcomes individualized to the client.

Standard   IV.   Planning. The nurse develops a plan of care that prescribes interventions to attain expected outcomes.

Standard   V.   Implementation. The nurse implements the interventions identified in the plan of care.

Standard   VI.   Evaluation. The nurse evaluates the client's progress toward attainment of outcomes.

"Standards of Professional Performance" describe a competent level of behavior in the professional role. . . . All nurses are expected to engage in professional role activities appropriate to their education, position and practice setting.

STANDARDS OF PROFESSIONAL PERFORMANCE

Standard   I.   Quality of Care. The nurse systematically evaluates the quality and effectiveness of nursing practice.

Standard   II.   Performance Appraisal. The nurse evaluates his/her own nursing practice in relation to professional practice standards and relevant statutes and regulations.

Standard   III.   Education. The nurse acquires and maintains current knowledge in nursing practice.

Standard   IV.   Collegiality. The nurse contributes to the professional development of peers, colleagues, and others.

Standard   V.   Ethics. The nurse's decisions and actions on behalf of client are determined in an ethical manner.

Standard   VI.   Collaboration. The nurse collaborates with the client, significant others, and health care providers in providing client care.

Standard   VII.   Research. The nurse uses research findings in practice.

Standard   VIII. Resource Utilization. The nurse considers factors related to safety, effectiveness, and cost in planning and delivering client care.

Reprinted, with permission, from *Standards of Clinical Nursing Practice*,[12] pp 2-3, 7-10, 13-17.

Supplement 2. Code for Nurses
American Nurses Association

1. The nurse provides services with respect for human dignity and the uniqueness of the client, unrestricted by considerations of social or economic status, personal attributes, or the nature of health problems.

2. The nurse safeguards the client's right to privacy by judiciously protecting information of a confidential nature.

3. The nurse acts to safeguard the client and the public when health care and safety are affected by the incompetent, unethical or illegal practice of any person.

4. The nurse assumes responsibility and accountability for individual nursing judgments and actions.

5. The nurse maintains competence in nursing.

6. The nurse exercises informed judgment and uses individual competence and qualifications as criteria in seeking consultation, accepting responsibilities, and delegating nursing activities to others.

7. The nurse participates in activities that contribute to the ongoing development of the profession's body of knowledge.

8. The nurse participates in the profession's efforts to implement and improve standards of nursing.

9. The nurse participates in the profession's efforts to establish and maintain conditions of employment conducive to high quality nursing care.

10. The nurse participates in the profession's efforts to protect the public from misinformation and misrepresentation and to maintain the integrity of nursing.

11. The nurse collaborates with members of the health professions and other citizens in promoting community and national efforts to meet the health needs of the public.

From *Code for Nurses with Interpretive Statements*, © 1985 American Nurses Association, Washington, DC. Reprinted with permission.[13] (ANA, 600 Maryland Av SW, Suite 100 West, Washington, DC 20024-2571)

PREAMBLE

Acknowledging the diversity of laws and conditions under which school nurses practice, NASN believes in a commonality of moral and ethical conduct.

1. **CLIENT CARE.** The school nurse is an advocate for students, families and members of the school community. The school nurse provides health services, while recognizing each individual's inherent right to be treated with dignity and confidentiality, and works to support the client's active participation in health decisions. All clients are treated equally regardless of race, gender, or socioeconomic status.

INTERPRETIVE STATEMENT

A.   School nurses uphold a moral obligation to recognize human existence as the only prerequisite for all persons to be worthy of dignity, respect and justice.

B.   School nursing services support and promote individuals' and families' ability to achieve the highest quality of life as understood by each individual and family.

C.   School nursing services are delivered with nonprejudicial behavior. Clients' value systems are represented at all times.

D.   School nurses safeguard client's rights to determine their own health care decisions with the use of accurate and complete information. School nurses safeguard their client's right to privacy through confidentiality.

2. **PROFESSIONAL COMPETENCY.** The school nurse maintains the highest level of competency by enhancing professional knowledge and skills, and by collaborating with peers, other health professionals and community agencies, adhering to the Standards of School Nursing Practice.

INTERPRETIVE STATEMENT

A.   The profession of nursing is obligated to provide competent nursing care. The school nurse must be aware of the need for continued professional learning and must assume personal responsibility for currency of knowledge and skills.

B.   It is necessary for school nurses to have knowledge relevant to the current scope of practice. Since individual competencies vary, nurses consult with peers and other health professionals with expertise and recognized competencies in various fields of practice. When in the client's best interest, the school nurse refers to other health professionals and community health agencies.

C.   Nurses are accountable for judgments made and actions taken in the course of nursing practice. *Standards of School Nursing Practice* reflects a practice grounded in ethical commitment. The school nurse is responsible for establishing a practice based on these standards.

3. **PROFESSIONAL RESPONSIBILITIES.** The school nurse participates in the profession's efforts to advance the standards of practice, expand the body of knowledge through nursing research and improve conditions of employment.

INTERPRETIVE STATEMENT

A. The school nurse is obligated to demonstrate adherence to the profession's standards by monitoring the standards in daily practice and participating in the profession's efforts to improve school health services.

B. The school nurse recognizes and promotes research as a means to advancing school health services and adheres to the ethics that govern research as follows:

   1. Right to privacy and confidentiality.
   2. Voluntary and informed consent.
   3. Awareness of and participation in the mechanisms available to address violation of the rights of human subjects.

C. The school nurse recognizes conditions of employment impact the quality of client care and is cognizant of working with others to improve these conditions.

4. **PROFESSIONAL ENDORSEMENTS.** The school nurse acknowledges personal accountability when endorsing products, programs or services. School nurses may not infer action as an agent of NASN.

INTERPRETIVE STATEMENT

The school nurse addresses health issues in a variety of settings. Informed studies of product design, testing and efficacy are mandatory if product acceptance or recommendation is made. The school nurse will enhance consumer awareness to minimize misinformation and misrepresentation; professional accountability is necessary to ensure licensure protection and to support the integrity of NASN.

Authored by the NASN Professional Rights and Responsibilities Committee.

Reprinted, with permission, National Association of School Nurses, 1990.[14]

Supplement 3. Standards of School Nursing Practice, 1983

American Nurses Association, American Public Health Association, American School Health Association, National Association of Pediatric Nurse Associates and Practitioners, National Association of School Nurses, National Association of State School Nurse Consultants

"Standards represent agreed-upon levels of quality in practice. Standards characterize, measure, and provide guidance in achieving excellence in care.

"Standards stimulate the development of peer review, guarantee the documentation of the benefits and outcomes of school nursing practice, inspire research to validate practice, generate research questions that lead to improvement of the health delivery system to students and families.

"The purpose of school nursing is to enhance the educational process by the modification or removal of health-related barriers to learning and by promotion of an optimal level of wellness" (pp. 1—2).

Each Standard includes a rationale, and structure, process and outcome criteria.

Standard I. Theory
The school nurse applies appropriate theory as a basis for decision making in nursing practice.

Standard II. Program Management
The school nurse establishes and maintains a comprehensive health program.

Standard III. Nursing Process
The nursing process includes individualized health plans which are developed by the school nurse.

Standard IV. Interdisciplinary Collaboration
The school nurse collaborates with other professionals in assessing, planning, implementing, and evaluating programs and other school health activities.

Standard V. Health Education
The nurse assists students, families, and groups to achieve optimal levels of wellness through health education.

Standard VI. Professional Development
The school nurse participates in peer review and other means of evaluation to assure quality of nursing care provided for students.

The nurse assumes responsibility for continuing education and professional development and contributes to the professional growth of others.

Standard VII. Community Health Systems
The school nurse participates with other key members of the community responsible for assessing, planning, implementing and evaluating school health services and community services that include the broad continuum of promotion of primary, secondary, and tertiary prevention.

Standard VIII. Research

The school nurse contributes to nursing and school health through innovations in theory and practice and participation in research.

General Guidelines for School Nurse Staffing Patterns:

school nurse-to-student ratio

1 : 750 in general school populations

1 : 225 in mainstream populations

1: 125 in severely/profoundly handicapped populations (Addendum, p. 19)

Reprinted, with permission, from *Standards of School Nursing Practice,* © 1983, American Nurses Association, Washington, DC. [7] Note: The National Association of School Nurses is authoring a revised Standards of School Nursing Practice expected to be available in 1993 and will be based on the new format in the American Nurses Association, Standards of Clinical Nursing Practice, 1991. (See Supplement 1.)

Using Nursing Diagnosis in the School Setting

Ruth Ellen Luehr

The nursing process, the cornerstone to nursing practice, is described in the previous chapter. The first step in the nursing process, assessment, is complete when the nursing diagnosis has been developed. In this chapter, nursing diagnosis is defined, the development of nursing diagnoses is described, and applications and advantages in the specialty practice of school nursing are suggested.

"Nurses diagnose and treat [human] responses [to health problems]—not the health problems themselves. The human responses are often multiple, episodic, or continuous, fluid, and varying, and are less discrete or circumscribed than medical diagnostic categories."[1]

Definition

Nursing diagnosis is the nurse's judgement or decision, the statement of the nurse's perception of a client's health status and needs. The nurse derives her/his decisions from the data gathered in the assessment phase of the nursing process. The information is then analyzed according to basic theories in nursing, physical and social sciences—theories such as understandings of wellness and illness, change and coping theory, principles of self-care, role theory, systems theory, fam-

ily theory, child/adolescent/adult development and learning theory. A nurse's way of knowing, the intuition grounded in knowledge and experience, influences the nursing diagnosis. The client, too, is a partner in the formation of a diagnosis. Through development of the diagnosis, the client can come to an understanding of his/her health status and needs, thereby gaining an investment in and developing expectations for the plans, actions, and outcomes that follow.

Nursing diagnosis is the nurse's opinion of a condition, behavior, or situation. This nursing diagnosis does not identify a specific pathology as in medical diagnosis, but rather, focuses on the effects of a given situation—the response of the client, the meaning or impact of the situation on the client's life, the lifestyle effects.[2] In most interactions between nurses and clients, more than one nursing diagnosis is needed to fully describe the complex situation.

A written nursing diagnosis contains several elements (see Table 1). The nursing diagnosis identifies the current state (often a concern), identifies the etiology (underlying or precipitating cause), relates to signs and symptoms collected in the assessment process, and indicates the client's response to the concern. Here are two examples: Ineffective family coping related to new diagnosis of HIV positive

Table 1. Components of the Nursing Diagnosis Statement

1. Problem or Positive Statement of the Issue or Concern
   connecting phrase "related to/associated with"
2. Etiology—anatomical, physiological, psychological, environmental
   connecting phrase "manifested by/evidenced by"
3. Signs and Symptoms (optional)
   connecting phrase "resulting in"
4. Response—meaning or impact in a person's life (optional)

status of adolescent daughter (evidenced by denial—noncommunication among family members about the diagnosis for four days) [resulting in lack of internal support for the grieving process/ lack of access to immediate medical intervention]; Adequate accident prevention practices due to integrated parent/student injury prevention program [resulting in child being granted increased privileges to ride bike in neighborhood].

The professional literature offers several definitions of nursing diagnosis. Those selected by the North American Nursing Diagnosis Association (NANDA) reflect various conceptual approaches:

A nursing diagnosis is a clinical judgement about an individual, family or community which is derived through a deliberate, systematic process of data collection and analysis. It provides the basis for prescriptions for definitive therapy for which the nurse is accountable. It is expressed concisely and it includes the etiology of the condition when known.[3]

Nursing diagnosis is a concise phrase or term summarizing a cluster of empirical indicators representing patterns of unitary man.[4]

Nursing diagnosis made by professional nurses describes actual or potential health problems that nurses, by nature of their education and experience, are capable and licensed to treat.[5]

A nursing diagnosis is a concise phrase or term summarizing a cluster or set of empirical indicators, representing normal variations and altered patterns (actual or potential) of human functioning which nurses by virtue of education and experience are capable and licensed to treat.[6] (Reprinted, with permission, *North American Nursing Diagnosis Association,*[7])

In 1990, NANDA agreed on this definition of nursing diagnosis:

A nursing diagnosis is a clinical judgement about individual, family or community reponse to actual or potential health problems/life processes. Nursing diagnoses provide the basis for selection of nursing interventions to achieve outcomes for which the nurse is accountable.[8]

While nurses individualize their diagnoses to each client or group they serve, it is important to have standardized statements that are valid and have meaning from one nurse to another—from one community to another within a specialty field of nursing and across nursing specialties. Therefore, in the written nursing diagnosis statement, the initial phrase is a standardized phrase drawn from an ever-increasing list of approved categories. The etiology and other phrases of the statement reflect the unique situation of the client at a given time. Nursing diagnoses statements are being standardized through an evolutionary scientific process involving nursing theorists and practitioners. The major work is being orchestrated by NANDA.

Development and Organization

For more than twenty years the term nursing diagnosis has been used in professional journals and has been incorporated in the publications defining the profession, the Standards of Nursing Practice (ANA, 1973). It was purposely chosen to label the intellectual, problem-solving process of nurses in determining their interactions with individual clients or client groups. The term also acknowledges the importance and accountability of nurses' autonomous clinical judgements—different than, separate from, independent of, yet interdependent with the practice of medicine and other disciplines.

In 1973 nurses met to take the following steps regarding nursing diagnoses: outline a process, identify the scope of nursing's interaction with clients, develop consistent nomenclature that describes these interactions, and group or classify the descriptive statements. A final step was to assign numerical values to each diagnosis to facilitate research on validating the diagnostic statements, description of nursing practice and client effects.[7] Note: The authors of this book have listed the applicable NANDA numerical numbers in the Nursing Diagnoses section in each of the Individualized Healthcare Plans. (Early work has begun on coding nursing diagnoses into a version for possible inclusion in the World Health Organization International Classification of Disease (ICD-10) system.) New and clarified nursing diagnoses are regularly approved by ballot vote of NANDA members, having met the scrutiny of the submission process. The process requires definition of the diagnosis, defining characteristics and evidence of validity in clinical practice. Guidelines

for submission may be obtained from NANDA, St. Louis University School of Nursing, 3525 Caroline St, St. Louis, MO 63014 (telephone 314/577-8954).

At first the approved nursing diagnoses were published in alphabetical order. Then under NANDA sponsorship, theorists clustered nursing diagnoses in a framework that is consistent with and descriptive of nursing as an art and science. Ways of organizing the diagnoses are called taxonomies, sometimes called theoretical frameworks. Each school nurse may find it beneficial to select a taxonomy or framework and use it regularly in assessment until she/he is familiar with and skilled in the use and formulation of nursing diagnoses. Then she/he should examine a second taxonomy, assessing the strengths, weakness, and applicability to her/his own school nursing practice. Four taxonomies or frameworks are briefly described here.

Framework 1

NANDA Taxonomy I Revised— Human Response Patterns

The original alphabetical list of NANDA-approved nursing diagnoses was reorganized to reflect what nurses do and how they think. "The purposes of a taxonomy are to provide a vocabulary for classifying phenomena in a discipline, provide new ways of looking at the discipline and play a part in concept derivation."[8] In the taxonomy NANDA selected, called Taxonomy I—Human Response Patterns, a person's whole way of being—his/her way of experiencing health and life—can be described by nine patterns (see Table 2). These patterns can be a guide to ensure all important areas of a client's health experience are considered when a nurse is conducting an assessment. These patterns can also be used when making sense of the assessment data obtained. (The NANDA list was first reorganized in 1986 and called

Taxonomy I. Edited in 1989, the list was renamed and is now called Taxonomy I Revised Human Response Patterns. Another edition will be published in September 1992.)

The first of the nine patterns in the [Taxonomy I Revised] Human Response Patterns is exchanging, a category that focuses on body functioning, physiological processes of giving and receiving or adaptation that occur in taking in and using nutrition; adjustments in physical regulation such as the immune response and body temperature; bowel, urinary and skin processes of elimination; vascular and cardiac functioning; oxygenation; and physical integrity including injury potential and skin and tissue integrity. The second pattern, communicating, deals with sending messages verbally and nonverbally. The third is relating, focusing on socialization, establishing roles and sexuality. Next, valuing, which includes the spiritual realm and includes assigning worth or establishing meaning in life. The choosing pattern has as a theme selecting from alternatives—coping, compliance, decision making, conflicts, and health-seeking behaviors. Activity is the theme of the moving pattern: physical mobility, rest and recre-

ation, health and home maintenance through activities of daily living, capacity for self-care, and growth and development. The next pattern, perceiving, deals with self-awareness including self-concept and also sensory functions. An important pattern is knowing—meaning associated with information, the processes of learning. The ninth and final pattern is feeling, the focus being the subjective nature of information or emotional responses and integrity.

In the implementation of [Taxonomy I Revised] Human Response Patterns, the nurse and client review a given situation, including information from the client's environment and information about how the client has dealt with a similar situation in the past. Together the nurse and client recognize or discover an emerging pattern—a description of the phenomenon that leads to greater insight and guides the next steps of action. Next steps may include further exploration, new skills development, problem solving, developing a support system, and so on.

See Supplement 1 at the end of this chaper for the current NANDA-approved diagnosis in Taxonomy I Revised-1990, Human Response Patterns.

Table 2. Human Response Patterns (NANDA Taxonomy I Revised)

1. Exchanging	physical/physiological—giving and receiving
2. Communicating	sending messages
3. Relating	establishing bonds; roles
4. Valuing	assigning worth; spiritual state; meaning
5. Choosing	selecting alternatives, participating
6. Moving	activity
7. Perceiving	receiving information, sensory, self-awareness
8. Knowing	meaning associated with information, learning
9. Feeling	subjective awareness of information, emotional integrity

Adapted from NANDA, 1990,[8] and Moberg, 1988.[16]

Framework 2

Hierarchy of Needs

The familiar Maslow's Hierarchy of Needs is a framework used by nurses and clients to set priorities when a number of goals are outlined. In order to sustain life and health, a person must meet basic physiological needs (identified as survival and stimulation by Kalish) before higher level needs can be addressed. If basic needs are unmet, the client may be unwilling or unable to attend to higher level, more abstract concepts.[9]

The levels of need include the physiological survival level, including needs for food, water, rest, and avoidance of pain. At the next level, a person requires stimulation in the form of manipulation, exploration, novelty, sexual pleasure, and diverse activity. Next, the safety needs include security, safety, and protection. Higher still is love and belonging, including a sense of connectedness and caring, closeness. Self-esteem includes a sense of self-worth, dignity, privacy, respect for self and others, recognition, usefulness, and freedom. In self-actualization, a person has a lifestyle that is congruous with his/her value system—an integrated, satisfying state of accomplishment and fulfillment.[9, 10]

School nurses have found this framework to be helpful in setting priorities with a student and family. Student's needs are often complex, including at a minimum physical health status, health practices, an impact on growth and development, and an impact on learning. Especially in times of crisis, a person's coping ability and energy for taking action are extremely limited. Recognizing that the student is fulfilling basic, low-level needs on the Hierarchy of Needs framework, the school nurse would help him/her set reasonable expectations for action so that the student and family do not feel overwhelmed and defeated before they take any action. This framework is particularly useful in dealing with crisis, stress and coping agendas with students and families. The framework also provides a challenge for the nurse and the student to always strive for higher levels of satisfaction and fulfillment.

An advantage in school nursing is that students and their families have a long term relationship with the nurse—a school year or perhaps the entire school career for a child, and the opportunity for school nurses to sometimes intervene from one generation to the next. This Hierarchy of Needs framework can guide long-term nursing interventions—stress and crises are normal and will cause clients to focus on basic needs from time to time, but the goal is to enhance the development of a child or youth and to assist the family to achieve higher goals.

The nursing diagnoses have been arranged according to the Maslow's framework in Table 3.

Table 3. Nursing Diagnoses and Maslow's Hierarchy of Needs

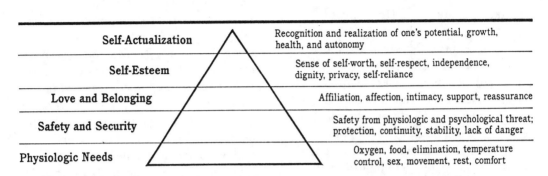

Self-Actualization	Recognition and realization of one's potential, growth, health, and autonomy
Self-Esteem	Sense of self-worth, self-respect, independence, dignity, privacy, self-reliance
Love and Belonging	Affiliation, affection, intimacy, support, reassurance
Safety and Security	Safety from physiologic and psychological threat; protection, continuity, stability, lack of danger
Physiologic Needs	Oxygen, food, elimination, temperature control, sex, movement, rest, comfort

Because human beings respond in a variety of ways to establish and maintain the self, health problems are much more than simply physical. Maslow's hierarchy of needs, diagrammed above, is a system of classifying human needs based on the idea that lower-level, abstract needs can be met. By considering these differing levels of need when trying to understand and resolve client problems, you'll be better able to provide more holistic care.

For nurses, Maslow's hierarchy has special significance in decision-making and planning for care. If a client is short of breath, for example, he's probably not interested in or capable of discussing his spirituality. Similarly, a client who demands frequent attention for a seemingly trivial matter may be exhibiting self-esteem needs. These need categories vary from person to person, so you'll need to be vigilant in assessment, diagnosis, planning, and intervention to meet the client's changing needs.

Read the descriptions of each category in the schematic above, and then see how you'd relate them to nursing diagnoses. Below we've categorized the nursing diagnoses according to this framework. Be sure to assess clients for potential problems at all levels of the pyramid, no matter what their initial complaint.

Categorization of Nursing Diagnoses Using Maslow's Hierarchy of Needs

Nursing Diagnoses	Maslow's Hierarchy of Needs	Nursing Diagnoses
Growth and Development, Altered • Health-seeking Behavior • Knowledge Deficit		Spiritual Distress
Adjustment, Impaired • Coping: Defensive, Denial, Ineffective Family, Ineffective Individual • Decisional Conflict • Diversional Activity Deficit		Hopelessness • Knowledge Deficit • Noncompliance • Post-trauma response • Powerlessness • Rape-Trauma Syndrome • Self-Concept • Violence, Potential
Coping: Family, Ineffective • Knowledge Deficit	**Self-Actualization** **Self-Esteem** Love and Belonging Safety and Security Physiologic Needs	Parenting, Altered • Parental Role, Conflict • Self-esteem Disturbance, Chronic Low, Situational Low • Social Interaction, Impaired • Social Isolation
Communication, Impaired Verbal • Disuse Syndrome • Dysreflexia • Fear • Grieving, Anticipatory • Grieving, Dysfunctional		Health Maintenance, Altered • Home Maintenance Management • Infection, Potential • Injury, Potential • Knowledge Deficit • Neglect, Unilateral • Sensory-Perceptual Alteration • Thought Processes, Altered
Activity Intolerance • Airway Clearance, Ineffective • Aspiration, Potential • Body Temperature, Potential Alteration • Bowel Elimination, Altered: Colonic Constipation, Constipation, Diarrhea, Incontinence, Perceived Constipation • Breastfeeding, Ineffective • Breathing Pattern, Ineffective • Cardiac Output, Decreased • Comfort, Altered: Pain, Chronic Pain • Fatigue • Fluid Volume Deficit: Actual or Potential • Fluid Volume Excess • Gas Exchange, Impaired • Hyperthermia • Hypothermia • Incontinence: Functional		Incontinence: Reflex, Stress, Total, Urge • Knowledge Deficit • Mobility, Impaired • Nutrition, Altered • Oral Mucous Membrane, Altered • Self-Care Deficit (specify) • Sexual Dysfunction • Sexuality Patterns, Altered • Sleep Pattern Disturbance • Swallowing, Impaired • Thermoregulation, Ineffective • Tissue Integrity, Impaired • Tissue Perfusion, Altered • Urinary Elimination Pattern, Altered • Urinary Retention

Reprinted, with permission, from Taylor. [10]

Framework 3

Functional Health Patterns

Marjory Gordon thought the direction of nursing diagnosis development had a problem orientation. She wanted a framework that would include the range of nursing actions—health promotion and health protection as well as problem intervention. She developed the functional health patterns to the whole health experience. The patterns apply to clients in various states of health or illness, across the age span, and to nursing in a number of practice settings. Gordon's system for organizing nursing diagnoses also lends itself well as a guide to the assessment process.[11] This type of health promotion framework can readily be used by public health and school nurses who work with healthy populations and who often use anticipatory guidance as an intervention strategy. This positive-oriented model can facilitate documentation of improvement in a client's already healthy state.[12]

The first pattern is health perceptions and health management and includes health status, health practices, worries or concerns about health issues, and personal responsibility. Nutrition and metabolic patterns are second and include food and fluid intake, appetite, healing of wounds, and general body functioning. Elimination focuses on bowel, urinary, and skin elimination. The activity and exercise pattern includes energy, exercise, and ability for activities of daily living. Sleep and rest is another pattern. Then the cognitive/perceptual pattern includes sensory functioning memory including pain or discomfort, and judgement/mental status. The self-concept pattern focuses on feelings, body image, and one's emotional state. The role-relationship pattern includes several family variables including living situation, members of the family, communication, roles in the family socialization, finances and roles/relationships in school or play group. Sexuality/reproductive pattern includes pubertal changes, sexual relations, satisfaction, and contraceptive practices. The coping pattern emphasizes stress tolerance including an understanding of stressors, including life change events, coping strategies, and problem management skills. The value or belief pattern has spiritual and religious elements at the core and also includes satisfaction with life.[11, 13]

Framework 4

Nursing Diagnosis for Wellness

A similar viewpoint reflecting nursing's role and expertise in health promotion and injury prevention is supported by Houldin, and associates.[14] Their focus is assessing and supporting the strengths of an individual and family to enhance health. The authors ascribe to Bircher's definition of nursing diagnosis, "a statement of the client's unique health status . . . based on factors affecting his[/her] wellbeing, dignity, rights, recovery maintenance, promotion of health and attainment of a meaningful lifestyle." Not only can health-promotion-oriented nursing diagnoses more fully describe a person's health and life experience, the positive diagnoses can increase a client's sense of mastery. Through this affirmation the client can more readily anticipate that prescribed actions will happen and that he/she is capable of achieving the outcomes.[12]

The authors selected the Functional Health Patterns of Gordon (described earlier) as the framework. They then selected and modified the nursing diagnoses to capitalize on clients' strengths. Some examples include changing body image disturbance to positive body image; changing self-care deficit to independent self-care, spiritual distress to spiritual support.

The nursing diagnoses organized according to this Functional Health Patterns framework are in Table 4.

Table 4. Nursing Diagnosis List Grouped Under Functional Health Patterns

Functional Pattern	Diagnosis
1. Health perception/ Health management	Health maintenance, appropriate Accident prevention practices, adequate
2. Nutritional/ Metabolic	Nutritional status, optimal Fluid volume, adequate Immune response, effective Skin integrity, adequate
3. Elimination	Bowel elimination, adequate Bladder elimination, adequate

4. Activity/
    Exercise
	Activity tolerance
	Physical fitness, optimal
	Respiratory function, effective
	Cardiac functioning, effective
	Home maintenance management,
	    effective
	Self-care, independence

5. Sleep, rest	Sleep pattern, adequate

6. Cognitive/
    Perceptual
	Developmental progression, efficient
	Potential for successful satisfaction of
	    developmental needs
	Comfort, adequate

7. Self-perception	Stress response, adaptive Self-concept, positive Body image, positive Self-esteem, adequate
8. Role/ Relationship	Coping, effective family Social interaction, satisfactory
9. Sexuality/ Reproductive	Sexual function, adequate
10. Coping/ Stress tolerance	Crisis resolution, effective Coping, effective individual
11. Value/Belief	Spiritual support

Table 4. cont. Commonly Identified Factors That Contribute to Wellness

Realistic self-concept
Acceptance of self
Accurate perception of reality
Autonomous functioning
Strong ethical sense
Responsibility for own actions
Self-direction
Adaptability
Creativity
Ability to express feelings
Effective problem-solving ability
Capacity for abstract thought
Sense of industry
Self-respect
Respect for needs of others
Scholastic (work) achievement
Insightful behavior
Role satisfaction
Effective social involvement
Satisfying interpersonal relationships
Ability to cope with illness
Ability to accept need for dependency
Positive role models
Physical capability
Effective management of disabilities
Accurate and sufficient information
Ability to accept the independent/dependent needs of others
Feelings of competence
Effective management of stressors ex. divorce, separation, illness, death.
Ability to grieve appropriately
Appropriate sense of humor
Adequate support systems
Availability of adequate resources (financial, cognitive, educational, and physical)
Sense of well-being
Political awareness and associated activities related to health and safety concerns
Desire to learn
Internal locus of control

Reprinted, with permission, from Houldin et al,[14] pp 22-24.

The work of NANDA and other nursing theorists and practitioners is ongoing and certain areas have not been fully addressed to date, including several arenas essential to school nursing—health promotion and wellness, family functioning, health in relation to education, community health focus, and others.[15] School nurses can be involved at two levels—the selection and use of a framework that is particularly suited to the school nursing specialty and development and submission of nursing diagnoses that are more descriptive of school nursing and the students as clients.

Components of the Nursing Diagnosis Statement

The first phrase of the diagnosis states the concern—a stage, phase, or level of problem or condition. (Refer to Table 1). As described, this is usually selected from the standardized list; however, as the emerging nature of the validation process has been noted, some situations require school nurses to develop new diagnostic statements. The first phrase in the diagnosis statement describes an alteration in health status—not necessarily negative or positive—for example, Alteration in individual coping. The alteration could be an actual (current/present) or potential change. Sometimes qualifiers are used to tailor the diagnosis to the client, for example, Potential for ineffective individual coping, or Acute ineffective denial. Care should be taken to avoid descriptors that connote value judgements and may lead to invalid conclusions.[15] To aid in communication, common definitions for these qualifiers were accepted by the NANDA conference attendees in 1986. Qualifiers for high-risk and wellness diagnoses were added in 1990 (see Table 5). Wellness diagnoses can be one-part statements.

A phrase "related to" links the concern to the etiology. The etiology is the reason phrase—the basis or cause for the alter-ation or problem, the underlying or precipitating cause. Etiology sources may be anatomical, physiological, psychological, environmental (physical environment, educational environment, social systems, and so on). The etiology may be a medical diagnosis, another nursing diagnosis, or another factor of a conceptual nature. The etiology is not data. Some examples include: Acute ineffective denial related to current intoxication; Acute ineffective denial related to parent also denying ____; Ineffective individual coping related to recent multiple losses in family support systems. For diagnoses that specify a client is at high risk, the etiology includes risk factors that may, with nursing interventions, reduce the likelihood of or prevent the problem. For wellness diagnoses, etiology statements are not required.

At times the related signs and symptoms (as collected in the assessment process) are included in the diagnostic statement. In this way the manifestation or evidence found in the data justifies the decisions about the first phrase, the diagnosis problem statement, and to the second phrase, the etiology. Frequently, for simplicity, the signs and symptoms are not included in the diagnosis statement, especially when the diagnostic statement is in the same record where the evidence—the assessment data—is documented. However, when working with the multi-disciplinary special education team, complete nursing diagnoses statements would aid other team members in understanding the nature and complexity of how health issues impact a child's ability to learn and function.

The phrase "resulting in/associated with" leads to the client's or student's response to the concern. More recently in the refinement of the nursing diagnosis statement, this phrase has been considered optional. However, this lifestyle impact or result for the individual client/student can

Table 5. Diagnosis Qualifiers

Actual:	Existing at the present moment; existing in reality.
Potential:	Can, but has not yet, come into being; possible.
Ineffective:	Not producing the desired effect; not capable of performing satisfactorily.
Decreased:	Smaller; lessened; diminished; lesser in size, amount, or degree
Increased:	Greater in size, amount, or degree; larger, enlarged.
Impaired:	Made worse, weakened; damaged, reduced; deteriorated.
Depleted:	Emptied wholly or partially; exhausted of.
Deficient:	Inadequate in amount, quality, or degree; defective; not sufficient; incomplete.
Excessive:	Characterized by an amount or quantity that is greater than is necessary, desirable, or usable.
Dysfunctional:	Abnormal; impaired or incompletely functioning.
Disturbed:	Agitated; interrupted, interfered with.
Acute:	Severe but of short duration.
Chronic:	Lasting a long time; recurring; habitual; constant.
Intermittent:	Stopping and starting again at intervals; periodic; cyclic.

Potential for enhanced _____ (wellness diagnosis)
    made greater, to increase in quality or more desired. *

High risk for _____
    client is more vulnerable to develop the problem than others in
    the same or similar situation; supported by risk factors that
    support interventions or reduce or prevent occurence *

Note: This list of modifiers or qualifiers is not exhaustive.

Reprinted, with permission, from McLane,[6] p. 470.

*NANDA, *Taxonomy I Revised, 1990 with Official Nursing Diagnoses*, 1990, pp. 116–117.

dictate the plans of action for the nurse and client. It is in this final phrase that the meaning or essence of the issue for the client is determined.

Relationship to Goal and Objective Statements

The nursing diagnosis summarizes the present status of a client. This can be followed by goals (global phrases) or objectives (precise, measurable phrases) that are positive and future oriented—offering a focus of working toward something rather than making up a deficit or working against something. For a given diagnosis, there may be several goals/objectives statements that break the varied hopes or solutions into incremental, achievable steps.

Student outcomes are the result of the goals or objectives, the result or impact. To compare, the nursing diagnosis is a statement of a present condition, a judgement of the situation at a given time. Goals and objectives are process- or progress-oriented and describe the steps to be taken through time. Student outcomes reflect the anticipated condition to be achieved, the changes in the student/client's health or life as a result of the nurse-client interaction and partnership. In addition to student outcomes, there may be nursing outcomes that deal with supporting the client in achieving his/her outcomes.

Application of Nursing Diagnosis in School Nursing Practice

School nurses use nursing diagnoses in a wide variety of situations. Their clients include several sets of individuals or groups: an individual student and/or the whole cluster of students in a classroom or school, family members of a student with a special health problem, faculty and support staff in a school building and/or throughout a school district, and the community as a whole of which the school is but one part. Each of these individuals vary by age, developmental status, size and type of community, and have many other variables that make each situation unique.

In each case, school nurses approach the actual and potential health needs of these "clients" using the nursing process as the framework for assessing needs and determining plans of action. In each situation, nursing diagnoses can summarize the situation and direct the plan of action. Some examples include diagnosing a student having trouble coping with an acute health problem or another student trying to deal with a chronic health problem, a family that is experiencing stress due to an economic crisis or a different well-functioning family that is anticipating change related to relocating, the school staff who are anxious about a health problem in their building or staff who need an update on a current issue to be included in the curriculum, or the community where a major public health initiative is under way.

In situations where individuals or the community has no apparent immediate problem, the school nurse uses a wellness-diagnosis approach and can determine several courses of intervention. For instance, all children grow and develop, so the role of the school nurse is anticipatory guidance—predicting and preparing for the changes ahead for the child, teacher and classroom, and the family. This would pertain if the child were healthy or if the child had a chronic health problem that was currently managed well. Second, an intervention that is always appropriate for individuals, schools, families, and communities is health education to increase knowledge and skills in a wide variety of topics. Third, programs that promote the health of the public are a regular part of school nurses' role—safety and injury-prevention programs, monitoring of environmental problems, and so on.

Advantages for Use of the Nursing Diagnoses— Implications

Scope of practice. As described in the historical development section, the standardizing of the nursing diagnostic statements will help to define the scope of practice by determining when nursing is responsible and accountable for diagnosing and treating conditions and by clarifying which activities are and are not nursing functions. The taxonomies or frameworks are a way to describe the independent aspects of practice, globally, and ensure that omissions are recognized. Having the taxonomies based on nursing theory also stimulates research that will validate current practice and describe or develop new arenas of nursing practice. For research purposes, the numerical system assigned to nursing diagnoses in a framework can be very useful in data manipulation and retrieval.[11, 16]

Quality assurance. Standards of practice and nursing theory guide nursing practice. Adherence to the standards and clinical practice guidelines by each practicing nurse can improve quality of care for clients. Accurate use of nursing diagnosis is one measure of compliance with the standards. School nurses could use the standards in self-assessment and/or peer review, measuring whether the nursing diagnoses reflect assessment data and also correlate with the action plans. Nursing diagnosis assures quality care in another way, by providing a common language within the school nursing specialty and across specialties within the discipline. This common, precise language increases the accuracy of communication and provides for continuity of care for students and families.[11] Finally, the use of pro-

jected nursing diagnosis outcomes can become a basis for outcome evaluation.

Fee for service and third party payment issue. With rising healthcare costs and diminishing public and private resources to meet the needs, different ways are being examined to fund independent nursing services. State and federal laws are being sought to provide payment for nursing (and school nursing) services from indemnity insurance plans, health maintenance organizations, and larger business with self-insured plans, in addition to the federal-and-state-subsidized payment systems. Sometimes clients pay nurses directly for services (well-child clinics, health education, primary healthcare). In all cases nurses must clearly articulate the need for service, the goal, the services offered, and the expected outcome. On a state and national level, standardized nursing diagnoses will expedite this process of validating nursing practice.[2, 11]

Staffing patterns. How nursing personnel staff are allocated and used in clinical settings and educational settings has often been arbitrary, at best. Nursing diagnoses can be a tool to delineate the type and amount of services required of an individual client or for a population. A medical diagnosis may give direction to the type and amount of nursing service required, but the client's response as described in the nursing diagnosis is a better indicator. The nursing diagnosis points to the interventions that are necessary, the level of expertise of healthcare provider required, and time and resources needed. The health and educational experience of a twelve-year-old student with asthma is significantly different than that of another student, whether eight or eighteen. The same way that the IEP defines the type of staff and the amount and level of service required for special education students, the nursing diagnoses for a student and related elements of the IHP can be used as a vehicle to determine school nurse staffing patterns.[2, 11]

Challenges for School Nurses

Incorporating nursing diagnoses into one's practice may be difficult—especially in the autonomous and isolated practice of school nursing. There is the immediate hurdle of learning the rhetoric of taxonomies, theories, and the diagnostic statements themselves—sometimes without anyone around who can help interpret or who understands the frustrations of an emerging framework in a profession. And there may be no fellow practitioners who encourage and insist in the daily use of nursing diagnoses. When supported, school nurses find nursing diagnosis brings increasing precision to their practice—brings clarity to the problems and ease in setting priorities for action.

Children and youth are presenting increasingly complex situations. There may be a tendency to expect one nursing diagnosis statement to summarize the issues, but several diagnostic statements may be needed. Again, the multiple diagnoses can bring clarity to the problems and set priorities for action. The school nurse functions in the role of planner and coordinator when determining the scope of the interventions for the client.[17]

One of the essential roles of school nurses is that of communicator.[17] This often includes interpretation and/or translation of medical diagnoses and treatment protocols to other educators, students and parents, and vice versa—translation of educational rhetoric and priorities to physicians and other health team members. Do nursing diagnoses add another element that needs translating? Newman [18] and Gordon [13] argue that the nursing diagnosis can describe for clients the phenomena they are experiencing, an emerging pattern, and help them make sense of what is

happening. Yes, the rhetoric of nursing diagnosis may need some interpretation but the nursing diagnosis process should offer an essential step—gaining consent or agreement that the diagnosis is accurate and that subsequent goals are desirable and attainable.

Selecting nursing diagnosis can aid in the difficult task, in the school setting, of documenting the nursing interactions. First, the nursing diagnosis' official language and requirement for the nurse to make a precise judgement call reaffirms/confirms the importance of each nursing interaction with students. Next, the nursing diagnosis can assist by focusing on the questions of where do I begin? what do I write? A key principle to remember is that documentation is NOT paperwork; it is an essential problem-solving and communicating process. Use of the nursing diagnosis can also ensure the record offers a nonjudgmental, unbiased view and the record does not ascribe blame to the client or to the nurse, but rather describes a situation with precision and reflects assessment data.

Some school nurses, due to the autonomy and isolation and hectic pace of the practice, wane in their attention to precision in judgements or nursing decisions, and in the documenting of these decisions. Few others in the educational setting realize the scope of responsibility and of liability of nurses in the independent practice of school nursing, so they may not support or encourage the use of nursing diagnosis or respect the time investment necessary for accurate documentation. Yet each nurse is accountable by state laws, the Code of Ethics and the Standards of Practice for all assessments, decisions and actions, and increasingly, the documentation of the same. The nursing process and nursing diagnosis step offers a method and guidelines for meeting the responsibilities.[11]

Summary

This chapter begins with definitions of nursing diagnosis and traces the development of the nursing diagnoses approval process directed by NANDA (North American Nursing Diagnosis Association). Several taxonomies or frameworks are presented that arrange the approved diagnoses or present alternative diagnoses. The components of the nursing diagnosis statement are described. Examples of use in school nursing are offered. Rationale are offered to assist school nurses in overcoming challenges to implementing nursing diagnosis in everyday practice for every client.

REFERENCES

1. American Nurses Association. *Nursing, a Social Policy Statement.* Washington, DC: American Nurses Association, 1980. (publication no. NP-63).
2. Luehr RE. Nursing process as applied to school nursing practice. In: Iverson, Carol, ed. *Health and Developmental History Assessment Skills Manual.* Scarborough, ME: National Association of School Nurses, 1983.
3. Shoemaker J. Essential features of nursing diagnoses. In: Kim MJ, McFarland GK, and McLane, AM, eds. *Classification of Nursing Diagnoses: Proceedings of the Fifth National Conference.* St. Louis: CV Mosby, 1987: 94-115.
4. Roy C. Theoretical framework for classification of nursing diagnosis. In: Kim MJ, Moritz DA, eds. *Classification of Nursing Diagnoses: Proceedings of the Third and Fourth National Conferences.* New York: McGraw-Hill, 1982: 215-221.
5. Gordon M. Nursing diagnosis and the diagnostic process. *Am J Nurs,* 1976; 76: pp. 1298-1300.
6. McLane AM, ed. *Classification of Nursing Diagnosis.* St. Louis: CV Mosby, 1987.
7. North American Nursing Diagnosis Association. Taxonomy I Revised - 1989 - with Official Diagnostic Categories. St. Louis: North American Nursing Diagnosis Association, 1990.
8. North American Nursing Diagnosis Association. Taxonomy I Revised—1990—with Official Nursing Diagnoses. St. Louis: North American Nursing Diagnosis Association, 1990. (NANDA, 3525 Caroline St, St. Louis, MO 63104; 314/577-8954)
9. Iyer PW., Taptich BJ, Bernocchi-Losey D. *Nursing Process and Nursing Diagnosis.* Philadelphia: WB Saunders, 1986.
10. Taylor CM, Cress S. *Nursing Diagnosis Cards.* Springhouse, PA: Springhouse Corporation, 1989.
11. Gordon M. *Nursing Diagnosis: Process and Application.* New York: McGraw Hill, 1982.
12. Lyons JF, Hester NO. Research-generated nursing diagnoses for healthy school-age children. *Compr Pediatr Nurs* 1987; 10: 149-159.
13. Gordon, M. *Manual of Nursing Diagnosis.* New York: McGraw-Hill, 1982.
14. Houldin, AS, Saltstein S, Ganley K. *Nursing Diagnosis for Wellness; Supporting Strengths.* Philadelphia: JB Lippincott, 1987.
15. Stolte K. A contemporary view of nursing diagnosis. *Public Health Nursing,* 1986; 3(1): 23-28.
16. Moberg MK. *Evolutionary Process of Nursing Diagnoses.* St. Paul, MN: College of St. Catherine, 1988, Aug (lecture and handouts).
17. Proctor ST. *Guidelines for a Model School Nursing Services Program.* Scarborough, ME: National Association of School Nurses, 1990.
18. Newman M. Nursing's emerging paradigm: The diagnosis of pattern. In: McLane, AM, ed. *Classification of Nursing Diagnosis.* St. Louis: CV Mosby, 1987.

Supplement 1. NANDA Taxomony I Revised—1990
Human Response Patterns, NANDA Approved Nursing Diagnoses

PATTERN 1: EXCHANGING

1.1.2.1	Altered Nutrition: More than body requirements
1.1.2.2	Altered Nutrition: Less than body requirements
1.1.2.3	Altered Nutrition: Potential for more than body requirements
1.2.1.1	Potential for Infection
1.2.2.1	Potential Altered Body Temperature
1.2.2.2	Hypothermia
1.2.2.3	Hyperthermia
1.2.2.4	Ineffective Thermoregulation
1.2.3.1	Dysreflexia
* 1.3.1.1	Constipation
1.3.1.1.1	Perceived Constipation
1.3.1.1.2	Colonic Constipation
* 1.3.1.2	Diarrhea
* 1.3.1.3	Bowel Incontinence
1.3.2	Altered Urinary Elimination
1.3.2.1.1	Stress Incontinence
1.3.2.1.2	Reflex Incontinence
1.3.2.1.3	Urge Incontinence
1.3.2.1.4	Functional Incontinence
1.3.2.1.5	Total Incontinence
1.3.2.2	Urinary Retention
* 1.4.1.1	Altered (Specify Type) Tissue Perfusion (Renal, cerebral, cardiopulmonary, gastrointestinal, peripheral)
1.4.1.2.1	Fluid Volume Excess
1.4.1.2.2.1	Fluid Volume Deficit
1.4.1.2.2.2	Potential Fluid Volume Deficit
* 1.4.2.1	Decreased Cardiac Output
1.5.1.1	Impaired Gas Exchange
1.5.1.2	Ineffective Airway Clearance
1.5.1.3	Ineffective Breathing Pattern
1.6.1	Potential for Injury
1.6.1.1	Potential for Suffocation
1.6.1.2	Potential for Poisoning
1.6.1.3	Potential for Trauma
1.6.1.4	Potential for Aspiration
1.6.1.5	Potential for Disuse Syndrome
#1.6.2	Altered Protection
1.6.2.1	Impaired Tissue Integrity
* 1.6.2.1.1	Altered Oral Mucous Membrane
1.6.2.1.2.1	Impaired Skin Integrity
1.6.2.1.2.2	Potential Impaired Skin Integrity

PATTERN 2: COMMUNICATING

2.1.1.1	Impaired Verbal Communication

Note: The authors of this book have listed the applicable NANDA numerical numbers in the Nursing
Diagnoses section in each of the Individualized Healthcare Plans.

PATTERN 3: RELATING

3.1.1	Impaired Social Interaction
3.1.2	Social Isolation
*3.2.1	Altered Role Performance
3.2.1.1.1	Altered Parenting
3.2.1.1.2	Potential Altered Parenting
3.2.1.2.1	Sexual Dysfunction
3.2.2	Altered Family Processes
3.2.3.1	Parental Role Conflict
3.3	Altered Sexuality Patterns

PATTERN 4: VALUING

4.1.1	Spiritual Distress (distress of the human spirit)

PATTERN 5: CHOOSING

5.1.1.1	Ineffective Individual Coping
5.1.1.1.1	Impaired Adjustment
5.1.1.1.2	Defensive Coping
5.1.1.1.3	Ineffective Denial
5.1.2.1.1	Ineffective Family Coping: Disabling
5.1.2.1.2	Ineffective Family Coping: Compromised
5.1.2.2	Family Coping: Potential for Growth
5.2.1.1	Noncompliance (Specify)
5.3.1.1	Decisional Conflict (Specify)
5.4	Health Seeking Behaviors (Specify)

PATTERN 6: MOVING

6.1.1.1	Impaired Physical Mobility
6.1.1.2	Activity Intolerance
6.1.1.2.1	Fatigue
6.1.1.3	Potential Activity Intolerance
6.2.1	Sleep Pattern Disturbance
6.3.1.1	Diversional Activity Deficit
6.4.1.1	Impaired Home Maintenance Management
6.4.2	Altered Health Maintenance
*6.5.1	Feeding Self Care Deficit
6.5.1.1	Impaired Swallowing
6.5.1.2	Ineffective Breastfeeding
#6.5.1.3	Effective Breastfeeding
*6.5.2	Bathing/Hygiene Self Care Deficit
*6.5.3	Dressing/Grooming Self Care Deficit
*6.5.4	Toileting Self Care Deficit
6.6	Altered Growth and Development

PATTERN 7: PERCEIVING

* 7.1.1	Body Image Disturbance
* 7.1.2	Self Esteem Disturbance
7.1.2.1	Chronic Low Self Esteem
7.1.2.2	Situational Low Self Esteem
* 7.1.3	Personal Identity Disturbance
7.2	Sensory/Perceptual Alterations (Specify) (Visual, auditory, kinesthetic, gustatory, tactile, olfactory)
7.2.1.1	Unilateral Neglect
7.3.1	Hopelessness
7.3.2	Powerlessness

PATTERN 8: KNOWING

8.1.1	Knowledge Deficit (Specify)
8.3	Altered Thought Processes

PATTERN 9: FEELING

* 9.1.1	Pain
9.1.1.1	Chronic Pain
9.2.1.1	Dysfunctional Grieving
9.2.1.2	Anticipatory Grieving
9.2.2	Potential for Violence: Self-directed or directed at others
9.2.3	Post-Trauma Response
9.2.3.1	Rape-Trauma Syndrome
9.2.3.1.1	Rape-Trauma Syndrome: Compound Reaction
9.2.3.1.2	Rape-Trauma Syndrome: Silent Reaction
9.3.1	Anxiety
9.3.2	Fear

New diagnostic categories approved 1990
* Categories with modified label terminology

North American Nursing Diagnosis Association,[8] pp. 6-8. Reprinted with permission.

3 | Individualized Healthcare Plans

Marykay B. Haas

PURPOSE

The Individualized Healthcare Plan (IHP) is a variation of the time-honored nursing care plan adapted specifically for the school setting. Nursing care plans originally served several purposes. First, care plans were a means of communication among hospital nurses. The nursing care plans detailed the complex care that a patient required. However, it was not unusual for patients with routine care to have only doctor's orders instead of a written care plan. Similarly, not every student's needs are complex and/or require daily nursing care, so every student will not require an IHP.

Second, care plans served as a teaching vehicle. Nursing students from every level of preparation—vocational through master's level programs—were expected to produce care plans or case studies to detail the nursing process that was used to arrive at the conclusions about the nature of the client's nursing needs.

Third, care plans, especially in public health nursing, were necessary to document needs and to claim third-party reimbursement.

With the increase in the complexity of care delivered in the community, many nurses began to see the benefits of using standardized care plans that could be adapted to individual client needs. Hospi-

tals and community health agencies began to have standardized care plans as well as policies and procedures as a means to ensure quality care. Besides saving a nurse time, a standardized care plan can trigger a nurse's memory as to the whole range of possible nursing interventions, thereby improving the comprehensiveness of care.

In addition, as the practice of school nursing expands in complexity, the need to communicate the outcomes of the care provided becomes more acute. School nurses will be in a better position to maintain a professional practice when they can articulate the care and the outcomes expected.

The current economics of healthcare and education indicate that future reimbursement for school health services may be influenced by the opportunities to access third-party reimbursement. School nurses are in an ideal situation to become case managers for children with chronic health conditions. Professional school nurses often see the child with a chronic health condition on a daily or weekly basis. They are aware of subtle changes in the child's condition and resulting needs for medical intervention. School nurses are also knowledgeable about the local healthcare community and resources available. Finally, school nurses are not as likely to overlook the health promotion needs of children with chronic health problems. They are likely to be involved when immunizations are not up-to-date or when health teaching is needed. All of this points to an increase in the ability to become case managers for these children. However, case management skills are complex and require a high level of involvement with families. School nurses are challenged to develop such case management models and share them with colleagues. Standardizing the school nursing care through IHPs will help to move school nurses to the next level of professional practice: case management.

School nurses have unique needs for constructing IHPs distinct from the nurse-to-nurse communication that usually transpires in hospitals. School nurses need to communicate nursing care needs to regular and special education administrators and teachers, health aides, and parents. Due to this diverse audience it can be difficult to produce a single care plan entity that will be useful for every purpose. Nevertheless, this author believes that only by being clear at the professional nursing level about student needs and desired outcomes, can school nurses then simplify and interpret to the various publics how professional school nurses contribute to the educational process and the health status of child.

Relationship to the Special Education Process

Individualized healthcare plans are frequently associated with the special education process, but this is not their only purpose. Any child, with a relatively complex health condition or a need for modifications in the school environment due to a health condition, could have an IHP.

When participating in the special education Individualized Education Plan (IEP) process, school nurses need a method to describe the health needs as they relate to the educational process of the student. An IHP is an important preparation for participating in an IEP meeting. School psychologists have reports of test scores. Occupational and physical therapists have reports based on testing and both formulate recommendations based on the testing. School nurses should use the IHP as a first step toward formulating special education recommendations and student goals. When appropriate, sections of the IHP should be incorporated into the IEP during the special education child study process.

Individualized Healthcare Plans (IHP) can be used as input into the interdisciplinary team of the special education child assessment process. In this case the school nurse would get permission from the parent to assess the child. After reviewing and updating the child's health history, gathering current assessment data, such as vision, hearing, height, weight, nutritional status, and so on, the school nurse could summarize the data and develop a list of recommendations based on the child's needs. This report, consisting of summary data and recommendations, could then be shared with the special education team as the school nurse's assessment report during the team conference. The planning phase would then be carried out by the entire team. It is advisable to have nursing care needs and services documented on the child's IEP, especially if special education "related services" funding is being accessed. Table 1 gives some parameters on which to compare an IEP, IHP, and emergency plan.

Use of an IHP in Chronic Illness

Children who are not special education eligible may also need an IHP. Children with chronic illness usually require some additional monitoring and modifications in the educational program. The formulation

Table 1. Comparison of IEP, IHP, and Emergency Care Plan

	IEP	IHP	Emergency plan
Mandated by special education law	Yes	No	No
Required by Professional Standards (ANA)	No	Yes	Yes
Used for student who may have a life-threatening episode	No	Yes	Yes
Contains student goals	Yes	Yes	No
Requires parent permission and/or signature	Yes	No	No
Must be eligible for special education	Yes	No	No

of an IHP helps to ensure that all necessary information, needs, and plans are considered to maximize the child's participation and performance in the school setting.

Emergency care plans are frequently confused with IHPs. Emergency care plans are necessary and may even be formulated as part of the IEP or IHP process. These emergency plans are usually procedural guidelines indicating who to call and other information to be used when a predictable emergency occurs. For example, a child with seizures may need a particular medication and transportation to a particular medical facility if the medication is ineffective. Emergency care plans usually do not give sufficient information to meet all the child's needs, but may give some procedural guidance to paraprofessionals or educators working with a particular student when a life-threatening incident occurs.

These children should have both an emergency care plan and an IHP. The IHP would then cover other aspects of their care, such as a child's knowledge about his/her condition, self-care abilities, and any modifications needed during the school day to enhance learning or to prevent emergencies if possible. For a sample emergency care plan see this book's Appendix.

Benefits of IHPs

School nurses can experience many benefits from using IHPs for students with complex nursing care needs. First, by documenting the student's needs and care, the school nurse establishes the type, amount, and intensity of nursing care required by a particular student. The number and type of IHPs in a particular school district could serve as a program needs assessment when proposing additional staffing needs.

Second, documented IHP needs can also serve as important school nursing staff information within a school district. If a school nurse in one school has six students with documented IHP nursing care needs of four hours per day and another school nurse has ten students with documented IHP needs of six hours per day, a rational decision can be made about how much nursing staffing is needed in each school. This is a much more complex way of assigning staff than a simple ratio of 1 nurse per 800 students. Other healthcare settings have similar acuity measures that determine staffing. However, we must not forget that this method does not take into account the ongoing public health screening and education program that all students need whether or not they have an IHP.

A third important benefit is to ensure the quality of school nursing services. When current nursing care standards are used to develop an IHP, administators, parents, and students can be assured that the student will be appropriately cared for at school. The ANA Standards of School Nursing Practice [1] require a school nurse to have an IHP for a student when significant health needs exist.

A school nurse whose practice includes written IHPs based on the most current standards and information on nursing care is more likely to deliver a higher standard of nursing care and to be recognized for that expertise by peers, parents, and school administrators. Beyond the obvious public relations benefits, parents are likely to feel more comfortable with their child's care when it appears in writing and clearly addresses the child's needs.

On a practical level a written IHP commits the school nurse to carry out the IHP services. Some school nurses may shy away from this commitment. After all, if a student needs asthma education and this is indicated on the IHP, the school nurse must find the time to deliver the service. IHPs may help some school nurses develop better ways to prioritize school nursing services.

By creating a written IHP, the school nurse is establishing a rational basis for practice. This written document could serve as a legal protection by showing that proper plans and safeguards were in place even if a bad outcome occurred.

The documentation of care plans by an IHP can also help to ensure continuity of care as students move from school to school or new school nurses are assigned to schools. How much valuable time is wasted when a student moves and the next school nurse has nothing in writing and must start over gathering a complete data base?

Finally, IHPs can help to create a safer process for delegation of nursing care in the school setting. The delegation of a particular task can be specifically described. More importantly the delegation of a particular task can be seen within the context of all of the student's needs.

As the complexity of nursing care delivered in schools increases, it is essential that a second-rate, inferior system of nursing care is not substituted for the adequate professional school nursing care that students may need. It is hoped that this book will help school nurses efficiently take on the special challenges of today's students with special healthcare needs.

REFERENCES

1.   American Nurses Association, in cooperation with APHA, ASHA, NAPNAP, NASN, and NASSNC. *Standards of School Nursing Practice.* (Publication no. NP-66) Washington, DC: American Nurses Association, 1983.

Constructing an Individualized Healthcare Plan

Marykay B. Haas

OVERVIEW AND CASE STUDY

Individualized Healthcare Plans (IHPs) should have the following identifiable parts: history, assessment data, nursing diagnosis, goal of care, student/family goals, selected nursing actions or interventions, and expected client outcomes. The components recognized by the *ANA Standards of School Nursing Practice* include: data collection, nursing diagnosis, planning, intervention, and evaluation. These components make up phases of the nursing process.[1] The IHP becomes the set of directions that the nurse constructs to direct the nursing care needed by a particular student. The plan itself may take one or all of several forms: a nursing care plan, an emergency care plan, or an integrated plan along with the Individualized Education Plan (IEP) or with the Individualized Family Service Plan (IFSP).

In order to be useful to school nurses, the IHP should be descriptive of the usual types of nursing interventions that are appropriate for students with similar conditions. The types of interventions should also reflect the unique ambulatory pediatric care setting of schools. Finally, the finished IHP should be individualized to reflect the data and needs of a particular student at a particular point in time. Plans should be updated periodically.

Standardized IHPs should reflect the "best practices" of school nurses as they interact daily with students, families, educators, and other members of the medical community. Healthcare plans must be specific enough to describe what will be done, what results are expected, and what parameters are important to keep track of. Individualized Healthcare Plans should not be confused with the more specific emergency care plans. This book's appendix contains a sample emergency care plan. Emergency care plans may be incorporated as a part of the IHP, but emergency plans just provide specific directions about what to do in a particular emergency situation. The emergency care plan never should be considered a substitute for a full IHP that addresses all of the student's relevant needs. In fact, if only an emergency care plan is used, it can give the false impression that a student's needs are being met when in fact there may be steps that can be taken to prevent emergencies if a more complete assessment of the student had taken place and been documented in an IHP.

History

History is sometimes considered a part of the assessment process. As the school nurse uses the nursing process to assist the student s/he must review the course of the condition prior to the nurse's involvement, including any medical care received, any related self-care practices, and any significant family and lifestyle factors. This information may be different from what is currently observable and provides a broad understanding of the student's current health status. This information then becomes a part of the essential data base. Most school nurses use a standardized health history form for each child and then update the information periodically as needed. An important part of history taking is knowing what questions to ask. Consequently you will find examples of questions to ask and topical areas to cover addressed in each IHP example.

Assessment

The school nurse must make some decisions about what essential data is needed in order to determine the student's health status and to make an appropriate nursing diagnosis. From there the healthcare plans are formulated. Usually the essential data base includes: physical findings, strengths, social and emotional relationships, coping strategies, family issues, and resources available. The ability to narrow the data base is a skill based on clinical judgement, knowledge of the usual course of the condition(s) involved and of the usual nursing interventions. For example, a student with diabetes requires particular attention to nutritional status. Therefore the dietary assessment would be more extensive than for a student with a seizure disorder.

Nursing Diagnoses (N.D.)

As stated in the chapter on nursing diagnosis, although the current work in the NANDA classification system[2] focuses primarily on the illness process rather than the wellness process, it is necessary that the school nurse sort and organize the data to come to some conclusion about the nature of the student's needs and what nursing might do to meet them. As school nurses become more familiar with nursing diagnosis terminology it will become easier to sort data along the parameters of nursing diagnosis. Note: The authors of this book have listed the applicable NANDA numerical numbers in the Nursing Diagnoses section in each of the Individualized Healthcare Plans. If a nurse chooses not to use nursing diagnoses, the nurse must still come up with some kind of problem statement that allows the nurse to summarize the student's problem or need.

Individual pieces of data by themselves have no meaning. It is the method of organizing the data about a particular individual or family and the process of conclusion drawing that separates professional school nursing knowledge and expertise from that of the lay person. For example, the following data describes a student: hasn't seen a doctor for over a year, medications are frequently missed at home and school, one week passed before parent supplied school with medication for at-school administration. In nursing diagnosis framework this situation could be described as: Altered or Impaired Health Maintenance related to lack of health insurance. Nursing diagnosis is one method of organizing data to assist in this process.

A nursing problem statement is another way of organizing and summarizing nursing data. For example, a student with a seizure disorder may have data that indicate poor control: misses medications regularly, hasn't seen a physician for over a year, increase in seizure activity while at school, and evidence of increasing school difficulties. This data could be summarized by saying that the student is experiencing poor medication control and needs to return to the doctor for reevaluation of seizure medication.

Nursing Interventions

Nursing interventions are the actions that the school nurse will take to achieve a desired client outcome. They are necessarily goal-oriented.

Nursing interventions are the "what" the nurse does about the information the nurse has concerning a particular student's needs. Carrying out nursing interventions provides the student with "school nursing services." The appropriate nursing interventions can vary across settings. For example, while it may be appropriate for a nurse to administer anesthesia in a hospital under the direction of a physician, it would not be appropriate in a school clinic. Education about medications may be more appropriate in the school setting than in the recovery room of outpatient surgery suites. Many areas also overlap. As schools increasingly become more involved in delivering primary care, schools will need to hire or educate school nurses with good physical assessment skills and advanced technical skills and abilities.

Goals

The nursing literature is not always clear about the nature of goals. Sometimes the term goal is used to refer to nursing interventions or nursing outcomes. Other times the confusion is in relation to student goals and outcomes. Each type of goal can be useful. A student goal is more useful when the purpose of the IHP is to integrate information and needs into the IEP. A nursing goal is more useful when the purpose of the IHP is to provide a written

plan for a paraprofessional to follow in the nurse's absence. Examples of each are found within this book. Some authors used only nursing goals while others used only student goals and a few IHPs have both student and nursing goals.

Regardless of the type, goals are generally broad statements and are not as situation-specific as interventions. A school nurse working with a child with a headache and an emergency room nurse comforting a child after a cast application might have the same goal of "relieving pain." However, the appropriate nursing interventions are likely to be quite different.

Expected Client Outcomes

Expected client outcomes are statements that describe how the student's situation will be "different" or "healthier" as a result of the nursing care received. Stating student outcomes is an important skill to learn. As more and more of education turns to outcome-based education, school nurses are in an ideal situation to use the language of "outcomes." Student outcomes can be long- or short-range. Student outcomes can reflect emotional, physical, or social changes or adaptation to a chronic condition. Student outcomes are usually stated as the most desirable state for the student to achieve. There can be some overlap between IEP\IFSP objectives and IHP outcomes.

Putting It All Together

In summary, standardized nursing care plans such as IHPs are a starting point for reviewing and organizing school nursing practices. IHPs are a framework that must be individualized in order to give the most benefit to the student. Only after the school nurse has determined the student's needs through the history and assessment phases can a nursing diagnosis and plan of care be formulated. The plan of care can then be used to formulate IEP\IFSP objectives, to create an emergency plan, to direct health aides, or to collect data and make recommendations about staffing needs.

Once a school nurse has completed the thinking process involved in planning an IHP and has all the necessary student data, the question arises as to what is the best way to write up an IHP. One approach might involve using a structure that takes each area of functioning and addresses it separately. *Responding with Support: An Individualized Health Plan for a Student with AIDS Virus Infection*[3] is a good example. This document goes through the most likely diagnoses and addresses how each area would be relevant to a student with AIDS. This format may be most useful when a school nurse is dealing with a student with complex healthcare needs that require significant accommodation in the school setting. This process is also useful when a student is being assessed by the school nurse for health needs as a part of the Special Education Child Study process. Every student who qualifies for special education on the basis of a "related health need" or "other health impaired" should have a complete IHP.

REFERENCES

1. American Nurses Association, American Public Health Association, National Association of Pediatric Nurse Associates and Practitioners, National Association of School Nurses, and National Association of State School Nurse Consultants. *Standards of School Nursing Practice.* 1983. Available from the American Nurses Association, 2420 Pershing Rd, Kansas City, MO 64208.
2. North American Nursing Diagnosis Association. 1989. 3525 Caroline St, St. Louis, MO 63104.
3. School Nurse Organization of Minnesota and Minnesota Department of Education. *Responding with Support: An Individualized Health Plan for a Student with AIDS Virus Infection.* (Prepared by Cyndy Schuster, Marykay Haas, Mary Villars, and Ruth Ellen Luehr.). 1988.

CASE STUDY

By presenting a case study this next section shows how to use the IHP format. In addition, it provides examples of health components of an Individual Education Plan (IEP) and an emergency care plan. This example is intended to show the differences between these type of tools as well as to give a specific application. These are not the only acceptable formats, nor are the examples as detailed as an actual case might be. The information is for illustration only. For additional illustration this book's Appendix presents sample forms for an IHP and an emergency care plan.

Your school district may have different forms or you may wish to experiment until you find a way of organizing the information that works best for you. Do add your district logo, school nurse name and phone number, or other identifying information so that if a student moves the new school nurse knows who to contact. More important than the format is the thinking process that the nurse follows and the interventions that the nurse selects.

Try to imagine yourself in the following situation:

You are the school nurse in a rural district of 2,000 students. You have a part-time health aide that helps you every morning from eight to noon. You have three school buildings, including two elementary schools and a combination junior/senior high school. You have four diabetic students in the district, one at the elementary and three at the combined high school. It is the second week of August and you get a call from the principal asking you to give a call to a parent of an elementary student. He says that a 12-year-old student, Judy, has been diagnosed with diabetes over the summer. The principal mentions that you should figure out what the school needs to do. The principal says she is particularly concerned that the other students not see Judy using a needle at school and that the teachers will not know what to do in an emergency.

You call the parent and learn the following:

Judy is a 12-year-old sixth grade student at North Elementary. She was diagnosed with diabetes about two months ago. She lives with her mother, father, and two brothers on a farm. She has about a 10-mile bus ride to school. Judy did well in school until last year when her attendance was poor and she had difficulty keeping up in the classroom. She had started a special education program during the last year. She is on a three-dose schedule of medication. She will need to have insulin at school before lunch. She has been learning to test her own glucose level using a glucometer and is learning to keep her own records. Her food intake and exercise patterns are difficult to regulate because she has started her growth spurt.

Judy plays basketball with her brothers and is on a recreation league team. In summer she helps out on the farm. She has been anxious about starting school this fall because she is afraid that the other girls will tease her about the diabetes. Judy has had several insulin reactions during the past weeks and has been back to the doctor twice for blood tests.

What can you do to help Judy and her family make a successful adaption this school year? Who else needs to be involved? What should you do first? What kinds of nursing care will Judy require this year? What additional data do you need? What kinds of outcomes do you want to achieve? How should Judy's IHP look? Does she need an emergency care plan as well?

Using the nursing process the school nurse decides that she needs more data. She calls the parent to set up a time to meet with Judy's mother about Judy's needs at school. The school nurse also asks the parent's permission to get information from Judy's physician. Finally, she suggests that Judy might like to come to school, bring her equipment, and go through her usual activities before school starts so that she will be comfortable when school starts. The school nurse also talks with the principal about reserving a 30-minute time block on a teacher in-service day before school starts to talk about Judy's needs and two other new students with chronic health conditions.

After meeting with Judy and her mother and reviewing the physician's information, orders, and recommendations, the school nurse develops the following Individualized Healthcare Plan(IHP):

Organizing Framework

Assessment Data:

Physician Information: Judy has Diabetes, Type I. Her insulin is being regulated carefully as she continues to have reactions. Doctor's orders include: Blood glucose check at noon. Report levels over 200. Assist Judy to self-administer insulin as necessary. Treat insulin reactions with oral glucagon. Transport to emergency room if unconscious or unable to arouse.

Nursing Assessment data:
*   history of insulin reactions
*   no sensory impairments upon screening
*   has grown 2 inches since last year, has lost 2 pounds
*   no signs of infection
*   needs to learn appropriate self-care for diabetes
*   is concerned about peer relations
*   knows major concepts about diabetes but doesn't have a good understanding of the effects of diet and exercise
*   states she is embarrassed by need to give insulin at school

Nursing Diagnoses:
1. Knowledge deficit related to recent onset of diabetes, need to balance diet and exercise and give insulin.
2. Potential for self-esteem disturbance due to embarrassment about need for medication and concerns about social stigma.
3. Potential for physiologic imbalance due to metabolic changes.

Nursing Interventions: (See Chapter 22 on Diabetes for more detail.)
1. Develop an emergency care plan with student and family.
2. In-service school staff to intervene appropriately.
3. Set up with student a schedule for blood testing and insulin injection. Monitor student's ability to draw up medication correctly and use good injection technique.
4. Initially, meet with student weekly to go over adjustment to diabetes. Within two months invite Judy to join the student support group of students with diabetes.

Outcomes expected:

1. Insulin reactions will be identified early by Judy and/or teachers and appropriate action will be taken.
2. Judy will demonstrate increasing knowledge and skill in diet, exercise, and medication management.
3. Judy will demonstrate good coping skills by feeling less embarrassed and better able to handle questions and concerns of friends.

In all cases it is important to develop the IHP with input from the parents and student. This school nurse decides to use the IHP as a means of contracting with Judy to increase Judy's ability to participate in her care. Especially with older students it is important to their self-esteem to be a partner in the planning process. The school nurse writes up a draft of the plan and gives Judy a copy to go over with her parents. Both Judy and her parents are asked to sign the IHP as a indication of their agreement and willingness to participate. (See Appendix for sample IHP forms.)

Judy's IHP

Name: Judy Smith   Birthdate:

Address: Emergency Phone:

Doctor: Phone:

School: Teacher:

Review dates:

Goals:
1. Increase Judy's information and skills in the management of her diabetes.
2. Increase Judy's level of comfort in talking with friends about her diabetes.
3. Create an emergency plan to assist Judy during insulin reactions and other emergencies.

Assessment Data	Nursing Diagnosis	Nursing Interventions	Outcomes
1. Frequent Insulin 2. New diagnosis	Potential for physiologic imbalance	1. Monitor blood sugar testing 2. In-service teachers on early identification of reactions	All insulin reactions will be treated promptly and reported to parent
1. Judy has difficulty understanding relationship between diet, exercise, and medication 2. Growth spurt in progress	Knowledge deficit related to new diagnosis	1. Set up a schedule to monitor blood sugar testing and insulin management skills with Judy 2. Build teaching sessions into daily contacts	Judy will increase her skill and ability to manage her diabetes
1. States that she is embarrassed by discussion of diabetes with friends	Potential for self-esteem disturbance	1. Give Judy opportunity to discuss her feelings 2. Encourage Judy to attend weekly support group 3. Meet with nurse weekly	Judy will feel comfortable about asking for help and sharing information with friends about her diabetes

JUDY'S INDIVIDUALIZED EDUCATION PLAN (IEP)

IEP Recommendation based on IHP assessment:
Current Health/Physical Status: Judy has diabetes, Type I. She continues to have insulin reactions and she needs assistance in monitoring glucose and administering insulin. Her general health status is good. She has no vision, hearing, or other sensory impairments. Judy should have preferential seating so the teacher is aware of her mental status, especially during the late morning.

Special Education Recommendation: Judy needs teaching regarding disease process and its influence on her physical and mental status. Judy needs monitoring of blood glucose and insulin administration before lunch. Teachers need to observe Judy for insulin reactions, especially before lunch. Proper regulation of insulin is an important factor in Judy being able to concentrate on schoolwork. Judy should not have physical education immediately before lunch until her insulin is better regulated.

The following may be inserted directly into the IEP after there is agreement from the IEP team at the IEP planning process.

IEP Goal 1: Judy will learn to monitor blood glucose, administer insulin, and recognize and report insulin reactions.
IEP Goal 2: Judy will increase her understanding of diabetes and increase her ability to cope with its requirements.

Short-term Instructional Objectives:

1. Judy will demonstrate proper use of glucometer and recording of insulin at least 75% of the time.
2. Judy will draw up insulin dosage and inject at rotating sites with 100% accuracy.
3. Judy will identify the relationship between diet, exercise, and insulin requirements as it applies to her school activities.
4. Judy will attend diabetic support group twice monthly.

Weekly nursing time required:

Daily 10-minute blood glucose check and insulin administration x 5 days = 50 minutes.

Weekly teaching conference with Judy on diet, exercise, medication and general adjustment = 30 minutes.

Classroom observation and discussion of progress with teacher approximately 10 minutes per week.

Total weekly nursing needs: 1.5 hours

JUDY'S EMERGENCY CARE PLAN

Remember that the emergency care plan should be as brief and yet as complete as possible. It should make it possible for a medically untrained person such as a teacher to take appropriate action quickly. Too much detail could slow down the teacher, principal, playground monitor, secretary, or bus driver from taking appropriate action.

Date: ___September 12,1992___   ID # _____

Student name:___Judy Smith___   Birthdate: ___August 4, 1979___   Grade: _____

Parent: ___Pat Smith___   Emergency phone numbers: _____

Doctor: _____Bob Jones_____   Hospital: _____Children's_____

Medical insurance (optional): ___Blue Cross-Blue Shield_____

****

Medical condition: Diabetes, Type I: body doesn't produce insulin, so insulin is injected into the body daily. Sometimes Judy gets too much insulin and needs extra sugar.

Usual treatment: Gets blood sugar test before lunch. Goes to nurse's office at 11:30. Takes insulin before lunch. Judy doesn't always know when low blood sugar is happening. She always carries oral glucagon in a tube in her pocket .

Signs of emergency:

Unconscious: true emergency

Tired, confused, headache, nausea, sweating: probably needs glucose immediately

Actions for teacher/secretary/aide to take:

Step 1: If unconscious call 911

Step 2: Ask Judy if she needs glucagon, get it for her if necessary. A glass of juice may be substituted.

Step 3: If no response to glucagon or if Judy has forgotten it, call nurse to get glucagon or sugar.

Note Judy's response to emergency action taken and tell nurse.
Principal notified _X_   School nurse notified   _X_
Doctor notified _X_   Parent notified   _X_

Chronic Health Conditions:
Indicators of the Need for Planned School Nursing Services

Cynthia K. Silkworth

According to the National Health Interview Survey on Child Health done in 1988, 30.8 percent of children and 31.5 percent of adolescents had one or more chronic health conditions.[1] Among all children with a chronic health condition, approximately 10 percent have severe conditions which have daily impact on the child's life.[2] Advances in healthcare technology have saved many children who, ten to twenty years ago, would have died. Many times these children have significant chronic health conditions. Most of the conditions will persist for years and will have a variable course, some improving, some remaining stable, and some becoming worse. Many of the children are dependent on medications and/or specific healthcare procedures at home and at school to maintain their health and ability to grow, develop, play, and learn.

A general definition of a chronic health condition is: a condition that interferes with daily functioning for more than three months in a year, causes extensive hospitalization or home health services, or (at time of diagnosis) is likely to do either of these.[2, 3]

Dealing with chronic health conditions is considerably different than dealing with acute conditions. Chronic health conditions require that we focus on the child as an individual rather than on a specific symptom or illness. The entire physical and social environment is relevant in management of the condition. As the child develops and as the chronic health condition changes or progresses, different pieces of management of the condition will take on the major focus. It creates a need for skill in decision making, self-care, and management planning for several different environments.

Chronic health conditions include those identified in Public Law 94-142 and 99-457 as handicapping conditions and eligible for special education and related services (Education of Handicapped Children, 1975, 1986, and Individuals with Disabilities Education Act, IDEA, 1990.)

> Educable Mentally Handicapped
> Trainable Mentally Handicapped
> Profound Mentally Handicapped
> Emotionally Handicapped
> Learning Disabled
> Visually Handicapped
> Hearing Handicapped
> Orthopedically Handicapped
> Deaf/Blind
> Speech/Language Handicapped
> Autism
> Traumatic Brain Injury
> Other Health Impaired: chronic or acute health problems which adversely affect a child's educational performance

Other chronic health conditions may need health services, but not necessarily special education. These include, but **are not limited to** the following specific conditions:

Asthma
Attention Deficit Hyperactivity
    Disorder
Chronic Kidney Disease
Congenital Heart Disease
Cystic Fibrosis
Diabetes
Epilepsy/Seizure Disorders
Hemophilia/Hematologic
    Disorders
Immunologic Deficiencies
Juvenile Rheumatoid Arthritis
Leukemia/Neoplastic Diseases
Lupus Erythematosis
Muscular Dystrophy
Severe Allergies
Sickle Cell Anemia
Spina Bifida

For children with chronic health conditions, and their families, the interaction with the educational system is often complex. Opportunities for control, mastery, and accomplishment can be brought into the life of children who have little control over their own health. Special problems can also occur, such as episodic and/or lengthy absences from school, limited endurance or ability to concentrate, and daily health management requirements which may affect the child's academic success and development of social skills. How children with a chronic health condition are handled in the educational system can influence their future academic success and success in society.

The educational team, in cooperation with the parents/guardians and healthcare providers, must provide an appropriate educational and support service program based on the child's educational needs and potential, developmental status, and healthcare needs. Because children with chronic health conditions have unique needs and health considerations, individu-

alized assessments, planning, and placement decisions are critical.

For this to happen, there needs to be good communication with everyone involved—the student, family, healthcare providers, and educational team. Lack of accurate information about the child may result in inappropriate educational placement, denial of a necessary service, or overprotective attitudes and behaviors.[4] Information that is critical for developing good educational and health plans for a child with a chronic illness includes:

- What is the diagnosis?

- What is the prognosis?

- Is the child's health stabilized, getting better, getting worse?

- What is the child's understanding of his/her health condition and current status? How has it been explained to the child? Are further explanations or continued reinforcements needed?

- What medications is the child presently taking? How will these medications affect the child's behavior and ability to learn? Have the medications been increased or decreased recently? Are there any medications that will need to be administered in school routinely, episodically, or on an emergency basis? Is the child able to self-administer the medication at home?

- What specialized healthcare procedures is the child currently receiving? Are there any specialized healthcare procedures that will need to be administered at school? Is the child able to self-direct or perform the healthcare procedure at home?

- What is the child's physical endurance? Is there a need to modify the child's school day?

- Does the child need classroom modifications, such as preferential seating, special desk or table, special equipment, other?

- Does the child's present physical condition require any specific restrictions in classroom activities, physical education activities, or playground/recess activities? Can the child participate on sports teams?

- Does the child require a special or modified diet?

- Does the child require transportation or special transportation to and from school?

- Does the child have mobility problems? What equipment does the child use to assist with mobility (wheelchair, crutches, etc.)? Does the child need assistance with mobility at school? Does a building evacuation plan need to be developed?

- Does the child need assistance with toileting?

- Does the child have communication difficulties?

- Are there any medical emergencies that may occur because of the child's chronic health condition?

- What needs to be done to manage these emergencies?

- See this book's Appendix for the Academic Assessment Guide for additional developmental, social, and academic items.

Most children with chronic health conditions will benefit most from being placed in a regular education classroom that meets their academic abilities.[5] However, they may need modifications in their school schedule or physical environment, medications and/or specialized healthcare procedures administered during the school day, special transportation to and from the school, assistance with mobility, toileting, or using special equipment in the class-room, preferential seating in the classroom, and special training and support for their teachers.

Children with moderate and severe levels of disability may need to have some special education classroom placement, however, some of these children can be placed successfully in regular education classrooms if the necessary related set of services is provided.[4]

Recommendations

1. Children with chronic health conditions need to be identified on initial school enrollment and by annual health status updates.

2. An Individualized Healthcare Plan (IHP) should be developed for each student identified with a chronic health condition. The IHP should address the specific healthcare needs identified by a multidisciplinary team, which should include the student, the parents/guardians, and the student's healthcare providers. The IHP may also be included in the Individualized Educational Plan (IEP) for those students who also qualify for special educational services. The IHP should be reviewed annually and revised as necessary.

3. Parent conferences need to be held annually and more often if indicated to review the student's current health status.

4. Individual health conferences with each student with a chronic health condition should be held at least twice annually to monitor the student's health status, discuss and evaluate the effectiveness of the IHP, and revise the IHP if necessary.

5. Individual and group conferences to provide information regarding a student's health condition should be held with the student's teachers and

other school personnel who have a direct need to know the information. The discussion needs to include a description of the health condition, the effects of the condition on this particular student, activity and mobility limitations, medications and special healthcare procedures that need to be done in school, special transportation needs, classroom modifications that need to be made, and potential medical emergencies and how to manage them if they occur. The student's knowledge about his/her health condition and his/her ability to do self-management or care should also be discussed.

6. All students with chronic health conditions need to have a case manager who is responsible for establishing and maintaining communication and coordination with the student's parents/guardians, healthcare providers, community agencies, and school personnel. The school nurse is the most appropriate person within the school to provide case management for students with chronic health conditions. Those students who have special educational services, as well as related services, may have a special education teacher as a case manager with the school nurse as manager of the health-related components of the IEP.

7. To help ensure that all children with chronic health conditions receive effective and safe healthcare services, the school district should have clearly written policies and procedures in the following areas: medication administration, administration of specialized healthcare procedures, emergency medical care, and identification and tracking of students with chronic health conditions.

The Role of the School Nurse[6]

Manager:

- develop a system to identify students who have chronic health conditions.

- determine services needed to meet the health needs of students.

- develop procedures and provide training for carrying out the services to meet student health needs.

- coordinate and direct the implementation of services.

- monitor and evaluate the effectiveness of the services provided.

- supervise the healthcare services delegated to health assistants and other school personnel.

- participate as a member of the multidisciplinary/special education team.

- incorporate a health component to an IEP when it is determined that the student's chronic health condition(s) does interfere with ability to learn.

Healthcare Provider:

- assessment of past and present health status of the student (through a health history, physical assessment, classroom observation, home observation, medical reports, test results, student interview, parent/guardian interview, and so on).

- determine student's health needs.

- develop an Individualized Healthcare Plan to address and meet the student's needs.

- provide direct health services for the student (specialized healthcare procedures, administration of medications, etc.).

- refer students with educationally significant health problems to the multidisciplinary/special education team.

Counselor:

- provide emotional support to school personnel working with children with chronic health conditions.

- assist the student to develop decision-making skills.

- assist the student to develop self-care skills.

- assist the student, parents/guardians, and school staff to interpret medical information.

Educator:

- provide in-service education to teachers and staff who will be working with the student.

- provide educational opportunities for students and their families regarding the students' chronic health condition (individual or group).

- provide educational opportunities for all students to learn about chronic health conditions.

- provide educational opportunities for the community to learn more about chronic health conditions.

Advocate:

- form liaisons and/or coalitions with organizations, healthcare providers, and educators to address the issues and needs of children with chronic health conditions.

REFERENCES

1. Newacheck PW, Taylor W. *Childhood Chronic Illness: Prevalence, Severity and Impact.* Atlanta: Centers for Disease Control, Dec. 1990.
2. Hobbs N, Perrin J, eds. *Issues in the Care of Children with Chronic Illness.* San Francisco: Jossey-Bass, 1985.
3. American Academy of Pediatrics, Committee on Children with Disabilities and Committee on School Health. Children with health impairments in schools. *Pediatrics* 1990; 86(4): 636-638.
4. Walker DK, Jacobs FH. Chronically-ill children in school. *Peabody J Education.* 1984; 61(2):29-71.
5. Stein REK, ed. *Caring for Children with Chronic Illness: Issues and Strategies.* New York: Springer, 1989.
6. Wold SJ. *School Nursing: A Framework for Practice.* North Branch, MN: Sunrise River Press, 1981.

BIBLIOGRAPHY

Baird SM, Ashcroft SC. Education and chronically ill children: a need-based policy orientation. *Peabody J Education.* 1984; 61: 91-129.

Education of Handicapped Children: Implementation of Part B of the Handicapped Act, Rules, and Regulations, and Amendment—Part H: PL 99-457. *Federal Register* . 1977 & 1986.

Gortmaker SL, Sappenfield W. Chronic childhood disorders: prevalence and impact. *Pediatr Clin North Am* 1984; 31:3-17.

Larson G, ed. *Managing the School Age Child with a Chronic Health Condition: A Practical Guide for Schools, Families, and Organizations.* Wayzata, MN: DCI Publishing, 1988 (distributed by Sunrise River Press, 11481 Kost Dam Road, North Branch, MN 55056, 612-583-3239).

Nelms BC. More similar than different. *J Pediatr Health Care* 1988; 2(2): 55-56.

Newacheck PW, McManus MA, Fox HB. Prevalence and impact of chronic illness among adolescents. *Am J Dis Children.* 1991;145: 1367-1373.

Panza JA. The school nurses role in assisting children with disabling conditions. *J School Health* 1985; 55(7):284.

Walker DK, Chronically-ill children in schools: programmatic and policy directions for the future. *Rheum Dis Clin North Am.* 1987; 13(1): 113-121.

Yoos L. Cognitive development and the chronically ill child. *Pediatr Nurs* 1988; 14(5):375-378.

6 | Psychological Aspects of Chronic Health Conditions

Cynthia K. Silkworth

INTRODUCTION

Chronic illnesses can produce difficulties far beyond the physical symptoms and problems of the specific diseases. Some children and adolescents with chronic health conditions will develop emotional, psychological, social, behavioral, and/or learning problems secondary to their health conditions.

Studies of the child's and family's ability to cope with and adapt to chronic illness have found more similarities than differences among children with diverse chronic illnesses.[1,2] Similar factors that have been associated with chronic health conditions, which correlate with the development of secondary problems, include the following: [1,3]

- Age of onset of the condition—the earlier the condition is acquired, the more likely secondary problems will develop. Early disability can not only interfere with ongoing development, but also disrupt fundamental developmental processes, such as social relationships.

- Permanence of the disability—children who understand the nature of their condition and recognize that it is permanent may develop emotional or psychological problems as a result.

- Severity of the condition—the more severe the condition, the more it will interfere with developmental processes and daily living activities.

- Visibility of the disability—the greatest effect is on peer relations where the response of other people often varies depending on the extent to which the health condition can be seen.

- Number of chronic health conditions—children and adolescents with multiple chronic health conditions are more likely to experience behavioral problems than those with a single condition.

Factors affecting family and child adjustment to a chronic illness are:[4]

Child	*Family*	*Community*
• developmental stage	• communication pattern	• healthcare system
• temperament	• experience with stress	• school system
• health status	• parental coping skills	• legal and political system
• limitations imposed by condition	• family developmental stage	• community values
	• family configuration	• facilities for special needs
	• socioeconomic resources	• child care assistance
	• religion and culture	• support networks (formal or informal)

Management

Healthcare providers, teachers, counselors, social workers, and others who work with children and adolescents with chronic health conditions need to be aware that normal social and developmental events, challenges and transitions may be more difficult for these students than students without chronic health conditions.

Specific interventions need to be based on the needs of the student and his/her family and the nature and severity of the problem.

School interventions may include:

- providing anticipatory guidance prior to transition periods (changing schools or grades), social changes (school events), and developmental changes (physical, cognitive, sexual).

- encouraging student and parent involvement in decision making regarding health management in school and school programming.

- modifying the student's school program to facilitate academic and psychosocial achievement, as well as health needs.

- encouraging an appropriate school attendance pattern.

- encouraging interaction with peers—classroom, intramural, clubs, organizations, community activities.

- modeling and encouraging appropriate social behavior.

- developing and maintaining a supportive school environment.

- multidisciplinary teaming.

INDIVIDUALIZED HEALTHCARE PLAN

History

- when the diagnosis was made
- severity of the health condition
- student's current health status
- student's prognosis
- current health conditions management plan and its effectiveness
- student's participation in development and implementation of his/her health management plan
- family structure—genogram
- family communication patterns
- family members role responsibilities
- family values
- family's resources—economic, social, extended family, community, religious, cultural
- involvement with support persons/systems
- past experience with stress and crisis
- past experiences with loss (real, perceived, and grieving)
- methods of resolving or coping with stress, crisis, or loss
- concerns regarding potential losses
- past experience with the healthcare system: healthcare providers, healthcare facilities, and health insurance
- community values

Assessment

- knowledge about the health condition—student, parents/guardians, and teachers
- student's perception of his/her health and chronic health condition
- student's perception of his/her abilities and disabilities
- student's perception of current stressors
- parents'/guardian's perception of the student's health and chronic health condition
- parents'/guardian's perception of current stressors for the student and for themselves
- current developmental stage of the student—physical, cognitive, social, self, values/ moral, and sexual
- current developmental stage of the family
- communication skills—student and parents/guardians
- student's temperament
- coping skills—student's and parents'/guardian's
- student's locus of control—health, school, family, and activities of daily living
- student's self-care skills—especially those related to the specific chronic health condition
- student's decision-making and problem-solving skills
- student's ability to interact with peers and adults
- student's self-concept—including body image
- student's fears, anxieties, and concerns
- student's environment—home and school
- See Appendix for Academic Assessment Guide for additional developmental , social, and academic items.

Nursing Diagnoses (N.D.)

N.D. 1 Anxiety (NANDA 9.3.1)* related to an actual or potential change in physical health status related to his/her chronic health condition.

N.D. 2 (Potential for) ineffective individual coping (NANDA 5.1.1.1) related to inability to manage stressors (internal or external, physical or psychological).

N.D. 3 (Potential for) powerlessness (NANDA 7.3.2), related to :
- inability to perform—activities of daily living, needed healthcare procedures, school activities.
- hospitalization.
- chronic health condition.

N.D. 4 (Potential for) impaired social interactions with peers (NANDA 3.1.1) related to chronic health condition and:
- ability to participate in regular peer activities.
- inability to attend school regularly.

N.D. 5 (Potential for) social isolation (NANDA 3.1.2) related to:
- hospitalizations due to chronic health condition.
- homebound educational program due to chronic health condition or high-risk school environment.

N.D. 6 (Potential for) alteration in self-concept (NANDA 7.1.1, 7.1.2, 7.1.2.1 or 2) related to:
- chronic health condition.
- loss or impairment of body function(s).

*(See Chapter 2, page 38 for explanation of the NANDA approved numerical system.)

- perception of being different from peers (appearance, abilities, and so on).
- disturbance in body image.

N.D. 7 (Potential for) independence-dependence conflict related to normal psychosocial development and a health condition that requires assistance from others.

N.D. 8 (Potential for) grieving (NANDA 9.2.1.2) related to:
- real or perceived loss of physical or psychosocial well-being.
- anticipated loss of well-being.

N.D. 9 (Potential for) alteration in family process (NANDA 3.2.2) related to a family member having (chronic health condition).

Goals

Effectively communicate feelings to others. (N.D. 1-9)

Use positive, effective coping mechanisms to decrease stress/anxiety. (N.D. 1,2)

Decrease stress/anxiety. (N.D. 1,2)

Cope effectively with stress/anxiety. (N.D. 1,2)

Increase internal locus of control. (N.D. 3, 6, 7)

Utilize good decision-making skills. (N.D. 3)

Participate in his/her healthcare. (N.D. 3)

Develop and maintain meaningful social interactions with peers. (N.D. 4)

Attend school, except when contraindicated due to high health risk. (N.D. 4,5)

Participate in classroom and other school activities, with modifications made as necessary. (N.D. 4)

Decrease barriers to social contact with peers. (N.D. 5)

Participate in activities with peers.

Develop confidence in his/her ability to acquire and use new knowledge and skills. (N.D. 6)

Develop a realistic body image. (N.D. 6)

Increase awareness of abilities and disabilities, knowledge, and skills. (N.D. 6,7)

Make appropriate decisions on when to seek and accept assistance from others. (N.D. 7)

Express his/her grief. (N.D. 8)

Share his/her feelings of grief with significant others. (N.D. 8)

Develop and/or maintain effective family communication pattern. (N.D. 9)

Maintain family integrity and mutual support. (N.D. 9)

Nursing Interventions

Assist the student to identify his/her perception of his/her health status and the affects of having a chronic health condition on his/her life. (N.D. 1)

Encourage the student to ask questions about his/her health, chronic health condition, management plan, and prognosis. (N.D. 1)

Encourage the student to express how he/she feels and views him/herself. (N.D. 1-9)

Encourage the student to communicate his/her feelings and concerns to: family members, teachers, peers, healthcare providers, or others. (N.D. 1-9)

Facilitate communication between student and parents/guardians, teachers, and healthcare providers. (N.D. 1-9)

Assist the student to identify signs that he/she is coping effectively. (N.D. 2)

Assist the student to identify the signs that may indicate that he/she is not coping effectively: not able to problem solve, anxiety, decreased social participation, destructive behavior, not able to meet role expectations, feeling there is too much to deal with. (N.D. 2)

Assist the student to identify coping methods that have worked well in the past. (N.D. 2)

Assist the student to identify effective coping mechanisms that are positive and constructive. (N.D. 1,2)

- seeking information to help in answering questions

- identifying the cause of the stress/anxiety

- setting goals for decreasing or managing stress/anxiety

- identifying alternative ways to decrease feelings of stress/anxiety

- learning new methods to decrease feelings of stress/anxiety (relaxation techniques, reducing environmental stimuli, and so on)

- asking for assistance if he/she feels a need for it—family, school, community, healthcare provider

Provide health education opportunities: individual or group. (N.D. 1-3)

- constructive problem-solving technique—what is the problem, who or what is the cause of the problem, what are the possible options for solving the problem, and what are the advantages and disadvantages of each option?

- stress-reducing activities—such as relaxation exercises, exercise program, relaxing activities (listening to music), and so on

- decision-making skills

Provide positive reinforcement to the student when he/she utilizes positive, constructive coping methods. (N.D. 1,2)

Assist the student to identify persons who assist him/her if he/she feels a need for assistance. (N.D. 1,2,3,7)

Explore possible resources the student might use if he/she feels a need for help—home, school, commmunity, healthcare provider, other (N.D. 1,2,3,7)

Make a referral to school counselor, psychologist, healthcare provider, or community mental health resource, if needed. (N.D. 1-9)

Assist the student to: (N.D. 3)

- identify things that make him/her feel powerful

- identify things that make him/her feel powerless

- identify things he/she can control

- identify things he/she cannot control

Explore and discuss ways the student can increase (N.D. 3,6,7) internal locus of control over his/her:

- activities of daily living

- healthcare management

- schoolwork and responsibilities

- home responsibilities with the student, parents/guardians, teachers and healthcare providers.

Involve the student in planning his/her school activities: such as schedule, special assistance needs, mobility between classes, bathroom arrangements, etc. (N.D. 3)

Explain all school and healthcare procedures, rules, and options to the student and parents/guardians. (N.D. 3)

Allow time for the student and parents/guardians to ask questions. (N.D. 1,3)

Keep the student and parents/guardians informed about the student's health and academic status. (N.D. 1,3)

Provide opportunities for the student to make decisions and participate in his/her health care. (N.D. 3)

Identify and remove as many barriers to self-care as possible.   (N.D. 3,7)

Provide recognition to the student when he/she makes good decisions and/or participates in his/her healthcare. (N.D. 3)

Explore activities the student likes to do with peers. (N.D. 4,5)

Assist the student, parents/guardians, and healthcare providers and teachers to understand the social interactions with peers; Discuss: (N.D. 4,5)

- school—guidelines for attendance, modifications needed in the classroom, daily and weekly schedule, school environment considerations, extracurricular activities, etc.

- home—interaction with neighborhood peers, indoor and outdoor play, birthday parties, extended family (cousins), etc.

- community—church, organizations (scouting, YMCA, other)

Assist the student to develop social skills. (N.D. 4,5)

- individual and/or group learning experiences

- buddy system

Assist the student, parents/guardians, and healthcare providers to identify the barriers to social contact for the student. (N.D. 4,5)

Explore ways the student can interact with peers—in school, at home, and in the community. (N.D. 4,5)

Assist the student, parents/guardians, and healthcare providers to decrease the barriers to social contact and interaction. Discuss: (N.D. 4,5)

- guidelines for school attendance

- special health considerations or modifications that need to be addressed (such as, specialized healthcare procedures; medications; special transportation to and from school; mobility around school; special diet; assistance with mobility; toileting, eating, or school activities; modified school day or week; and so on)

- environmental changes needed (such as, handicapped accessible bathrooms, ramps, removing allergens, other)

- intermittent homebound or regular homebound program

- hospital-based education program

Assist parents/guardians and teachers to implement school modifications (academic, environmental, scheduling). (N.D. 4)

Assist the student to identify strengths and abilities—activities of daily living, home, school, health-care management, and decision making. (N.D. 6,7)

Assist the student to identify weaknesses and disabilities. (N.D. 6,7)

Explore ways the student can use his/her strengths and abilities to help with weaknesses and disabilities. (N.D. 6,7)

Assist the student, parents/guardians, and teachers to identify barriers to the student utilizing his/her strengths and abilities—at home, at school, in the community. (N.D. 6,7)

Explore ways to remove barriers that may prevent the student from using his/her strengths and abilities (for example, for a student with motor disabilities develop a schedule that has a short distance between classrooms and/or allows extra time for the student to get from class to class). (N.D. 6,7)

Remove as many barriers as possible. (N.D. 6,7)

Explore and discuss, with the student, ways he/she is alike and different from his/her peers: (N.D. 6)
- appearance—physical, clothes, hair, skin color
- abilities and disabilities
- knowledge and skills
- daily schedule
- interests and activities inside and outside of school

Assist the student to develop a realistic body image. (N.D. 6)
- discuss reasons for body changes—caused by normal human development and by his/her health condition
- discuss similarities and differences in his/her body from that of peers

Assist the student to identify activities he/she does independently, activities he/she needs assistance with, decisions he/she makes independently, and decisions that others need to make for him/her (N.D. 7)

Discuss, with the student, when it might be important to accept assistance from others (academic, mobility, emergency healthcare procedure, special environment, special activity, other). (N.D. 7)

Assist the student to ask for and accept assistance from others, when it is needed. (N.D. 7)

Assist the student to identify losses—real, perceived, or anticipated. (N.D. 8)

Provide opportunities for the student to express his grief, verbally and emotionally. (N.D. 8)
- private area
- grief group

Facilitate communication: (N.D. 9)
- between student and parents/guardians
- between student and siblings
- with extended family
- with healthcare providers

Provide anticipatory guidance to the student and family. (N.D. 9)
- effects chronic health conditions can have on a child and on a family
- effects of hospitalizations and absences from school
- effects a chronic health condition can have on family members' roles and responsibilities

Assist the student and family to recognize roles and responsibilities and develop a plan that would help to reduce stress. (N.D. 9)

Discuss, with the student and family, the importance of family members providing mutual support for each other. (N.D. 9)

Encourage the student and family to explore involvement with counseling or a support group (disease-specific or one that would address the needs of families with a child with a chronic health condition).

Expected Student Outcomes

The student will:

- describe his/her perception of his/her health status. (N.D. 1)
- identify and describe concerns about actual (or potential) changes in his/her health status. (N.D. 1)
- verbally communicate feelings and concerns to others: family members, teachers, peers, healthcare providers, others. (N.D. 1-9)
- list signs that indicate he/she is coping effectively. (N.D. 2)
- list signs that may indicate he/she is not coping effectively. (N.D. 2)
- identify current stressors, those he/she can control and those he/she cannot. (N.D. 2)
- identify ways to modify or reduce stress/anxiety. (N.D. 2)
- identify positive, constructive coping methods for dealing with stress/anxiety. (N.D. 2)
- demonstrate positive, constructive coping methods that decrease his/her feeling of stress/anxiety. (N.D. 2)
- demonstrate ability to constructively problem solve. (N.D 2)
- demonstrate use of effective stress-reducing activities. (ND 2)
- name persons or facilities in school, at home, and in the community who can assist him/her to cope with stress/anxiety. (N.D. 2)
- seek assistance from others to help reduce or deal with stress/anxiety, as needed. (N.D. 1,2)
- identify activities that make him/her feel powerful. (N.D. 3)
- identify activities that make him/her feel powerless. (N.D. 3)
- identify activities he/she has the power to control. (N.D. 3)
- identify activities he/she cannot control. (N.D. 3)
- describe ways he/she can control activities that are possible to control. (N.D. 3)
- demonstrate good decision-making skills. (N.D. 3,7)
- participate in his/her healthcare. (N.D. 3)
- demonstrate increase in control (in specific situation). (N.D. 3)
- lists activities he/she likes to do with peers. (N.D. 4)
- names his/her friends. (N.D. 4)
- identify his/her barriers to social contact. (N.D. 4)
- list ways to decrease the barriers. (N.D. 4)
- list ways to interact with peers—at home, in school, in the community, in the hospital. (N.D. 4)
- attend school regularly, unless contraindicated due to high health risk. (N.D. 4,5)
- participate in regular classroom activities, with modifications made as necessary. (N.D. 4,5)

- participate in activities with peers at home. (N.D. 4,5)

- participate in activities with peers in the community. (N.D. 4,5)

- identify his/her strengths and abilities. (N.D. 6,7)

- identify his/her weaknesses and disabilities. (N.D. 6,7)

- list ways he/she can use his/her strengths and abilities to help with weaknesses and disabilities. (N.D. 6,7)

- identify ways he/she can increase his/her internal locus of control over: activities of daily living, healthcare management, schoolwork and school responsibilities, and home responsibilities, (dependent on developmental level, knowledge, and skills). (N.D. 3, 6, 7)

- list ways he/she is like his/her peers, including appearance. (N.D. 6)

- list ways he/she is different from his/her peers, including appearance. (N.D. 6)

- describe body changes that have occurred (and/or will occur, normal development and disease-related changes). (N.D. 6)

- identify activities he/she does independently. (N.D. 7)

- identify decisions he/she makes independently. (N.D. 7)

- demonstrates good decision-making ability, (appropriate for developmental level and decision-making skills). (N.D. 7)

- identify and describe activities he/she needs assistance with from others. (N.D. 7)

- identify decisions he/she needs assistance with or others need to make. (N.D. 7)

- identify when it would be important to accept assistance from others. (N.D. 7)

- ask for assistance when he/she needs it. (N.D. 7)

- accept assistance from others, when it is needed. (N.D. 7)

- identify the loss he/she is experiencing—real, perceived, or anticipated. (N.D. 8)

- share his/her feeling of grief with: parents/guardians, or other significant people in their life. (N.D. 8)

- name persons or places in school, at home, and in the community that can assist him/her to cope with feelings of grief. (N.D. 8)

- describes his/her role and responsibilities in the family. (N.D. 9)

- describes role and responsibilities of his/her parents/guardians in the family. (N.D. 9)

- allow family members to play a supportive role in managing his/her health condition (based on student's age, self-care skills, knowledge about his/her health condition, and decision-making skills). (N.D. 9)

REFERENCES

1. Nelms, BC. More similar than different: children with chronic illness. *J Pediatr Health Care* 1988; 2(2): 55-56.
2. Pless IB, Perrin JM. Issues common to a variety of illnesses. In: Hobbs N, Perrin J, eds. *Issues in the Care of Children with Chronic Illness*. San Francisco: Jossey-Bass, 1985.

3. Newacheck PW, McManus MA, Fox HB. Prevalence and impact of chronic illness among adolescents. *Am J Dis Children* 1991; 145 (Dec):1367-1373.

4. Leonard BJ. Psychosocial Dimensions of Chronic Conditions in Childhood. In: Motts, Fazekas N, James S, *Nursing Care of Children and Families.* Menlow Park, CA: Addison Wesley. 1985: 977-980.

BIBLIOGRAPHY

Carpenito LJ. *Nursing Diagnosis: Application to Clinical Practice.* Philadelphia: JB Lippincott, 1989.

McGrab P, Lehr E. Assessment techniques in pediatric psychology. In: Tuma J, ed., *Handbook for the Practice of Pediatric Psychology.* New York: J Wiley, 1982.

Stein REK, ed. *Caring for Children with Chronic Illness.* New York: Springer, 1989.

Wong DL, Whaley LF. *Clinical Manual of Pediatric Nursing.* St. Louis: CV Mosby, 1990.

7 | IHP: Abdominal Pain

Wanda R. Miller

INTRODUCTION

Abdominal pain is a common complaint in school-age children, and its etiology can vary a great deal, which requires that the school nurse make initial determinations as to the cause and significance of the pain. Accuracy in determining the cause of abdominal pain is extremely difficult in children and in women of childbearing age[1]; therefore, the task of the school nurse in triaging or managing school-aged children and adolescent women with abdominal pain is extremely difficult. Although appendicitis is the most frequent emergent cause of abdominal pain, gastroenteritis and acute respiratory illnesses are more commonly reported in small children and require careful scrutiny by the school nurse. The ten most common diagnoses in patients with abdominal pain as seen by Reynolds[2] in a pediatric emergency care setting were, in order of their frequency, gastroenteritis, nonspecific abdominal pain, viral illness, constipation, urinary tract infection, pharyngitis, appendicitis, asthma, otitis, and pneumonia. These ten diagnoses were given to 83 percent of the patients complaining of abdominal pain in an emergency pediatric hospital department.[2] The two most frequent causes, gastroenteritis and nonspecific abdominal pain, accounted for 58.8 percent of the children, respiratory illnesses accounted for 12 percent, and only 6.5 percent of the children seen for abdominal pain were treated surgically.[2]

Pathophysiology

The following is a discussion of the pathophysiology of the most frequent causes of abdominal pain for the ten areas identified by Reynolds.

Gastroenteritis: May be caused by viral or bacterial agents, by parasites, or by food poisoning (see Table IA, IB). Onset varies but most episodes are accompanied by a low-grade fever, nausea, and vomiting that usually precedes abdominal pain, and is then followed by diarrhea. Most gastroenteritis episodes are self-limiting to two to seven days.[2, 3] Severe diarrhea or accompanying CNS symptoms indicate the need for urgent care. The most serious and urgent physiological results of gastroenteritis are dehydration, acid-base derangements with acidosis, and shock that occurs with severe dehydration.

Nonspecific abdominal pain:
Psychogenic recurrent abdominal pain (RAP) that lasts over a period of three months usually interferes with normal activity, occurs with variable frequency and duration during the day; nausea, pallor,

Table 1A. Enteropathologic causes of infectious gastroenteritis

Organism	Characteristics/manifestation	Comments
Viral agents		
Rotavirus Incubation period: 2-3 days	Abrupt onset Fever (38°C or above) lasting approximately 48 hours Associated upper respiratory tract infection Diarrhea may persist for more than a week	Incidence higher in cool weather (80% in winter) Affects all age groups; 6- to 24-month-old infants more vulnerable Usually mild and self-limited
Norwalk-like organisms Incubation period: 1-2 days	Fever Loss of appetite Nausea/vomiting Abdominal pain Diarrhea Malaise	Source of infection: drinking water, recreation water, food (including shellfish) Affects all ages Benign; seldom lasts more than 3 days Self-limited

Bacterial agents
Pathogenic
  Escherichia coli
    Incubation period: highly variable
	Onset gradual or abrupt
	Variable clinical manifestations
	Moist—green, watery diarrhea with mucus; becomes explosive
	Vomiting may be present from onset
	Abdominal distention
	Diarrhea
	Fever; appears toxic
		Incidence higher in summer
		Usually interpersonal transmission but may transmit via inanimate objects
		A cause of nursery epidemics
		With symptomatic treatment only, may continue for weeks
		Full breast-feeding has a protective effect
		Symptoms generally subside in 3-7 days
		Relapse rate approximately 20%

Salmonella groups (nonty-phoidae)—gram-negative,nonencapsulated, nonsporulating
   Incubation period:
    6-72 hours for intraluminal
    7-21 days for extraluminal
	Rapid onset
	Variable symptoms—mild to severe
	Nausea, vomiting, and colicky abdominal pain followed by diarrhea, occasionally with blood and mucus
	Chills not uncommon
	Hyperactive peristalsis and mild abdominal tenderness
	Symptoms usually subside within 5 days
	May have fever, headache, and cerebral manifestations, e.g., drowsiness, confusion, meningismus, or seizures
	Infants may be afebrile and nontoxic
	May result in life-threatening septicemia and meningitis
		Two thirds of patients are younger than 20 years of age
		Highest incidence in children younger than 9 years of age, especially infants
		More prevalent July through October, lowest from January through April
		Transmission primarily via contaminated food and drink
		Most common sources are poultry and eggs
		In children—pets, e.g., dogs, cats, hamsters, and especially pet turtles
		Communicable as long as organisms are excreted

S. typhi	Variable in infants Older children—irregular fever, headache, malaise, lethargy Diarrhea occurs in 50% at early stage Cough is common In a few days, fever rises and is consistent; fatigue, cough, abdominal pain, anorexia, and weight loss develop: diarrhea begins	Rapid invasion of bloodstream from minor sites of inflammation Decreased incidence in last decade Acute symptoms may persist for a week of more

Table 1A. Enteropathologic causes of infectious gastroenteritis—cont'd

Organism	Characteristics/manifestation	Comments
Bacterial agents—cont'd		
Shigella groups—gram-negative, nonmotile, anaerobic bacilli Incubation period: 1-7 days	Onset variable but usually abrupt Fever and cramping abdominal pain initially Fever—may reach 40.5°C Convulsions in about 10%—usually associated with fever Patient appears sick Headache, nuchal rigidity, delirium	Approximately 60% of cases in children younger than age 9 years with more than one third between ages 1 and 4 years Peak incidence late summer Transmitted directly or indirectly from infected persons Communicable for 1-4 years
Vibrio cholerae (cholera) groups Incubation period: usually 1-3 days; range from few hours to 5 days	Sudden onset of profuse, watery diarrhea without cramping, tenesmus, or anal irritation, although children may complain of cramping Stools are intermittent at first, then almost continuous Stools are whitish, almost clear, with flecks of mucus—"rice water stools"	Rare in infants younger than 1 year old Mortality high in both treated and untreated infants and small children Transmitted via contaminated food and water Attack confers immunity
Food poisoning *Staphylococcus* Incubation period: 4-6 hours	Nausea, vomiting Severe abdominal cramps Profuse diarrhea Shock may occur in severe cases May be a mild fever	Transferred via contaminated food—inadequately cooked or refrigerated, e.g., custards, mayonnaise, cream-filled or -topped desserts Self-limited; improvement apparent within 24 hours Excellent prognosis
Clostridium perfringens Incubation period: 8-24 hours	Moderate to severe crampy, midepigastric pain	Self-limited illness Transmission by commercial food products—most often meat and poultry
Botulism *Clostridium botulinum* Incubation period: 12 hr-3 days	Nausea, vomiting Diarrhea CNS symptoms with curare-like effect Dry mouth, dysphagia	Transmitted by contaminated food products Variable severity—mild symptoms to rapidly fatal within a few hours Antitoxin administration

Table 1B. Clinical Manifestations of Dehydration

	Isotonic (loss of water and salt)	Hypotonic (loss of salt in excess of water)	Hypertonic (loss of water in excess of salt)
Skin			
Color	Gray	Gray	Gray
Temperature	Cold	Cold	Cold or hor
Turgor	Poor	Very poor	Fair
Feel	Dry	Clammy	Thickened, doughy
Mucous membranes	Dry	Slightly moist	Parched
Tearing and salivation	Absent	Absent	Absent
Eyeball	Sunken and soft	Sunken and soft	Sunken
Fontanel	Sunken	Sunken	Sunken
Body temperature	Subnormal or elevated	Abnormal	Subnormal or elevated
Pulse	Rapid	Very rapid	Moderately rapid
Respirations	Rapid	Rapid	Rapid
Behavior	Irritable to lethargic	Lethargic to comatose; convulsions	Marked lethargy with extreme hyper-irritability on stimulation

Reproduced by permission from Wong, Donna L., and Whaley, Lucille F.; *Clinical Manual of Pediatric Nursing*, ed. 3, St. Louis, 1990, The C.V. Mosby Co., pp. 341-343.[5]

and faintness may be associated symptoms. Descriptions of pain are vague, and poorly localized to a specific area, and the pain seldom wakes the child at night.[2, 3] Between episodes there is complete resolution of pain and any associated symptoms.[2,4]

Viral hepatitis: History of exposure, fever, anorexia, darkening of the urine, clay-colored stools, jaundice, and liver tenderness.

Constipation: Bowel movements are infrequent, with a hard, pellet-like stool that is difficult to pass.

Urinary tract infection: The only symptom may be abdominal pain; may include fever, chills, frequency of dysuria.

Pharyngitis and post-nasal drip usually are associated with fever, cough, or sore throat.[2] The lymphadenitis that accompanies streptococcal throat infection may be a cause of the pain.[5]

Appendicitis: An acute condition that, when undiagnosed, progresses to perforation and peritonitis. It usually begins with migrating periumbilical pain, and anorexia, followed by nausea and vomiting, tenderness, rebound pain, localization of pain to the right lower quadrant, and fever as a result of the onset of peritonitis.

Fever and vomiting are the most consistent symptoms in children who receive appendectomies, followed by abdominal pain with guarding and tenderness.[2] The progression from simple to complicated appendicitis with peritonitis is more rapid in the young child than it is in the older child or the adult due to a thinner appendiceal wall in younger children.[6]

Asthma: After an asthma attack, muscle fatigue and increased use of the chest and abdominal muscles result in abdominal pain.

Otitis: Usually begins with fever, cough, or sore throat and can be determined on observation by otoscopy.

Pneumonia: Abdominal pain is secondary to diaphragmatic irritation or muscular pain caused by coughing.

In addition to these ten common causes of abdominal pain there are some other causes to rule out:

Peptic ulcer: Abdominal pain may be generalized or periumbilical but the abdomen is frequently tender to deep palpation in the midepigastric region. Pain is not always limited to mealtimes in children. The pain may be described as a burning or gnawing sensation in the epigastrium related to vomiting, obstruction, or bloody emesis or stool[5].

Parasites: History of contact or recent travel related to symptoms of chronic diarrhea.

Abdominal migraine and epilepsy: Family history of migraine, severe pain in upper half of abdomen, associated with nausea, vomiting, and photophobia.

Dysfunctional recurrent abdominal pain: Lactose intolerance, stool retention, and/or irritable colon.[3]

Intussusception: One of the most frequent causes of intestinal obstruction during infancy and occurs three times more commonly in males than in females.

Trauma: Nearly all abdominal injury is the result of blunt trauma. The spleen and the liver are the organs injured from blunt trauma. Both require emergent care for any indication of internal bleeding.

In the adolescent female pelvic inflammatory disease and ovarian cysts further complicate the diagnosis when abdominal pain is the presenting complaint.

INDIVIDUALIZED HEALTHCARE PLAN

History

The purpose of obtaining the history of abdominal pain as the chief complaint is to rule out organic causes of the pain, relieve discomfort, and attempt to determine the situations that precipitate attacks.

- When did the pain begin?
- Did the pain begin gradually or suddenly?
- What were you doing at the time the pain began, or what had you just been doing?
- How often does the pain occur?
- How hard is the pain, how sharp?
- Is the pain the same all the time or does the pain get worse and then better, and then worse again?
- Where is the pain located? Point to the spot with one finger. Does the pain start at one spot and move to another?
- What makes the pain worse?
- What makes it better?
- What else happens at the same time?
- Is this a single attack or has it occurred before?
- Does it happen every day? When in the day does it happen?
- Is the pain better, worse, or the same as it has been?
- How are you treating it?
- What kind of medicine are you taking to help the pain?
- What have you eaten in the past day?
- When did you have your last bowel movement? Describe the color and consistency of the stool.
- Is anything unusual happening at your house?
- What is happening at home?
- What is happening at school?

For females aged 10 and older:

- Are you menstruating?
- When was your last period?
- Has there been a change in the pattern of your menstrual periods?
- Have you had any vaginal bleeding between periods?
- Have you had any vaginal discharge?
- Are you sexually active?
- Are you pregnant?

Assessment

The age of the child, the status of the child's general health, and the socioeconomic environment are important factors in the assessment of abdominal pain.

Observe the skin for perspiration, cold touch, paleness, sallowness, or jaundice. Measure the child's temperature, blood pressure, pulse, and respirations. Determine any alteration in gait, guarding, or changes in posture that may indicate the child is favoring one side of the body. Observe the symmetry of the abdomen. Listen for bowel sounds in each of the four quadrants. Palpate the abdomen to determine any tenderness, or the existence of masses, distention, or rigidity. Gently press the lateral aspect of the abdomen and release to determine if the child has any rebound pain after the release.

Nursing Diagnoses (N.D.)

N.D. 1   Alteration in nutrition resulting in less than body requirements related to anorexia, diarrhea, knowledge deficit of fluid needs or low fiber or low motility. (NANDA1.1.2.2.)*

N.D. 2   Alteration in knowledge related to inadequate nutritional intake. (NANDA 8.1.1.)

N.D. 3   Alteration in bowel elimination, related to absence of routine bowel elimination pattern, constipation, diarrhea, or painful defecation. (NANDA 1.3.1.1,2, or 3)

N.D. 4   Coping, ineffective, related to stress or anxiety, deficit in problem-solving skills. (NANDA 5.1.1.1.)

N.D. 5   Alteration in comfort due to abdominal pain. (NANDA 9.1.1.)

Goals

Hydrate student adequately. (N.D. 1)

Restore adequate diet. (N.D. 1)

Student will maintain an adequate diet to sustain nutritional need and avoid hunger pains. (N.D. 2).

Student will reestablish a routine bowel elimination schedule. (N.D. 3.)

Student will identify the cause of stress and anxiety and be able to tell the school nurse or teacher when they are anxious. (N.D. 4)

Student will be able to identify a variety of behaviors that will alleviate stress and anxiety (N.D. 4)

Student will be pain-free. (N.D. 5)

---

*(See Chapter 2, page 38 for explanation of the NANDA approved numerical system.)

Nursing Interventions

For vomiting or vomiting with diarrhea, the child is given nothing by mouth depending on the age of the child (for infants, 2-4 hours; for children aged 1 to 5, 4 hours; and for older children, 6 to 8 hours), then start on teaspoons of clear liquids containing sugar (Pedialyte or Lytren) and/or ginger ale, Jell-O-water, and Popsicles for older children. Start at fifteen minute intervals; if there is no vomiting gradually increase amount to tolerance. If clear liquids are tolerated add bland soft foods such as, a BRAT diet of bananas, rice, applesauce, and toast.[6] (N.D. 1)

For diarrhea, discontinue solid food, follow above liquid regimen until diarrhea is absent for 24 hours; gradually add the BRAT diet. (N.D. 1).

Provide, if possible, crackers, milk, or fruit to reduce hunger. (N.D. 2).

Determine reason for student's lack of adequate nutrition. (N.D. 2).

- If related to lack of funds, assist in obtaining free or reduced-cost school lunch and/or breakfast.

- If related to lack of knowledge, review the immediate effects of missing meals on the body and the need for eating food routinely.

Develop a management plan: (N.D. 3)

- Consult with the child's healthcare provider to establish medical practice

- Engage the child and family in the treatment process

- Include the family, student, and physician in the development of a plan

- Assist the parent to establish a bowel evacuation protocol.

- Develop with the family and child a set of common language terms for the words bowel movement, urine, and anus.

- Explain defecation process to parent and review with child.

- Establish periods during the day when defecation is encouraged

Provide a quiet rest area at school for student having mild to moderate discomfort. (N.D. 4)

Assist student in developing relaxation methods (Use a combination of belly breathing exercises and a process of identifying pleasant images to focus on in times of stress.)(N.D. 4).

Notify parents if the child has vomiting, diarrhea, or a temperature greater than 100.5 degrees. (N.D. 5).

Refer for consultation to healthcare provider if pain is severe, sharp, and localized; is associated with fever greater than 100.5; is of 48-hour duration; increases in intensity; or is localized in the right lower quadrant. (N.D. 5)

Refer for consultation to healthcare provider if a female has pain in the lower abdomen, accompanied by vaginal discharge or fever, or is pregnant. (N.D. 5)

Refer for consultation to a healthcare provider if a child has pain following a recent injury to the abdomen; blood in the urine, stool or emesis; walks protecting the abdomen; has rigidity, localized tenderness, rebound tenderness or an abdominal mass.

Facilitate obtaining an appointment with a healthcare provider. (N.D. 5)

Assist in obtaining medical care if healthcare costs are too expensive for the family. (N.D. 5)

Expected Student Outcomes

Student will decrease the frequency of or stop vomiting and will be able to retain fluids. (N.D. 1)

Student will decrease the frequency of or cease to have episodes of diarrhea and will be able to retain fluid and eventually soft foods.(N.D. 1)

Student will eat at regular intervals during the day and be free from pain due to hunger. (N.D. 2).

The student will maintain routine bowel elimination. (N.D. 3)

The student will: (N.D. 4)

- identify anxiety-producing situations
- increasingly be able to use techniques of relaxation to reduce anxiety.

Student is free of pain or a specific diagnosis is established for the condition and appropriate medical intervention is in process. (N.D. 5)

REFERENCES

1. Bond GR, Tully SB. Use of the Mantrels score in childhood appendicitis: a prospective study of 187 children with abdominal pain. *Ann Emerg Med.* 1990;19(9):1014-1018.
2. Reynolds SL, Jaffe DM. Children with abdominal pain: evaluation in the pediatric emergency department. *Pediatr Emerg Care* 1990;6(1):8-12.
3. Sapala S. Pediatric management problems. *Pediatr Nursing* 1989;15(3):288-289.
4. Li BUK. Recurrent abdominal pain in childhood: an approach to common disorders. *Compr Ther* 1987;13(10):46-53.
5. Wong DL. Whaley L. *Clinical Manual of Pediatric Nursing.* St. Louis: CV Mosby, 1990.
6. Sperhac AM. Abdominal pain in pediatric patients: assessment and management update. *J Emerg Nursing* 1989;15(2):93-100.
7. Geist R. Use of imagery to describe functional abdominal pain as an aid to diagnosis in a pediatric population. *Can J Psychiatry* 1989; 34(8):506-511.

8 | IHP: Abuse and Neglect

Susan I. Simandl Will

INTRODUCTION

Child abuse and neglect represent a growing crisis in children's healthcare. Estimates indicate that up to 5,000 abused children die each year.[1] According to the National Association of Children's Hospitals and Related Institutions abuse and neglect continue to rise. Reports of abuse and neglect increased 55 percent between 1981 and 1985, sexual abuse reports increased 58 percent between 1983 and 1984 and then another 24 percent in 1985.[1] In the United States 1.5 million cases of child abuse are estimated annually.[2]

Child abuse is an act of omission or commission by a caretaker which endangers or impairs a child's physical or emotional health or development. There are five major categories of abuse: Physical abuse, physical neglect, emotional abuse, emotional neglect, and sexual abuse.

Physical Abuse: The deliberate infliction of injury.

Physical Neglect: Omission of caretaker acts or behaviors which results in detrimental effects on the child's physical status or development.

Emotional Abuse: Deliberate attempts to destroy or significantly impair the child's self-esteem, self-worth, or competence.

Emotional Neglect: Omission of caretaker acts or behaviors which results in failure to meet the child's needs for affection, nurturing, attention, and emotional security.

Sexual Abuse: Contacts or interactions between a child and an adult when the child is being used for the sexual stimulation or gratification of the adult. (Above definitions adapted from Wong and Whaley.[3])

School nurses are frequently in a position to be an important part of early identification of children who are victimized by any form of abuse. All fifty states have mandatory reporting requirements, the majority of these specifically cite nurses as required reporters. Legislation in most states includes liability protection for the reporter who reports in good faith.

INDIVIDUALIZED HEALTHCARE PLAN

Assessment

History

• Is there a history of parent(s)' being abused as a child?
• Is there a history of abusive relationships in family?
• Is there a prior report of abuse and/or neglect for this student?
• Is there a prior report of abuse and /or neglect for siblings?

Assessment for Physical / Emotional Neglect

• Student report of inadequate attention to physical and/or emotional needs by caregiver
• Evidence of failure to thrive:
>   growth and/or developmental delays
>   thin limbs
>   poor personal hygiene
>   inability to manage activity level appropriate for age
>   fatigue
• Enuresis
• Encopresis
• Inadequate healthcare
>   immunization status
>   untreated infections
>   untreated illnesses
• Frequent illnesses
• Frequent accidents or injuries
>   lack of supervision
>   unsafe environment
• Behavioral problems
>   inattention
>   depression
>   passivity
>   acting out (disruptive, inappropriate behavior)
>   frequent or unexplained long absences from school
>   alcohol or chemical use/abuse
>   legal encounters (shoplifting, stealing, vandalizing, truancy, other)
>   fearfulness
>   cruelty or aggression to peers
>   suicide attempts, gestures, or verbalizations
>   delays in socialization (withdrawn, uninvolved)
>   emotional or behavioral extremes
• Sleep disorders
• What are the home self-care and family responsibilities the child reports?
>   Are these appropriate to age and developmental level?
>   (May relate to cooking, food supply, sibling care, alone time and pattern, clothing supply and laundering, hygiene)

Assessment for Physical Abuse

- Student report of injuries inflicted by care provider adult
- Injuries inconsistent with child's report of occurrence
- Bruises, welts, burns, lacerations, abrasions: observe for identifiable characteristics of causing object
    belt buckle or strap
    cigarette
    hanger
    chain
    wooden spoons, spatula
    finger pinches or squeeze marks
    degloving burn pattern as from scalding liquid
    splash burn pattern from scalding liquid
    rope, electric cord
    iron
    fist, fingers, hand
    teeth
    pins, forks, hammers, screwdrivers
- Ritualistic (cult) symbols in burn, bruise, or laceration form
- Fractures
    repeated
    multiple
- Internal abdominal injury
    pain, swelling, or distension from impact of punching
- Behavioral indicators
    cautious or afraid of adults
    fear of environment (lying or sitting very still)
    inappropriate reactions to injuries (fearful of crying, anger, suppression of reaction)
    acting out or aggressive behavior toward peers or adults or younger children
    withdrawal
    depression
    suicide attempts, gestures or verbalizations
- Enuresis
- Encopresis

Assessment for Sexual Abuse

- Student report of sexual contact by adult
    touching any part of body which was not acceptable to the student
    touching genitalia, breasts, buttocks
    sexual penetration of any body orifice
    request from adult to handle or fondle their genitalia or to provide sexual stimulation
    kissing by adult in manner student perceives to be sexual
    adult verbal requests for sexual activities
    sexually suggestive conversation from adult

- Injury to genitalia, anus, mouth, throat, or breasts
    bruises
    bleeding
    lacerations
    inflammation or irritation
    abrasions
    burns
- Underwear semen-stained, torn, or bloody
- Pregnancy
- Sexually transmitted disease
- Vaginal discharge or penis discharge
- Urinary tract infection
- Genital pain, difficulty sitting or walking
- Genital odor
- Enuresis
- Encopresis
- Behavior problems
    depression, withdrawal
    suicide gesture, attempt, or verbalization
    peer conflicts or relationship problems
    regression (bedwetting, thumbsucking)
    phobias or fears
    running from home
    sexually-related problems (inappropriate sexual play, promiscuity, seductivity, public masturbation)
    alcohol or chemical use/abuse
    truancy or school attendance problems

Developmental/Academic/Social Supports

- Student's age and developmental level?
- What are age and developmentally appropriate sexual activities?
- What is student's knowledge level of sexuality issues?
- Is student currently involved in school club or athletic activities?
- What are student's support systems: family, friends, church, school groups, other?
- What are patterns of academic performance as indicated by review of academic or cumulative school record?
- What is teachers' perception of student's performance and classroom adjustment?
- How does student compare in behavior, social skills, academic performance to peer norms?
- What is school absence pattern—current and previous?
- Is there a potential need for special education (P.L. 94-142) services to adequately educate the student?
- What are student's intellectual abilities? Presence of learning disability or retardation?

Nursing Diagnoses (N.D.)

N.D. 1   Alteration in physical integrity (NANDA 1.6.2.1)* due to:
- Trauma
- Neurological, muscular, skeletal impairment
- Sexual penetration or force
- Tissue destruction
- Altered nutritional state

N.D. 2   Alteration in comfort (Physical pain and/or emotional distress) (NANDA 9.1.1, 9.3.1 or 2) due to:
- Trauma
- Neurological, muscular, skeletal impairment
- Sexual penetration or force
- Excessive disciplinary measures
- Unsafe physical environment
- Infection
- Tissue destruction
- Altered nutritional state
- Willful neglect
- Unmet needs

N.D. 3   Infection (NANDA 1.2.1.1) due to:
- Trauma
- Sexual penetration or force
- Tissue destruction
- Altered nutritional state
- Willful neglect
- Unmet needs

N.D. 4   Altered growth and development (NANDA 6.6) due to:
- Trauma
- Neurological, muscular, skeletal impairment
- Altered nutritional state
- Willful neglect
- Unmet needs

N.D. 5   Alteration in elimination (NANDA 1.3.1, 1.3.2) due to:
- Trauma
- Sexual penetration or force
- Infection

N.D. 6   Altered nutrition (NANDA 1.1.2.1 or 2) due to:
- Willful neglect
- Unmet needs

N.D. 7   Anxiety (Mild, moderate, or severe) (NANDA 9.3.1) due to:
- Emotional, physical, or sexual abuse
- Post-trauma response
- Disturbance in self-concept or self-esteem
- Powerlessness over life events
- Vulnerability
- Inadequate support systems

* (See Chapter 2, page 38 for explanation for the NANDA approved numerical system.)

- Unmet needs
- Threat of death or trauma
- Fear

N.D. 8   Ineffective individual coping skills (NANDA 5.1.1.1) due to:
- Emotional, physical, or sexual abuse
- Post-trauma response
- Disturbance in self-concept or self-esteem
- Powerlessness over life events
- Vulnerability
- Inadequate support systems
- Unmet needs
- Threat of death or trauma
- Fear

N.D. 9   Alterations in socialization (NANDA 3.1.1, 3.1.2) due to:
- Emotional, physical, or sexual abuse
- Post-trauma response
- Disturbance in self-concept or self-esteem
- Powerlessness over life events
- Vulnerability
- Inadequate support systems
- Unmet needs
- Threat of death or trauma
- Fear

N.D. 10   Alteration in role identity (NANDA 3.2.1) due to:
- Emotional, physical, or sexual abuse
- Post-trauma response
- Disturbance in self-concept or self-esteem
- Powerlessness over life events
- Vulnerability
- Inadequate support systems
- Unmet needs
- Threat of death or trauma
- Fear

N.D. 11   Altered parental or family coping (NANDA 5.1.2.1.1 or 2) due to:
- Parent history of abuse
- Chemical dependency
- Family crisis or unusual demands (mental, physical, social, economic)
- Unmet parental needs or developmental deficit
- Inadequate support systems

N.D. 12   Parental knowledge deficit (NANDA 8.1.1) due to:
- Ineffective or inadequate parenting skills
- Parent history of abuse
- Lack of knowledge of growth and development
- Inadequate support systems

N.D. 13   Altered parenting (NANDA 3.2.1.1.1) due to:
- Parent history of abuse
- Lack of knowledge of growth and development

- Chemical dependency
- Family crisis or unusual demands (mental, physical, social, economic)
- Unmet parental needs or developmental deficit
- Inadequate support systems

N.D. 14 Altered Parental emotional integrity (NANDA 5.1.2.1.1) due to:
- Ineffective or inadequate parenting skills
- Chemical dependency
- Family crisis or unusual demands (mental, physical, social, economic)
- Unmet parental needs or developmental deficit
- Inadequate support systems

Goals

Protect child from additional abuse or neglect. (N.D. 1-6)

Student will have support systems available and not demonstrate distress. (N.D 7-10)

Parent (family) will develop supports, knowledge, skills, and behaviors to safely and competently parent children without additional abuse. (N.D. 11-14)

Nursing Interventions

School Interventions

Coordinate access to child at school by police or social service agencies. (N.D. 1,2)

Coordinate and communicate with other involved agencies. (N.D 7,8,10)

Include student in any appropriate school-based support groups and counselling. (N.D 7-10)

Apprise teacher of student issues with abuse/neglect or identify as "significant health problem" if necessary for confidentiality purposes. (N.D 7-10)

Monitor for academic decline and arrange for assistance (tutoring, special education) as appropriate. (N.D 9,10)

Arrange for nurse's office to be "safe place" when stresses of abuse, reporting, continuing investigation, and court appearances cause dysfunctional behavior. (N.D 7,8)

Introduce student to other support sources within school, especially if nurse not at school full-time: (counselor, social worker, other). (N.D 7,8)

Student Interventions

Perform physical assessment of child: document head-to-toe findings.(N.D. 1,3-6)

Identify and provide first aid for any injuries requiring emergency management. Leave non-life-threatening injuries for hospital and/or physician management and additional documentation. Cover bleeding lacerations or abrasions with protective dressing without cleaning or disruption.(N.D. 1-3)

Report suspicion of abuse/neglect to authorities in accordance with child protection laws and school district policy. (All states have required reporting laws.) (N.D. 1,2)

Arrange for medical management of injuries. (N.D. 1-6)

Provide child with reassurance, comfort, and understanding. (N.D. 2)

Document:(N.D. 1-6)

Date, time, student name, age, birthdate, address, parent(s) name

Specifics of student's statement about abuse/neglect (use quotations if possible).

Detailed objective observations of any apparent injuries to child (use drawings).

Time, date of abuse/neglect incident(s).

Was student's report to nurse spontaneous or result of questioning?

Apparent emotional condition of student during disclosure (distress, reluctant, excited, fearful, trusting, calm, and so on).

Where, when, to whom initial disclosure was made.

When and to whom nurse reported the student's disclosure.

Any potential evidence obtained (torn, bloody, or semen containing clothing; objects used to inflict injury, other). Initiate "chain of evidence" record: what was obtained and to whom entrusted.

Assist in removing child from unsafe environment. (N.D. 1,2,7)

After initial report and interventions continue to monitor child for additional occurrences. (N.D. 1-6)

Develop and maintain open, trusting communication with student. (N.D 7,8,)

Provide reassurance, nurturing, and comfort. (N.D 7-10)

Be honest with student about to whom and why you will report the disclosures of abuse/neglect. (N.D 7,8,10)

Inform student of what will happen after report to authorities is made: additional interviews with police, social services. (N.D 7,8)

Stay with student during authority interview if desired by student and permissible. (N.D 7,8,10)

Be available to student and encourage communication as investigation proceeds. (N.D 9,10)

Seek appraisal of status of report/investigation/prosecution. (N.D 7,8)

Continue to be aware of child's living placement, permitted at home? placed in foster care? (N.D 7-10)

Assure student that abuse/neglect was not his/her fault and that she/he is not "bad." (N.D 7-10)

Refer student to community agencies for support group, counseling. (N.D 7,8,10)

Provide student with continued counseling and support as investigation and family treatment or prosecution proceeds. (N.D 7-10)

Encourage and assist student in maintaining contact with school friends and activities. (N.D 8-10)

Family Interventions

Develop supportive and nonthreatening relationship with parent (family). (N.D. 11,14)

Avoid judgmental, authoritarian, or negative messages to parent (family). (N.D. 11,14)

Identify, reinforce, and support positive parenting characteristics. (N.D. 11-14)

Support parent involvement in counseling, therapy, classes, and support groups. (N.D. 11-14)

Teach parents about expectations appropriate to student's age, cognitive, and developmental level. (N.D. 12,13)

Teach parents appropriate discipline methods for age and developmental level. (N.D. 12,13)

Be a role model and demonstrator of positive and appropriate student-adult interactions. (N.D. 12,13)

Encourage support systems which lessen family stress. (N.D. 11,14)

Refer family to community social service agencies for additional interventions. (N.D. 11,14)

Expected Student Outcomes

Student is in a safe environment. (N.D. 1,2,7,8)

Student's physical injuries receive medical treatment. (N.D. 1,2)

Student has medical, legal, and social service assistance initiated to stop maltreatment. (N.D. 1-8)

Student will maintain and expand support systems within the school environment. (N.D 7-10)

Student will maintain and expand trust of helping professionals within school. (N.D 7-10)

Student will maintain and expand social activities and peer contacts. (N.D 9,10)

Student will verbalize positive feelings about self. (N.D 9,10)

Student exhibits positive interactions with family. (N.D. 11-14)

Student shows no evidence of abuse or neglect. (N.D. 11-14)

Student involved in community support systems with family. (N.D. 11-14)

IHP Example

The following page contains an example of using the parts of an IHP: assessment data, nursing diagnosis, goals, and expected outcomes for a student with physical abuse concerns. Joyce, a 15-year-old high school student, reported to the school nurse that her father was physically hitting and restraining her and her younger two siblings. Several weeks later, the initial report to the county sherrif has been accomplished, Joyce is in a foster home, as are her younger siblings, and a court hearing is pending. Joyce is talking with the school nurse about feeling sick, not getting assignments completed for classes, and wanting to drop out of the drama club. Further inquiry identifies fear of the court appearance, anxiety about what will happen in court, and what will happen to her family. She shares anger because she isn't allowed home, even though her father promised he would not hit anyone anymore, and fear that everyone in the family is angry with her because she caused all this by talking to the police. On the basis of this data, the IHP related to Joyce's current situation is demonstrated on the following page.

SAMPLE INDIVIDUAL HEALTH PLAN FOR STUDENT WITH ABUSE/NEGLECT ISSUES

ASSESSMENT	NURSING DIAGNOSIS	GOALS	INTERVENTIONS	STUDENT OUTCOMES
Physical abuse reported 2 weeks ago	Ineffective individual coping skills due to post-trauma response & powerlessness over life events	Student will have support systems available	Coordinate and communicate with other agencies involved	Student attends school support group
Student living in foster home			Refer student to appropriate school-based support groups	Student decreases somatic complaints
Increase in complaints of illness			Arrange for nurse's office to be safe place when stresses of investigation and court cause dysfunctional behavior	Student can identify 2 school support staff to contact when distressed
Student expresses fear of court appearance			Introduce student to other support staff in building	Student attends counseling session
Student wants to drop out of school club			Develop and maintain open, trusting communication with student	
Previous competent student now not completing work and getting failing grades			Provide reassurance, comfort	
Anger related to foster placement			Refer student to counseling	
Fear that family is blaming her for family break-up			Encourage and assist student in maintaining school activities and friends	
			Assure student that abuse was not her fault and she is not "bad"	
			Encourage and assist in the continued verbalization of feelings	

REFERENCES

1. Jacobson E. The sad state of children's health includes a rise in abuse. *Am J Nursing* 1989; 89(9):1115.
2. Aleieri M. Child abuse: when to be suspicious and what to do then. *Postgrad Med* 1990; 87(2): 153-162.
3. Wong D, Whaley L. *Clinical Manual of Pediatric Nursing.* 2d ed. St. Louis: CV Mosby, 1990.

BIBLIOGRAPHY

Chadwick D. Preparation for court testimony in child abuse cases. *Pediatr Clin North Am* 1990; 37 (4): 955-970.

Johnson C. Inflicted injury versus accidental injury. *Pediatr Clin North Am* 1990; 37(4): 791-813.

Johnson S. *High-Risk Parenting: Nursing Assessment and Strategies for the Family at Risk.* Philadelphia: JB Lippincott, 1979.

Neff J, Scherb B. Standardized care plans: suspected abuse and neglect of children. *J Emerg Nursing* 1988; 14(1):44-47.

Newberger E. Pediatric interview assessment of child abuse. *Pediatr Clin North Am* 1990; 37(4): 943-955.

Stanley S. Child sexual abuse: recognition and nursing intervention. *Orthop Nursing* 1989; 8(1): 33-40.

Stanley S. Disclosure of sexual abuse: the secret is out—what now? *J Child Adolesc Psychiatr Ment Health Nursing* 1989; 2(4):154-160.

Waechter E, Philips J, Holaday B. *Nursing Care of Children.* 10th ed Philadelphia: JB Lippincott, 1985.

IHP: Acne

Kathleen M. Kalb

INTRODUCTION

Acne is a condition which affects from 75 percent to 85 percent of all adolescents.[1,2] The school nurse can be instrumental in helping the adolescent begin a successful course of care. Since this is a very common and potentially traumatic condition for the adolescent, concerns about acne should be addressed directly and knowledgeably by the nurse.

The initial appearance of acne is often one or two years prior to the onset of puberty.[1] Since there are a number of factors which contribute to the appearance and severity of the condition, the course is very individualized. The adolescent should be reassured that, although it may take some time, a variety of effective treatments are available and it is very likely that one can be found that will work for his or her particular case.

Pathophysiology

Hormonal activity on the sebaceous glands in the skin is the initiator of the acne process in an adolescent.[3] A complex interplay of genetic predisposition, hormone levels, bacterial activity, and stress response work together to determine the course of this condition.[1] The sebaceous glands, under hormonal stimulus, secrete a fatty substance known as sebum. Bacteria colonize in this substance and produce by-products which are responsible for the subsequent formations of comedones (blackheads and whiteheads). These lesions may go on to form papules, pustules, nodules, and/or cysts, depending on the patient's unique combination of the previously mentioned factors.

Usual treatment consists of topical and/or systemic agents which have various actions on the acne process. Common treatments may include those shown in Table 1.[1,2,4]

Table 1. Common Treatments for Acne.

Agent	Action	Usage
Benzoyl Peroxide	Limits bacterial activity, breaks up comedones, and increases blood supply to the area	Topical (available over the counter)
Retinoic Acid	Decreases hyperkeratosis, increases production of epithelial cells, and increases blood supply to the area	Topical (by prescription)
Antibiotics (tetra-cycline, erythromycin, clindamycin)	Decrease bacterial activity	Topical and systemic (by prescription)
Isotretinoin (Acutane)	Inhibits sebaceous gland activity, normalizes keratinization process	Systemic (severe cystic acne only)
Estrogens	Supress sebaceous gland activity	Systemic (used for females only)

Since many of these treatment approaches have marked and uncomfortable side effects, it is best for the patient to be monitored by a doctor or nurse practitioner familiar with the treatment of acne.

INDIVIDUALIZED HEALTHCARE PLAN

History

Update the student's history with particular emphasis on family history of acne. Following are questions addressing the most pertinent data.

- Does anyone else in your family have acne?
- Did either your mother or father have acne at your age?

  How severely did they have it?

  How does that compare to your case of it?

- Have you ever seen a doctor or nurse practitioner for your acne?

  If yes, what did that person do for it?

- What have you tried so far to treat it?
- Did anything seem to help?
- Is there anything that seems to make it worse?
- Generally, does it seem to be getting better or worse?
- How often are you washing your face every day?
- What are you using as a cleansing agent?

Assessment

Current status

- Discuss the student's current outbreak of acne and determine his or her emotional response to the condition.
- Ascertain whether this outbreak is fairly typical, and what treatments are currently being used.
- Note whether the student seems to be coping with the disfiguring aspects of the condition.

Physical assessment

- Describe lesions in terms of type, size, location, color, tenderness, configuration, and distribution.
- Note any areas of hyper- or hypopigmentation.
- Note edema.
- Note texture of skin.
- Note size of pores.
- Note any scars, bleeding or exudate.

Psychological/emotional assessment

- Ask the student how the outbreak of acne is affecting his or her life.
- Ask whether peers or family have called attention to the acne in any negative manner.
- Ask whether (s)he would be willing to seek professional guidance in the treatment of this condition.
- Note the student's affect, outlook and general attitude toward the condition.

Nursing Diagnoses (N.D.)

N.D. 1 Impairment of skin integrity (actual and potential) (NANDA 1.6.2.1.2.1, and/or 2)* related to altered hormonal activity
N.D. 2 Self-care deficit: grooming (NANDA 6.5.3)
N.D. 3 Self-concept disturbance—self-esteem (NANDA 7.1.2) body image (NANDA 7.1.1)

Goals

The school nurse will:
1. Assess skin condition and refer if necessary.
2. Monitor student's emotional responses to condition.
3. Educate student regarding normal course of acne as well as appropriate management and/or self-care techniques.

---

*(See Chapter 2, page 38 for explanation of the NANDA approved numerical system.)

Nursing Interventions

Update history as above to provide foundation for nursing assessment and information for referral. (N.D. 1–3)

Listen carefully to the student's primary concern(s) so that they may be addressed first. (N.D. 1-3)

Explain common treatments and how they work so that the student will understand the process. (N.D. 1,2)

Emphasize the need for patience and adherence to a treatment plan so that the student doesn't become discouraged with the time necessary for the lesions to heal. (N.D.1)

Refer for medical intervention if over-the-counter methods are proving ineffective. (N.D.1)

Educate the student regarding myths and noneffective treatments: (N.D. 1)

- Acne is not related to diet.
- Blackheads get their color from a keratinization process, not dirt, so excessive washing will not result in fewer comedones.
- Excessive washing (more than three times a day) may actually break down the integrity of the skin and make lesions more likely.
- Acne is not related to masturbation or other sexual activity.
- Drying and exfoliating agents (such as abrasive soaps, astringents, ultraviolet light, sulfur, resorcinol, and salicylic acid) may cause peeling and drying of skin oils, but do not prevent future lesions and may interfere with the action of more effective treatments.[2]

Discuss the effect of acne on the student's self-esteem so an assessment may be made regarding how well he or she is coping. (N.D. 3)

Discuss acne as a common condition of adolescence so the student has some perspective on the "normalness" of the attendant emotional response. (N.D. 3)

Discuss stress as a factor in the acne process and recommend and explain stress-reduction techniques to minimize its effect. (N.D.1-3)

Refer for additional professional counseling if the student seems to be coping unsuccessfully with body image concerns, or if she or he is preoccupied with being "ugly" or unacceptable to peers. (N.D. 3)

Follow up with student on a weekly or biweekly basis to determine effectiveness of treatment and student's emotional status. (N.D. 1-3)

Expected Student Outcomes

The integrity of the skin will be restored.

- The student will be compliant with prescribed treatment as shown by decrease in severity and number of acne lesions.

The student will demonstrate appropriate self-care.

- The student will cooperate with follow-up schedule as shown by keeping appointments with the nurse.

- The student will report consistent and suitable skin-grooming routines.

The student will experience increased self-esteem as demonstrated by:

- Ability to take part comfortably in group activities
- Ability to take social risks
- Appropriate eye contact when interacting verbally
- Affect reflecting comfort or positive emotional status
- Ability to express positive opinion of self

4. The student will express increased comfort with body image as demonstrated by:

- Appropriate dress and grooming as compared to peer group
- Ability to verbalize acceptance of body, especially face
- Lack of negative comments about physical features

REFERENCES

1. Hurwitz S: Acne vulgaris: its pathogenesis and management. *Adolesc Med: State of the Art Reviews* 1990; 1(2): 301-13.
2. Neinstein LS. Acne. In: Neinstein LS. *Adolescent Health Care: A Practical Guide.* Baltimore: Urban and Schwarzenberg, 1984: 221-231.
3. Goos SD, and Pochi, P E. Endocrine aspects of adolescent acne. *Adolesc Med: State of the Art Reviews* 1990; 1(2):289-99.
4. Abel EA. Isotretinoin (Accutane) therapy for acne in adolescents. *Adolesc Med: State of the Art Reviews* 1990; 1(2): 315-24.
5. Bates B. *A Guide to Physical Examination.* 2d ed. Philadelphia: JB Lippincott Co., 1979.

10 | IHP: AIDS/HIV Infection

Ruth Ellen Luehr

INTRODUCTION

Acquired Immunodeficiency Syndrome (AIDS) is a blood-borne, sexually transmitted disease. Human Immunodeficiency Virus (HIV), the virus that causes AIDS, enters the body through a portal such as a break or tear in the mucous membrane that provides access to the circulatory system. There HIV infects the key cells of the immune system—T-helper white blood cells (otherwise known as T-4 lymphocytes or CD4s). HIV attaches to receptor sites on the T-4 lymphocytes or CD4s and gains entry to its nucleus, turning them into a factory for producing more HIV. HIV also destroys the T-helper cells' function as the trigger that activates the immune system's attack on new infections.

The virus may lay dormant in the cells for more than ten years during which time a person feels and is healthy. Once HIV activates—the cofactors that trigger HIV action have not been clearly identified—the immune system is compromised, the infected person is vulnerable to routine illnesses and infections such as colds and flu. Infections occur with increasing frequency, severity, and duration. The person is also vulnerable to a long list of serious illnesses that would not be a threat to a person with a noncompromised immune system; these are known as "opportunistic" infections (OIs). In addition, there is an increased sus-

ceptibility to fungal infections and neoplasms.

HIV also invades other body cells besides the immune system, most notably the neurological system. The neurological impact can affect the brain, nerve tracts and muscle tone, personality and cognition. People with HIV infection and/or AIDS may have immune system problems and related illnesses, neurological problems, or both.[1-4]

HIV is transmitted by sexual contact and needle sharing, and prior to March 1985 through transfused blood or blood components. Another risk is maternal-child transfer during pregnancy or birth, and on rare occasions through breast milk. High-risk behaviors include sharing needles by using injected drugs and unprotected anal or vaginal intercourse and probably oral sex, particularly with multiple partners.

Inside the human host, HIV is a deadly virus. But HIV is fragile outside the body. The virus does not survive outside the human host, living only seconds to a minute, by most sources. There is no evidence of HIV transmission in casual contact settings, even where there may be exposure to saliva and urine of an infected person, such as schools, and most work and recreational settings, public places such as restaurants, or by nonsexual contact in homes.[5, 6]

Two major strains of the virus exist, HIV-1 being the most prevalent in the United States, and HIV-2 is more widely spread in African nations, with few cases in the Americas. The effects of the disease by both strains are nearly the same. The information in the remainder of this chapter pertains to HIV-1.

A person can learn if he/she is HIV-infected—even if there are no symptoms—by having a blood test (known as EIA or ELISA) which measures the level of antibodies to HIV. The body's immune system responds to all foreign substances (called antigens) with fighter proteins called antibodies that are specific to each antigen. These protein antibodies are larger and easier to detect than viruses, hence the test for HIV antibodies rather than HIV itself. If the HIV-antibody EIA test is positive, the EIA test is rerun and then confirmed with a Western Blot lab test. It takes from two to ten days for most counseling and testing sites to have results ready for worried clients. Just released by the Food and Drug Administration is a 10-minute test for HIV antibodies called SUDS HIV-I Test.[7]

A person is considered HIV-positive, or HIV+, if antibodies are present. It takes about two to three weeks from the time of exposure for the body to begin an antibody response. A sufficient number of antibodies are detectable in six weeks (EIA being 95 percent accurate) to six months (EIA being 99.9 percent accurate). This period from the time of exposure to accurate test results is sometimes called the "window period." Even though the virus and antibodies are present in small numbers during this early period, a person can pass the virus on to another person through engaging in high-risk behaviors.

A common question concerns the difference between HIV infection and AIDS. Once a person is infected with HIV (and confirmed by the antibody test), he/she is considered infected for life. The progression of the disease is from asymptomatic HIV infection to symptomatic HIV infection to AIDS. (See Table 1 for an illustration of the progression of the disease for a neonatally exposed child.)

When the blood tests show the presence of antibodies to HIV, the lab results are HIV+ (read: HIV positive). A person is then known as HIV-infected. This is usually a phase without symptoms, technically called "asymptomatic HIV infection," although people may use the label of "HIV-positive." It may be ten or more years from time of exposure and infection with HIV to the time of first symptoms. Denial of high-risk behaviors or naiveté regarding exposure to an infected person are still major factors in why people do not get tested during this asymptomatic period. A person who has HIV but is asymptomatic can transmit the virus to others through high-risk behaviors.

The diagnosis changes to "symptomatic HIV infection" when a person's immune system shows evidence of being affected, resulting in persistent, prolonged, or chronic infections. Neurological complications or wasting syndrome are other reasons for the diagnosis to change to symptomatic infection. A person may fluctuate from a status of symptomatic to asymptomatic if he/she recovers from an opportunistic infection. The term AIDS Related Complex (ARC) is no longer used for this phase of the disease in the scientific community because it had no precise definition as the status fluctuates.

A person is diagnosed as having AIDS if he/she has an opportunistic infection or in another way meets the criteria in the pediatric and adult definitions set by the CDC.[1,8] The definition has not included several problems noted by children and opportunistic infections unique to women. Therefore, a redefinition of the diagnostic

Table 1. HIV Infection—A Continuum.

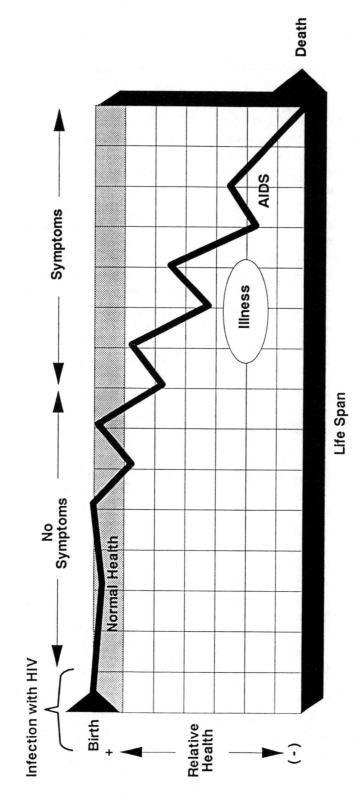

Reprinted, with permission, from Allbritten DJ,[21] p. 7.

criteria was under discussion for much of 1992. A proposal expected in the fall of 1992 is to use the T-4 or CD4 lymphocyte count as a diagnostic measure. A person in normal health has approximately 10,000 white blood cells per cubic centimeter of blood, about 1,000 of these being T-4 cells. When HIV destroys the T-4 cells the levels drop. A person with a T-4 count of 200 is vulnerable to opportunistic infections and neoplasms. So the new definition may be a T-4 count of 200, whether the person is asymptomatic or symptomatic, and a T-4 count of 400 if a person is symptomatic. A diagnosis of AIDS provides access to a number of federal programs that provide health subsidies and deal with work issues and housing support. A final note: due to effective treatments, a person may recover from the opportunistic infection and return to very good health, some people living, working, and running marathons for years with a diagnosis of AIDS. However, a person, once diagnosed with AIDS, continues to be considered as having AIDS even if his/her actual health status improves.

Research is under way in several arenas. Antiviral drugs (AZT, ddI, ddC, and others) have shown promising results in containing HIV and halting the decimation of the immune system. Early diagnosis of HIV status and positive results from early treatment are the rationale for early testing if a person realizes he/she has been exposed to HIV. At a testing site and at first diagnosis of HIV+, blood is drawn to measure the T-4 counts and close monitoring of the immune system response begins. Interventions are initiated as soon as there are signs of a compromised immune system. People are being treated by private practitioners when drugs have been released by the FDA (Food and Drug Administration) or through clinical trials programs under experimental drug protocols at some thirty-five research sites across

the nation. In many cases the progression from symptomatic HIV infection to AIDS has been slowed, but not without cost. Antiviral drugs affect core parts of all living cells, so they cause side effects that need be be monitored carefully. Clients may switch among several antiviral drugs if their tolerance decreases, or they may take low doses of two at a time.

A second focus of research is prophylactic treatments—to bolster the immune system, protect certain vulnerable body systems, and to prevent infections (antimicrobial therapy). For example, aerosolized pentamydine has been used extensively in adults and children to protect the respiratory system from the prevalent infection of *Pneumocystis carinii* pneumonia. Still another focus of research is nontraditional interventions, such as meditation, visualization, folk remedies, and therapeutic touch.[9] To date no effective vaccine has been developed, and it may be decades before one is available.[10]

Prevalence

As of September 1992, nearly 250,000 people were diagnosed with AIDS in the United States; the worldwide estimate was 502,000. Some 66.5 percent of people with AIDS have died.[11] The reported cases of AIDS represent perhaps 10 percent of the total population infected with the virus—1.5 to 2 million in the United States, or 1 in 250 people; 15 to 30 million worldwide. Approximately 40,000 new cases of AIDS are reported annually in the United States to the Centers for Disease Control.

The reported cumulative cases of AIDS in 0-19 year olds was 4,963, as of September 1992. There were 3,268 cases of 0-5 year olds; and 783 in 6-12 year olds. For these two groups, 574 were diagnosed in 1991 alone. The case fatality rate is 52.6 percent. For 13-19 year olds, the reported cases number 912. The number of cases for 20-29 year olds is 46,476, twenty percent of total cases, notable because many of these people were most likely infected as adolescents.[11] Data are tallied according to the age (and residence) at the time of diagnosis with AIDS. For the current age distribution and geographic distribution, the data need to be adjusted for the aging and mobility of people living with AIDS.

The numbers for women, children, and youth are growing faster than for those traditionally considered at greatest risk—gay and bixsexual men. The geographic distribution of AIDS continues to show significant problems in the states of New York, New Jersey, Florida, Texas, and California; however, major cities and rural areas across the nation are being affected. (See Figures 1-5, which depict the first decade of the epidemic.)

People of color are overrepresented in all age groups of people with AIDS. The pervasive poverty among minority groups perpetuates desperation, which influences intravenous drug use and lack of self-protective behaviors. Of the pediatric cases of AIDS, 80 percent are black or Hispanic; in contrast, 25 percent of all children in the United States are black or Hispanic. The Association for the Care of Children's Health reports that more than half of the adolescents with AIDS are people of color.[12]

Regarding pediatric cases of AIDS, nearly 80 percent are caused by maternal-child exposure. This is related to the spread of infection in the intravenous-drug using population where the mothers themselves are intravenous drug users or are sexual partners of intravenous drug users.[13, 14] The remaining children with AIDS are primarily cases resulting from exposure to contaminated blood or blood products prior to 1985, a stable number but decreasing percentage being children with hemophilia.[11]

Adolescents are at great risk because of their normal developmental characteris-

tics—risk taking, sexual identity exploration, fragile self-esteem, limited experience for developing a repertoire of decision-making and self-protection skills, vulnerability to peer pressure, and sense of invulnerability to risk. While the total number of adolescents with AIDS remains low (1 percent of the total AIDS cases), they have a high rate of increase of transmission. During the past two years, the number of teens diagnosed with AIDS (not HIV-infection) increased by 77 percent.[15]

Young gay males make up a substantial portion of adolescents with AIDS (64 percent of 13-24 year olds).[16] Communities and schools must begin to recognize the existence of and needs of young gay and bisexual men. They are highly vulnerable for HIV transmission due to unprotected, sometimes anonymous, sex. Too often chemical use may be involved, either injectable drugs (direct risk for HIV infection) or alcohol (indirect risk due to effects on decision-making and refusal skills). Depression is also a factor that affects self-esteem and the likelihood of using protection. Discounting these adolescents only increases their invisibility and vulnerability.[16] It is important to remember that the sexual partners of gay and bisexual youth are both young women and young men.[17]

The rate of heterosexual transmission is higher in adolescents than in adults, especially adolescent women, who are infected in proportionally greater numbers than adult women. This may be related to the high levels of sexually transmitted diseases (STD), so the virus has greater access through lesions from STDs. The nature of the cervical mucus itself may contribute to higher rates of infection (pH and progesterone levels in adolescence offer less protection from sperm and disease organisms than in adult women; location of transition zone [junction of cells

a. Total cases, cases among homosexual/bisexual men[†], and cases among women and heterosexual men reporting intravenous (IV)-drug use

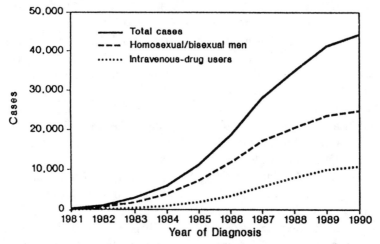

*Based on cases reported through March 1991 and adjusted for reporting delays.
[†]Excludes IV-drug users.

Figure 1. AIDS Cases by Year of Diagnosis—total cases, cases among homosexual/bisexual men and cases among women and heterosexual men reporting intravenous (IV)-drug use. (Reprinted from *MMWR*, [60] p. 360.)

b. Cases among persons reporting heterosexual contact with persons with, or at high risk for, HIV infection

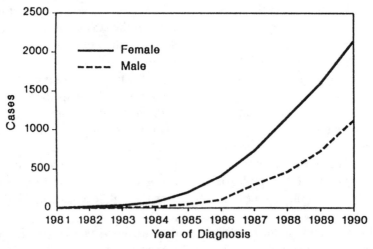

Figure 2. AIDS Cases by Year of Diagnosis—cases among persons reporting heterosexual contact with persons with, or at high risk for, HIV infection. (Reprinted from *MMWR*, [60] p. 360.)

c. Perinatally acquired pediatric AIDS cases

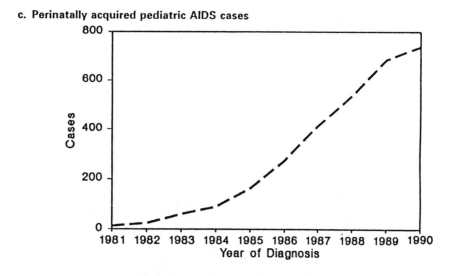

Figure 3. AIDS Cases by Year of Diagnosis—perinatally acquired pediatric AIDS cases. (Reprinted from *MMWR*, [60] p. 361.)

d. Cases among recipients of transfusions of blood or blood products

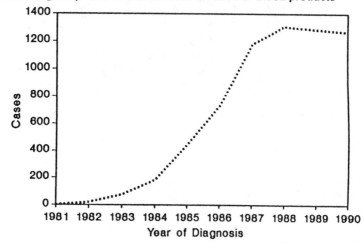

Figure 4. AIDS Cases by Year of Diagnosis—Cases among recipients of transmissions of blood or blood products. (Reprinted from *MMWR*, [60] p. 361.)

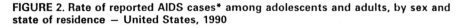

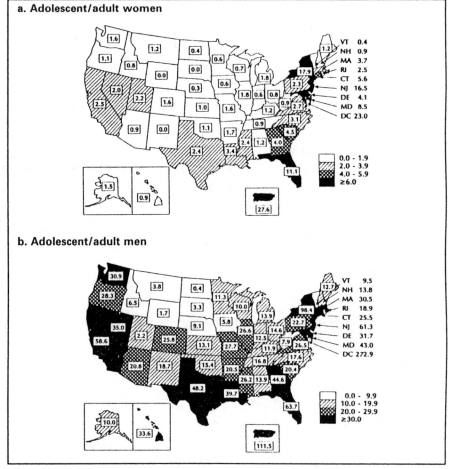

*Per 100,000 population.

Figure 5. Rate of reported AIDS cases among adolescents and adults, by sex and state of residence—United States, 1990. (Reprinted from *MMWR*, [60] p. 363.)

that line the vagina and the more fragile cervical cells] is further into the vagina allowing greater exposure of organisms to more fragile cells).[18, 19] Finally, the self-esteem and body image of young women are fragile, too, and need to be considered when defining risk.[20] At great risk as well are disenfranchised youth—runaway/street young people—who may have to sell sex for survival, for food, or for a place to sleep.[19]

Course of the Disease

The pediatric and adolescent course of HIV infection and AIDS differs from adults in several ways: Pediatric infection is usually an intergenerational problem (maternal-child transfer; mother exposed through IV drug use or heterosexual contact, often with an IV drug user); Sources outside the family are called on to be primary care providers; Children and youth who are Black or Hispanic are disproportionately affected; Children and families whose very limited resources are stressed and stretched, precipitating other problems; and, Federal funds are disproportionately footing the bill for total services, more evidence that the most needy families are most affected by HIV.[21]

For infants, the first problem is correct identification of antibody status. Because of maternal antibody interference, an accurate diagnosis may not be possible until the child is 15 months of age.[2, 21] Clinical signs of AIDS are usually present, however, within months of birth, rather than years after exposure to HIV as in adults. Neurological involvement and/or developmental delays occur in most cases (up to 90 percent), although children being treated with antiviral drugs (AZT) have shown remarkable improvement in immune status, and a halt—even reversal—of developmental delays.[13] *Pneumocystis carinii* pneumonia is the most common

serious illness for young children, diagnosed in 39 percent of pediatric cases. And it is the most deadly, causing death in 1 to 4 months from the first infection, often during the first year of life. Guidelines now call for early and aggressive use of prophylactics.[22]

For children who acquired HIV through transfusions or blood factor VIII for treatment of hemophilia prior to 1985, the period between exposure and symptoms is years, perhaps up to ten years. One of the early and prevalent manifestations of HIV in children is neurological problems, present in one-half to nine-tenths of children (two to three out of five in adults). Some of the problems include delayed brain development, encephalopathy, impaired attention, slowing motor speed, and academic problems. Besides the obvious problems with learning, three other issues compound the potential for effective education with these children—sporadic attendance due to illnesses and medical treatments, stress and anxiety of the child and parents, and fatigue.[23, 24]

The course of the disease varies in adolescents, and is complicated by factors like STDs, chemical use, denial, depression, problems with compliance with medical regimes, and the normal invincibility and invulnerability of youth. The common misconception continues, especially among youth, that an HIV+ test result means "the end." Contrary to attitudes prevalent in the mid-1980s, there is hope and there are interventions—monitoring and treatment should begin immediately. Early monitoring of the immune status through measuring CD4 counts is important. As described, low doses of antiviral drugs such as AZT, antimicrobial drugs such as prophylactic aerosolized pentamydine, and TB chemoprophylaxis may be initiated.

The federal Office of Civil Rights has determined that a person with HIV is protected from discrimination under Section 504 of the Rehabilitation Act of 1973. This is supposed to provide guarantees that a person with AIDS/HIV should not be excluded or denied an equal opportunity to maintaining a job or accessing services. Also, due to the debilitating and neurological problems of many of the children, they may be eligible for special education and related services under PL 99-457 and PL 94-142.[24-26]

The impact on the families of children with HIV/AIDS is significant. As described, parents may be dealing with their own infection and mortality at the same time as nurturing an infected child. Or, for adolescents, the problem may be disenfranchisement due to parents' difficulty in dealing with the risky behaviors and/or sexual behavior and identity issues. Some family responses that can be expected include the psychological stresses of chronic illness (for parent and child), grief and mourning at each stage of what should be normal developmental stages for the child and the family, guilt and shame at having direct transmission (maternal-child exposure) or inability to prevent the disease, feelings of isolation, and lack of support due to fear of discrimination.[25]

For the student with HIV infection, the priorities set by the school nurse and the student/family vary greatly. Some of the critical variables that will direct the assessment, planning, and interventions include the progression (or nonprogression) of HIV infection; frequency and duration of regular infections and/or of opportunistic infections, neoplasms, blood descretias or neurological effects; the age of the child/adolescent at the time of infection and developmental phases as he/she grows; the family resources (fiscal, psychosocial, spiritual, coping skills); and the community response.

Continuum of Response for Schools—Prevention to Intervention

Schools are presented with several challenges due to the AIDS/HIV epidemic (See Table 2). While the focus of this sample IHP is the child or adolescent who is known to have AIDS/HIV infection, it is important to recognize that school nurses are also called on to deal with several related situations. There are students and staff who are worried about their own risk for HIV infection, or are anxious about a family member—for example, the student who fears his/her parent may be at risk for HIV because the parent has more than one sexual partner, and/or is gay/bisexual. There are students who have a parent, sibling, or extended family member with AIDS/ HIV and who need to deal with all of the issues of loss and death, and sometimes carry the burden of secrecy about AIDS. There are staff members with AIDS/HIV, or staff members whose family members have AIDS/HIV. Embedded in the fear of AIDS/HIV is anxiety about potential negative responses in the community to issues related to sexuality, including sexual identity/orientation, drug use issues, and fear of death itself. Dealing with AIDS/HIV means school nurses need to be prepared to respond to these issues, also. Some important questions that help the school nurse assess his/her readiness for dealing with AIDS issues are in Table 3.

A comprehensive response to AIDS/ HIV requires several foci from school leaders and staff. These include policy development, instruction, in-service, counseling, and community networking (see Table 4).

The first assignment for the school nurse is being involved in the design and delivery of *prevention programs*—effective classroom health education,[27] one-to-one counseling and small group counseling, and community prevention efforts. Programs require work of multi-disciplinary

Table 2. Policy Statement: The AIDS Challenge

As educators, parents and leaders, there are three reasons why we need to educate ourselves about AIDS. First, to ensure that we know the facts about AIDS so that people understand when they are at risk and when they are not at risk of contracting the AIDS virus. Second, to prevent the transmission of the AIDS virus by providing clear information about high-risk behaviors and encouragement to minimize the risks. And third, to provide support for those with the disease, their family members and friends, as we would in any case where a person has a chronic or acute health problem that is life threatening. We need to respond with support and understanding.

This will require that each one of us in the educational community know the facts about AIDS—and that each one of us walk through our own fears raised by the disease.

The issues that AIDS raises challenge us as educators and parents to deal with our reluctance to provide sexual health and responsibility curriculum including information about heterosexuality and homosexuality, to discuss our fear of death, and to address people's right to privacy, right to know and right to work. It is a violation of our stewardship, our responsibility as educators, not to address these issues with our students—for these are issues they are facing as young people and will certainly need to face as adults.

Finally, it is our challenge in the educational community to provide the kind of honorable and moral leadership that will reduce the anxiety and fear that can so readily erode the dignity of others.

Nan Skelton, Assistant Commissioner, Division of Development and Partnership, Minnesota Department of Education, April 2, 1986. In: *Preventing AIDS Through Education*,[28] p7.

Table 3. Preparation for Counseling and Support

What is your knowledge of AIDS/HIV?

What are your feelings—concern or comfort—about AIDS/HIV?

What do you know and what are your attitudes about adolescent sexual activity?

What do you know and what are your feelings about the spectrum of sexual orientation—from heterosexual to bisexual to homosexual?

What do you know and what are your attitudes about injectable drug use?

How comfortable are you talking about sexuality with students? With adults?

What resources are available for information and referral for people who need assistance in dealing with issues related to sexuality, chemical use and abuse and AIDS/HIV in your community?

What is your experience with death and dying, grief and loss?

Who is available to be in a supportive role to you?

Adapted, with permission, from Schuster, Luehr,[52] p7.
Reprinted, with permission, © 1988, Health Information Publications, Inc.

teams and linking school and community programs. This multidisciplinary approach offers several advantages. There are options so the educators who are most knowledgeable and comfortable are in key roles. The information and skills of learners can be reinforced by repetition in different subject areas. Different students relate better to different teachers, increasing the likelihood that students get the messages. This also shows learners that a single topic or issue has implications in several arenas. A network of educators provides more ideas, support, and problem solving. Including community educators provides valuable links to prevention, testing, and counseling resources.[28] In all prevention programs— classroom instruction, counseling, and community programs—the emphasis needs to be on building essential skills to enhance total well-being, building and sustaining self-esteem, and developing self-protection

skills. These need to be taught in concert with other risk issues for students, such as pregnancy prevention, AIDS/STD prevention and drug/alcohol use prevention initiatives. Specifically, the school nurse's role as educator includes general raising awareness of issues; reviewing the literature and obtaining current information; gathering curriculum resources and materials for instruction; assisting in curriculum development; review and revision; providing instruction—one-to-one, group, classroom, and community; developing and providing instructional resources; networking and collaborating with community resources to meet community education needs.[29, 30]

The focus of AIDS prevention programs is outlined in federal and national resources. In January 1988, the Centers for Disease Control suggested by age the content for instruction.[27] Educational administrators' national organizations have also suggested

Table 4. What is the School's Role?

- Providing awareness within the school and community of AIDS/HIV issues.

- Developing policies and procedures in the school setting for individuals with AIDS/HIV infection. These policies should be based on careful and open-minded weighing of the risks and alternatives according to current scientific information.

- Providing educational opportunities for learners of all ages, and utilizing a curriculum that is age appropriate, culturally sensitive, and integrated with the current curriculum in comprehensive health education and other subject areas.

- Providing in-service on policy, instruction, student services, and universal blood and body fluids precautions to all school personnel.

- Developing and providing a counseling/support services team for learners and staff that is multidisciplinary and well-prepared to deal with AIDS-related issues.

- Networking and collaborating with community education, public health, medical, human resource, religious and business resources to meet the needs of the community regarding AIDS and AFRAIDS (Acute Fear Regarding AIDS).

Adapted, with permission, from Schuster, [59] p 6.
Reprinted, with permission, © 1987, Health Information Publications, Inc.

model programs.[31-36] Some excellent resources for curricula and instructional materials are available from clearinghouses.[37-39]

An important role of the school nurse is developing and implementing policies, procedures, and in-service for all staff regarding *universal blood and body fluids precautions*. Although HIV does not survive outside the human host, the public must respect blood and other body fluids, assuming all fluids may be infected with HIV, or more likely, Hepatitis B Virus (HBV). All prudent actions must be taken to establish a barrier between a care provider and the body fluids of another—intact healthy skin is the first barrier, latex gloves, effective handwashing—are all protection measures.

(See the federal guidelines,[40-43] and also resources for school educators in the pamphlets list.[44, 45])

Another role for school nurses is *awareness of potential risk* for HIV infection and related issues in students—paying attention to the most subtle cues. This includes recognizing when students are vulnerable: 1) challenges to self-esteem and personal integrity—when they may be swayed to engage in sexual activity or drug/alcohol use, 2) victimized through child abuse/sexual abuse/partner abuse,[46] 3) students with learning disabilities, physical or mental handicaps (low self-efficacy).[47] Young men and women who are exploring ways to express their sexuality are at risk—particularly those adolescents who are clarifying their sexual identify as gay or lesbian.[48] Sharing the works for injection of drugs is an obvious risk; however, students do not always realize that using steriods or injecting any chemical also puts them at risk for HIV.[49]

While all of these children and young people could be directly exposed to HIV, it is important to remember that there is another potential circle of exposure, their affiliates—the often-naive present or future sexual partners or injecting partners. The denial runs deep—"*My* partner has never/would never shoot up drugs; never had another sexual partner; is not bisexual; never had anonymous sex; never had unprotected sex," and so on. Given this list, all students are vulnerable, and the school nurse needs to become very astute at identifying potential risk behaviors and opportunities for intervention.

The school nurse has an important role in *early determination of risk*. This requires open, effective interviewing skills that assist students in recognizing their own risk for HIV exposure, and identifying critical issues that increase vulnerability—for example, specific sexual and drug using risk behaviors, drug/alcohol use that influences sexual activity, a history of sexual victimization or exploitation, previous sexual risk situations (pregnancy, STDs), risk-taking characteristics (assess physical, social, and emotional risk-taking patterns), and emotional health.[30, 50]

The school nurse then facilitates *counseling and testing*. There are many questions regarding HIV antibody counseling and testing for adolescents at risk. If services are available and if they serve young people without parental permission, do the current public or private sites have the expertise or structure to serve adolescents?[32] Adolescents are suspicious of the promises of confidentiality, have difficulty with

the delay in getting HIV antibody test results and sometimes do not return for results, and may fear the testing process itself but also fear "knowing the truth" of a positive result. The school nurse is in a pivotal role to assist the student in his/her decision to get tested, to support the student in making testing arrangements, to provide support while waiting for results, and to be attune to the student's response to the results, positive or negative. Persistent and consistent support is essential with either.

Maintaining confidentiality remains a high priority for all people involved in AIDS/HIV—children, youth, parents, health providers, and school people. This need to have strict control of information is related to maintaining some sense of control, privacy, and dignity on the part of the person with HIV/AIDS, and to prevent the stigma and discrimination that continue to be linked to the disease.[2, 32] Federal law (Family Education Data Privacy Rights Act—FERPA) and state laws prohibit disclosing personal health information to anyone without the client's consent. Further, the state practice acts, licensure rules, and the ethical codes of educators and health providers reinforce practices that limit disclosure of data. School nurses have had and must continue to keep the secrets, be the confidant for family members—not even discussing information with building peers, nursing colleagues, or their own family members. In addition, school nurses are called on to write and clarify formal policies and informal practices on data disclosure. This includes asking colleagues to cease inappropriate discussion and to squelch rumors. This is a burdensome role, but the basic rights and fragile self-esteem of very vulnerable children, youth, and families are at stake.

INDIVIDUALIZED HEALTHCARE PLAN

Nursing Diagnoses (N.D.)

The nursing diagnoses in this IHP example address the following nine broad priorities for a student: 1) Knowledge of health condition, 2) Optimal activity level, 3) Optimal nutrition, 4) Positive health practices, self-management, self-care skills, 5) Medications and other special healthcare procedures, 6) Infectious disease transmission, 7) Age-appropriate psychosocial skills, 8) Coping and support, and 9) Healthy sexuality.[51-53]

Assessment

(Material adapted from Allbritten, [21] Bradley,[34] and Schuster,[54])

Physical health—physical assessment, health history, laboratory tests

- Immune system status—lymph nodes, etc.
- Susceptibility/pattern of recurring infections—viral, bacterial
- Hematologic disorders
- Cardiovascular system—cardiopathy, vasculitis
- Skin disorders
- Neoplasms—lymphoma (brain primary), lymphoma (non-Hodgkins, B-cell)
- Failure to thrive or wasting syndrome
- Growth (height and weight)

Nutritional status

- Chronic diarrhea
- Signs of malnutrition/malabsorption and dehydration
- Appetite variations
- Nutritional supplements and/or tube feedings

Neurological system functions

- Neuropathy
- Sensory function—vision and hearing
- Neuromuscular status and development

Developmental status—nature and progression of delays/alterations

- Cognitive ability/developmental level—ability to comprehend HIV infection,
- Mental/cognition
- Fine/gross motor, fatigue
- Speech/language
- Age-appropriate socioemotional state

Knowledge

- Health/disease/wellness/illness, infectious diseases, disease prevention
- Sexuality: anatomy/physiology, sexual practices/behaviors, STDs/AIDS/HIV, STD prevention and birth control, sexual identity development/sexual orientation spectrum, sexual behavior options
- Chemical use/abuse

Health behaviors, practices, skills

- Locus of control
- Physical activity pattern—exercise and play
- Nutrition
- Elimination
- Relaxation, rest, and sleep
- Personal hygiene, physical care
- Safety: home, bicycle, automobile; avoiding injury
- Chemical use/abuse and related skills; effect on sexual activity
- Sexual behavior and related skills
- Relationship skills
  - communication, assertiveness, decision making, negotiating
- Stress management
- Creativity and self-expression
- Resourcefulness—problem solving, accessing resources

Self-care and personal responsibility

- Health beliefs
- Perception of physical capacity, health status, health status changes
- Participation in routine health maintenance, including self-care of wounds
- Level of independence/dependence; self-control/self-efficacy/personal power

Coping skills

- Previous losses (real and perceived) and coping strategies (effective and ineffective patterns) (denial, anger/rage, submission to loss)
- Issues/situations that cause stress, anxiety, fear; coping strategies
- Support systems

Family and other support systems

- Availability of parent or other family members
  (e.g., HIV-infected parent(s), state of illness; disenfranchised youth may be living independently or may be in need of housing)
- Juggling logistics—transportation, appointments, etc.
- Stress, anxiety, grief and loss at developmental stages
- Financial resources—to maintain home, provide food, pay medical expenses
- Current roles and responsibilities within the family, with peers, at school
- Cultural variables affecting access to support systems, family resources
- Social networks to provide support, sustain treatment and/or behavior change
- Spiritual support
- School and community reaction/response to AIDS/HIV issues, people with AIDS/HIV

Selected Nursing Diagnoses
with related Goals, Outcomes, and Interventions

Nursing Diagnosis #1

Knowledge deficit (NANDA 8.1.1)* related to existing/new health condition.

Knowledge deficit (NANDA 8.1.1) related to lack of/or misinterpretation of information.

Goal

Increase knowledge of his/her health condition.

Outcome

Student will know and understand what HIV is, how it is transmitted, how to prevent transmission, and how to seek and access information in the community.

Intervention

Teach correct and current information about HIV/AIDS.

Provide an open, supportive environment that encourages student to ask questions, examine issues.

Assist student in identifying community resources that provide accurate information.

Nursing Diagnosis #2

Potential for alteration in activity tolerance (NANDA 6.1.1.3) related to active infectious process/fatigue/chronic health condition.

Potential for alteration in sleep/rest pattern (NANDA 6.2.1) related to active infectious process/fatigue/chronic health condition.

Goal

Achieve optimal activity level.

Outcome

Student will maintain activity level within tolerance level by modifying or substituting activities when required by physical condition.

Interventions

Monitor activity tolerance regularly.

Develop adaptive activities based on current activity tolerance level.

Teach about signs/symptoms that indicate:

> appropriate activity level
> activity tolerance level
> over-exertion

Assist parents in monitoring activity level.

Assist student to maintain appropriate sleep/rest pattern.

---

*(See Chapter 2, page 38 for explanation of the NANDA approved numerical system.)

Nursing Diagnosis #3

Potential for alteration in nutrition—taking in less than body requirements—(NANDA 1.1.2.2) related to debilitation from recurrent infections.

Potential for alteration in nutrition—less than body requirements—(NANDA 1.1.2.2) related to wasting syndrome.

Potential for fluid volume deficit (NANDA 1.4.1.2.2.2) related to repeated infections resulting in physiologic instability.

Goal

Achieve optimal nutrition.

Outcome

Student will understand nutritional principles and choose well-balanced meals and healthy snacks.

Interventions

Assess understanding of nutrition principles and teach as indicated.

Monitor growth.

Arrange for additional high-nutrition snacks.

Assess understanding of need for adequate nutrition intake and teach as indicated.

Arrange for frequent opportunities for fluid intake.

Nursing Diagnosis #4:

Potential for self-management deficit.

Potential for growth in health decision-making.

Potential for alteration in health maintenance (NANDA 6.4.2) related to ineffective family coping.

Goal

Develop self-directed management of a lifestyle that promotes health.

Outcome

Student will understand and participate in decision-making process as it relates to his/her health.

Interventions

Assist student in learning/recognizing options for wellness behaviors.

Encourage student to provide input on modifications in schedule or environment

Provide opportunities for student to choose and demonstrate positive health/ lifestyle.

Assist student to identify alternatives when faced with needs to modify routine health behaviors based on changing level of health.

Provide health screening services, health and safety education.

Nursing Diagnosis #5

Potential for alteration in health management (NANDA 6.4.2) related to change in health status.

Potential for self-care deficit (NANDA 6.5.1, 2, 3 and/or 4) related to treatment regime.

Potential for noncompliance (NANDA 5.2.1.1) related to inability to perform task, nontherapeutic environment, knowledge deficit, poor self-concept, complex regime.

Potential alteration in comfort (NANDA 9.1.1) related to inflammation process/fatigue/ elevated temperature.

Goal

Participates in self-management.

Outcome

Student will actively participate in healthcare procedures and administration of medications.

Interventions

Assist student and family in identifying community health resources/services.

Assist student to identify/develop self-care skills, including decision-making skills.

Teach correct administration of medication or other healthcare procedures, including rationale, correct steps and documentation.

Monitor medications/health procedures when self-administered by student.

Teach student self-assessment of pain/discomfort including descriptions of pain/altered body comfort to enable appropriate intervention.

Teach stress management/relaxation/meditation for pain control.

Design medication/health procedures so the student is invoved in the decision-making, directive position regarding:

> Nutrition/Feeding
> Elimination/Toileting
> Respiratory Care
> Ambulation/Mobility
> Rest
> Medication

Nursing Diagnosis #6

Potential for infection (NANDA 1.2.1.1) related to alteration in immune response.

Potential for transmission of infection to others (NANDA 1.2.1.1) related to infectious agent.

Goal

Know and follow procedures to prevent transmission of infectious diseases.

Outcome

Student will understand and demonstrate positive personal health practices that decrease his/her risk of acquiring infections and risk of transmission of HIV to others.

Interventions

Teach and reinforce good personal hygiene practices, examples:

> Handwashing to reduce nosocomial infection (check technique and supplies)
> Avoiding rubbing eyes to reduce infection
> Oral hygiene to reduce likelihood of infection

Reinforce ability to choose clothing appropriate to weather and environment.

Teach about infections that are of increased threat due to diminished immune response; teach about infection control, ways to reduce exposure.

Plan to survey for and notify of communicable diseases (e.g., chicken pox).

Teach injury control strategies, including environments: classroom, bus, playground, gym, bike and safety rules.

Teach proper procedures for cleaning and bandaging minor wounds, disposal of wound care products.

Nursing Diagnosis #7

Potential for change in role performance (NANDA 3.2.1) related to changing self-perception, physical capacity, or usual patterns of responsibility.

Potential for independence-dependence conflict related to normal psychosocial development and health condition requiring assistance from parent and healthcare providers.

Potential for impaired social interactions (NANDA 3.1.1) related to HIV infection resulting in experiencing fear, discrimination, denial/avoidance from others.

Potential for alteration in self-concept (NANDA 7.1.2) related to perceptions of self as different because of having AIDS/HIV infection.

Potential for disturbance in self-concept (NANDA 7.1.2) related to having a life-threatening infectious disease.

Goal

Develop age-appropriate psychosocial skills.

Outcome

Student will sustain/develop age-appropriate roles, independence and social interactions and will sustain/develop positive self-concept.

Interventions

Assist student in identifying roles and expectations.

Assist student in identifying skills and abilities needed to meet role expectations.

Provide opportunities for the student to make independent decisions and develop skills needed for management of activities and care.

Provide opportunities for student to develop and maintain peer relationships.

Encourage active participation in school and extracurricular activities.

Nursing Diagnosis #8

Potential for ineffective individual coping (NANDA 5.1.1.1) related to inability to manage internal and external stresses—physical/psychosocial.

Potential for alteration in family process (NANDA 3.2.2) related to illness of family member.

Potential for social isolation (NANDA 3.1.2) related to alteration in wellness/inability to engage in satisfactory peer relationships/hospitalizations.

Potential for disturbance in body image. (NANDA 7.1.1)

Potential for powerlessness (NANDA 7.3.2) related to nature of disease.

Potential for powerlessness (NANDA 7.3.2) related to inability to control situations.

Grieving (NANDA 9.2.1.2) related to perceived potential loss of well-being.

Goal

Develop coping skills to deal with self, family, peer and social reactions.

Outcome

Student will identify current problems, concerns, and stressors.

Student will actively participate in identifying coping skills and strategies to assist in addressing and managing them.

Interventions

Assist student to identify stressors.

Provide a supportive environment that encourages the student to express feelings and concerns.

Assist student to identify support systems in school, community; may include conducting support groups.[32]

Monitor school attendance, classroom participation.

Assist student in identifying and utilizing coping strategies.

Assist student in addressing grief and loss.

Provide resources to meet these psychosocial needs:
  Informational needs: medical status and prognosis, epidemiological trends, research on treatment options, guidelines for reducing transmission, services (medical, mental health, alternative therapies, social services) psychological adaptation trends.
  Concrete services: financial assistance, transportation, legal assistance, educational planning, mental health, planning for emergency services, support.
  Substance abuse services: treatment for recovering drug users and alcoholics, support to reduce drug use.
  Services for neuropsychiatric complications: (30 to 75 percent of people with AIDS may experience some degree of cognitive impairment).

Nursing Diagnosis #9

Knowledge deficit (NANDA 8.1.1) related to risk of transmission of HIV to others.

Alteration in sexual patterns (NANDA 3.3) related to physical condition and risk of transmission of HIV to others.

Alteration in sexual patterns (NANDA 3.3) due to anxieties about development of sexual identity.

Goal

Develop sexual attitudes and behaviors that will prevent HIV transmission.

Outcome

Student will know and understand how to prevent HIV transmission to others and adopt attitudes and personal sexual behaviors that will prevent transmission to others.

Interventions

Provide meaningful learning opportunities to gain knowledge about sexuality, AIDS/HIV/STDs, STD prevention and birth control.

Assist student in clarifying issues—sexual identity, intimacy, and relationships.[55]

Assist student in identifying sexual behavior alternatives.[56]

Assist student in building effective relationship and decision-making skills.

Nursing Goals

Review local school district policies for inclusion of these issues[54, 57, 58]
    attendance of student or faculty member with AIDS/HIV
    support for curriculum/instruction on AIDS/HIV
    support for healthy sexuality and drug use prevention curriculum
    access to health and counseling services
    nondiscrimination/harassment of people with AIDS/HIV
    confidentiality/data privacy
    community/parenting programs
Assess one's own knowledge, attitudes, and counseling skills,[52, 54] for example:
    comfort with adolescent sexuality, sexual orientation, sexual expression
    awareness of and comfort with drug/alcohol use intervention
    communication skills regarding sex and drug issues—with adults, students
    resources for referral
    own systems for problem solving and support
Design strategies to prepare and support faculty for prevention and intervention initiatives[29, 32, 54]
    comprehensive school health education/HIV education[27]
    skills to deal with disclosure by students of AIDS/HIV, sexual abuse,
      parent/family member with HIV
    coordinating with the full range of support services for student infected or affected by
      AIDS/HIV
    reinforce universal precautions, safeguards for bloodborne pathogens [6]

Assist faculty and students in coping/grieving
 grief/loss for student, staff, family members with AIDS/HIV
 grief/loss of the regular/normal classroom role for teachers
 grief/loss of the "loss of innocence" for children/youth
Design/coordinate community support systems
 referral and coordination of services[32]; clarify the roles and linkages of
  case managers[2]
 awareness, counseling for AIDS/AFRAIDS (Acute Fear Regarding AIDS)[58]
 community network for prevention education efforts
 programs for parental skills in communicating with children and youth community
 network for support for people with AIDS/HIV
Participate in/follow the nursing research priorities [9]
 physiologic aspects of nursing care
 psychosocial aspects of nursing care
 delivery of nursing care
 prevention of transmission
 ethical issues

REFERENCES

1. Revision of the CDC Surveillance Case Definition for AIDS. *Morbidity and Mortality Weekly Report (MMWR)* 1987; 36 (Aug 14):1-15S.
2. Thurber F, Berry B. Children with AIDS: issues and future directions. *J Pediatr Nursing* 1990; 5(3): 168-177.
3. Healy RM, Coleman T. A primer on AIDS for health professionals. *Health Education* 1988/1989; Dec/Jan: 4-10.
4. Harvey DC, Decker DL, Imhof AM. HIV Infection and Developmental Service Provider Liability: An Introduction to Tort Principles. Technical Report on Developmental Disabilities and HIV Infection, 5. Washington, DC: National Association of Protection and Advocacy System, Apr 1990.
5. Educational and Foster Care of Children Infected with HTLV-III/LAV. *Morbidity and Mortality Weekly Report (MMWR)* 1985;34 (34): 517-521.
6. Rogers MF, White CR, Sanders R, Schable C, Ksell T, Wasserman RL, Bellanti JA, Peters SM, Wray BB. Lack of transmission of Human Immunodeficiency Virus from infected children to their household contacts. *Pediatrics* 1990;85(2): 210-214.
7. American Public Health Association. New HIV test gets results in 10 minutes. *The Nation's Health* July 1992, 24.2.
8. Guidelines for Effective School Health Education to Prevent the Spread of AIDS. *Morbidity and Mortality Weekly Report (MMWR)* 1988; 37 (Jan 29): 1-14S.
9. National Nursing Research Agenda. *HIV Infection: Prevention and Care, A Report of the NCNR Priority Expert Panel on HIV Infection.* Bethesda, MD: National Institutes of Health, National Center for Nursing Research, 1990. (NCRC, Building 31, Room 5B25, Bethesda, MD 20892; 301-496-0207).
10. Philadelphia Sciences Group. AIDS vaccine development. In: *AIDS 91 Summary: Practical Synopsis of the VII International Conference, 1991.* Reprinted in AIDS Reference Guide, Atlantic Information Services (May 1992). (1050—17 St. NW, Suite 480, Wash. DC 20036, 202-775-9008.)
11. Centers for Disease Control. *HIV/AIDS Surveillance Report.* Atlanta: Centers for Disease Control, Sept 1992.
12. *Building Systems of Care for Children with HIV Infection and Their Families.* Bethesda, MD: Association for the Care of Children's Health, 1989 (20 pg. booklet).
13. Pizzo PA. Emerging concepts in the treatment of HIV infection in children. JAMA 1989; 262 (14): pp. 1989-92.
14. Government Accounting Office. *Pediatric AIDS: Health and Social Service Needs of Infants and Children.* Report to the Chairman, Committee on Finance, US Senate. US GAO Health Resources Division (GAO/HRD-89-96), May 5, 1989.

15. Select Committee on Children, Youth and Families. *A Decade of Denial: Teens and AIDS in America.* Washington, DC: US House of Representatives, Select Committee, May 1992.

16. Reynolds SG, Remafedi G, Yoakam J, Cwayna K. *Surviving AIDS: Simple Answers to Complex Questions about AIDS and Adolescent Homosexuality.* Minneapolis, MN: University of Minnesota Youth and AIDS Project, 1991 (Youth and AIDS Project (YAP), Adolescent Health Program, 428 Oak Grove St, Minneapolis, MN 55403; 612/627-6820).

17. Chu SY, Petersman TA, Doll LS, Buehler JW, Curran JW. AIDS in bisexual men in the United States: epidemiology and transmission to women. *Am J Public Health* 1992; 82 (2):220-224.

18. Hein K. AIDS in adolescents: a rationale for concern. *NY State J Med* 1987; May: 290-295.

19. HIV infection among adolescents: falling between the cracks of services and prevention. *National AIDS Network Multi-Cultural NOTES on AIDS Education and Service*, 1989;2(6): 1-4.

20. Bower B. Teenage turning point: does adolescence herald the twilight of girls' self esteem? *Science* 1991; Mar 23: 184-6.

21. Allbritten DJ. *Children with HIV/AIDS: A Sourcebook for Caring, A Guide for Establishing Programs for Children.* Alexandria, VA: National Association of Children's Hospitals and Related Institutions, 1990.

22. Centers for Disease Control. Guidelines for prophylactics against *Pneumocystis carinii* pneumonia for children with human immunodeficiency virus. *MMWR* 1991; 40 (RR-2, Mar 15): 1-13.

23. Cohen SE, Mundy T, Karassik B, Lieb L, Ludwig D, Ward J. Neoropsychological functioning in Human Immunodeficiency Virus Type 1 seropositive children infected through neonatal blood transfusion. *Pediatrics* 1988; 88 (1): 58-67.

24. Byers J. AIDS in children: effects on neurological development and implications for the future. *J Special Education* 1989;23 (1): 5-13.

25. Rudigier AF, Crocker AC, Cohen HJ. The dilemmas of childhood HIV infection. *Children Today* 1990; Jul-Aug: 26-29.

26. Office of Civil Rights. Fact Sheet: Your Rights as a Person with HIV Infection, AIDS, or Related Conditions (H-21). Washington, DC: US Department of Health and Human Services, Office of Civil Rights, Aug 1990.

27. Guidelines for Effective School Health Education to Prevent the Spread of AIDS. *Morbidity and Mortality Weekly Report (MMWR)* 1988; 37 (Jan 29): 1-14S.

28. *Preventing AIDS Through Education* (Instructional Resources for Teachers). St. Paul, MN: Minnesota Department of Education, 1988.

29. Schuster C. AIDS update: AIDS education—the key strategy. *Community Nurse Forum* 1988; (5)2: 6.

30. Brainerd E. HIV in the school setting: the role of the school nurse. In: American School Health Association. *Implementation Guide for the Standards of School Nursing Practice* . Kent, OH: American School Health Association, 1991.

31. American School Health Association. *Sexuality Education within Comprehensive School Health Education* . Kent, OH: American School Health Association, 1991 (ASHA, 7362 State Route 43, PO Box 708, Kent OH 44240; $12).

32. American Association for Counseling and Development (ASCD), American School Health Association, National Association of School Nurses, National Association of School Psychologists, National Association of Social Workers (Education Commission), National Association of State School Nurse Consultants, National Coalition of Advocates for Students (NCAS). *Guidelines for HIV and AIDS Student Support Services* . Boston, MA: National Coalition of Advocates for Students, 1990 (NCAS, 100 Boylson St, Suite 737, Boston, MA 02116; $2.00).

33. Burger JE, Williams JH, Rivera RO, eds. *Responding to HIV and AIDS, A Special Publication for NEA Members* . Washington, DC: National Education Association Health Information Network, 1992 (NEA Professional Library, PO Box 509, West Haven, CT 06516; $3; # A501-00100-1).

34. Bradley BJ. *HIV Infection and the School Setting: A Guide for School Nursing Practice* . Kent, OH: American School Health Association, 1990 draft (ASHA, PO Box 708/7363 State Route 43, Kent, OH 44240; 216-678-1601).

35. Freudenberg N. *Preventing AIDS , A Guide to Effective Education for Prevention of HIV Infection.* Washington, DC: American Public Health Association, 1989 (APHA, 1015 Fifteenth St NW, Washington, DC 20005).

36. Keough K. *Dealing with AIDS, Breaking the Chain of Infection , A Guide for Developing an AIDS Education Program.* Arlington, VA: American Association of School Administrators, 1988 (American Association of School Administrators, 1801 N. Moore St, Arlington, VA 22209-9988; 703/528-0700).

37. National Guidelines Task Force. *Guidelines for Comprehensive Sexuality Education, K—12 Grade.* New York, NY: SIECUS, 1991 (SIECUS, 130 W. 42nd St Suite 250, New York, NY 10036; $5).

38. Quackenbusch M, Nelson M, Clark K, eds. *The AIDS Challenge , Prevention Education for Young People.* Santa Cruz, CA: Network Publications, a division of ETR Associates, 1988.

39. Quackenbusch M, Villareal S. *Does AIDS Hurt? Educating Young Children About AIDS.* Santa Cruz, CA: Network Publications, a division of ETR Associates, 1988.

40. Recommendations for Prevention of HIV Transmission in Health Care Settings . *Morbidity and Mortality Weekly Report (MMWR)* 1987; 36(Aug 21): 1—18S.

41. Update: Universal Precautions for Prevention of AIDS and Hepatitis B Virus and other Blood Borne Pathogens in Health Care Settings. *Morbidity and Mortality Weekly Report (MMWR)* 1988; 37(Jun 24): 377-388.

42. Recommendations for Preventing Transmission of Human Immunodeficiency Virus and Hepatitis B Virus to Patients During Exposure-Prone Invasive Procedures. *Morbidity and Mortality Weekly Report (MMWR)* 1991; 40 (RR-8–Jul 12): 1-9.

43. OSHA Regulations on Bloodborne Pathogens (29 CFR 1910 Subp. Z-Ammended). *Federal Register* 1991; No. 56 (235): 64175-64182.

44. Infectious Disease (AIDS/HIV, Hepatitis-B) in the School Setting. Merced, CA: Classroom Connections, revised 1992. (Classroom Connections, PO Box 2208, Merced, CA 95344; 202-383-1008).

45. It's Up to You—Building A Safer Approach to Universal Hygiene. (poster/video) American Federation of Teachers, no copyright date. (AFT AIDS Education Project, 1-800-238-1133 x4490; $8.00 for video).

46. Moore KA, Nord CW, Peterson JL. Nonvoluntary sexual activity among adolescents. *Fam Plann Perspect* 1989;32(3): 110-114.

47. Bartel N, Meddock TD. AIDS and adolescents with learning disabilities: issues for parents and educators. *Reading, Writing Learning Disabilities* 1989; 5: 299-311.

48. Remafedi G. Fundamental issues in the care of homosexual youth. *Adolesc Med* 1990; 74(5): 1169-1179.

49. Buckley WE, Yesalis C III, Friedl KE, Anderson WA, Streit AL, Wright JE. Estimated prevalence of anabolic steroid use among male high school seniors. *JAMA* 1988;260(23): 3411-3445.

50. Luehr RE. *Student Services AIDS/HIV Prevention Project—Interviewing Guidelines.* St. Paul: Minnesota Department of Education, 1990. (Available from AIDS/HIV Program, MDE, 550 Cedar St, St. Paul, MN 55101; 612/296-5825).

51. Schuster C, Will S, Luehr RE, Erickson Connor MJ. AIDS in children and adolescents—learning to cope with a harsh reality. *School Nurse J* 1986; Nov/Dec: 14-25.

52. Schuster C, Luehr RE. AIDS update: AIDS virus infection—responding with understanding and support. *Community Nurse Forum* 1988;5(3): 7.

53. Luehr RE. Helping the student with AIDS virus infection. Chapter 10. In: Larson ed. *Managing the School Age Child with a Chronic Health Condition: A Practical Guide for Schools, Families and Organizations.* Wayzata; MN: DCI Publishing, 1988 (distributed by Sunrise Rivers Press, 11481 Kost Dam Rd, North Branch, MN 55056, 612-583-3239).

54. Schuster C, Haas MK, Villars M, Luehr RE. *Responding with Support, An Individualized Health Plan for A Student with AIDS Virus Infection.* St. Paul, MN: School Nurse Organization of Minnesota and Minnesota Department of Education, May 1988 (AIDS/HIV Prevention Program, Minnesota Dept of Education, 550 Cedar St, St. Paul, MN 55101; 612-296-5825).

55. Gibson P. Gay male and lesbian youth suicide. In: *Report of the Secretary's Task Force on Youth Suicide.* Volume 3: Prevention and Intervention in Youth Suicide (Marcia R. Feinleib, ed.) Washington, DC: Alcohol, Drug Abuse and Mental Health Administration, 1989 (DHHS pub. lication No. (ADAM) 89-1623).

56. Shernoff M. Integrating safer-sex counseling into social work practice. *Social Casework: J Contemp Social Work* 1988; Jun: 334-339.

57. Schuster C. AIDS update: policy foundation for school programs. *Community Nurse Forum* 1988; 5(4): 4.

58. *The First 24 Hours, A Suggested Guide for Responding to Students Infected with the AIDS Virus by the Northeast Metropolitan Intermediate School District Learners at Risk Committee.* St. Paul, MN: Minnesota Curriculum Services Center, Jan 1988.

59. Schuster C. AIDS update: Issues—impact on schools. *Community Nurse Forum* 1987; 4 (3): 6.

60. Centers for Disease Control. Update: Acquired immunodeficiency syndrome-United States, 1981-1990. *MMWR* 1991; 40 (22):358-363,369.

BIBLIOGRAPHY

American Academy of Pediatrics. Guidelines for HIV-infected children and their foster families. *Pediatrics*, 1992;89(4): 1992; 681-3.

American Public Health Association. *Pediatric HIV Infection*, A Report of the Special Initiative on AIDS of the American Public Health Association. Washington, DC: Oct 1989 (APHA, 1015 Fifteenth St, NW, Washington, DC 20005; 202/789-5688).

Centers for Disease Control. Selected behaviors that increase risk for HIV infection among high school students—United States, 1990 *MMWR* 1992; 42(14): 236-239.

Centers for Disease Control. Sexual behavior among high school students—United States, 1990. *MMWR* 1992; 40 (51-52): 885-888.

Hein K. AIDS in adolescence, exploring the challenge. *J Adolesc Health Care* 1989; 10: 10S—35S.

Koop C. *Surgeon General's Report on Acquired Immune Deficiency Syndrome.* Bethesda, MD: US Department of Health and Human Services, 1986.

Luehr RE. *Healthy Sexuality: Understanding Sexuality, Communicating About Sexuality.* St. Paul: Minnesota Department of Education, 1990 (Available from AIDS/HIV Program, MDE, 550 Cedar St, St. Paul, MN 55101).

Public Health Service (PHS). *Report of the Surgeon General's Workshop on Children with HIV Infection and their Families.* Washington, DC: US DHHS, 1987 (DHHS publication No. (HRS) D-MC-87-1).

Seidel J. The development of a comprehensive pediatric HIV developmental service program. *Technical Report on Developmental Disabilities and HIV Infection*, No. 7, December, 1991.

RESOURCE TEXTS

Benenson AS, ed. *Communicable Diseases in Man* . 15th Ed. Washington, DC: American Public Health Association, 1990.

Cornish J, coordinator and Johnson S, ed. *Caring for Children with HIV Infection , A Handbook for Foster Parents.* Minneapolis, MN: Human Service Associates, 1992 (MN Human Resources Associates, 570 Asbury St,#306, St. Paul, MN 55104; $14; 612-645-0688).

Crocker AC, Cohen HJ, Kastner TA. *HIV Infection and Developmental Disabilities , A Resource for Service Providers.* Baltimore, MD: Brookes Publishing Company, 1992 (Brookes Publishing Company, PO. Box 10624, Baltimore, MD 21285-9945; 800-638-3775).

Fraser K. *Someone at School Has AIDS , A Guide to Developing School Policies for Students and School Staff Members Who Are Infected with HIV.* Alexandria, VA: National Association of State Boards of Education, 1989 (National Association of State Boards of Education, 1012 Cameron St, Alexandria, VA 22314).

Hochhauser M, Rothenberger JH. *AIDS Education*, Dubuque, IA: Wm. C. Brown Publishers, 1992.

Pohl M, Deniston K, Toft D. *The Caregivers' Journey: When You Love Someone with AIDS.* Center City, MN: Hazelden Foundation, 1990.

Schools Face the Challenge of AIDS . Newton, MA: Education Development Center, 1990.

Schuster C, Haas MK, Villars M, Luehr RE. *Responding with Support, An Individualized Health Plan for A Student with AIDS Virus Infection.* St. Paul, MN: School Nurse Organization of Minnesota and Minnesota Department of Education, May 1988 (AIDS/HIV Prevention Program, Minnesota Dept of Education, 550 Cedar St, St. Paul, MN 55101; 612-296-5825).

FEDERAL DEFINITIONS and GUIDELINES

US DHHS Public Health Service Centers for Disease Control

Classification System for HTLV-III/LAV Infections. *Morbidity and Mortality Weekly Report (MMWR)* 1986; 35(20): 334-339.

Classification System for HIV Infection in Children Under 13 Years of Age. *Morbidity and Mortality Weekly Report (MMWR)* 1987; 36 (Apr 24): 225-36.

Revision of the CDC Surveillance Case Definition for AIDS. *Morbidity and Mortality Weekly Report (MMWR)* 1987; 36 (Aug 14):1-15S.

Human Immunodeficiency Virus (HIV) Infection Codes and New Codes for Kaposi's Sarcoma—Official Authorized Addenda ICD-9-CM, No. 2. *Morbidity and Mortality Weekly Report (MMWR)* 1991; 40(RR-9, Jul 26): 1-19.

Revision in the Case Definition for HIV infection and AIDS expected Fall 1992.

Educational and Foster Care of Children Infected with HTLV-III/LAV. *Morbidity and Mortality Weekly Report (MMWR)* 1985;34 (34): 517-521.

Recommendations for Prevention for HIV Transmission in Health Care Settings . *Morbidity and Mortality Weekly Report (MMWR)* 1987; 36(Aug 21): 1-18S.

Update: Universal Precautions for Prevention of AIDS and Hepatitis B Virus and other Blood Borne Pathogens in Health Care Settings. *Morbidity and Mortality Weekly Report (MMWR)* 1988; 37(Jun 24): 377-388.

Recommendations for Preventing Transmission of Human Immunodeficiency Virus and Hepatitis B Virus to Patients During Exposure-Prone Invasive Procedures. *Morbidity and Mortality Weekly Report (MMWR)* 40 1991; 40,(RR-8—Jul 12): 1-9.

OSHA Regulations on Bloodborne Pathogens (29 CFR 1910 Subp. Z—Ammended). *Federal Register* 1991; No. 56 (235): 64175-64182.

Guidelines for Effective School Health Education to Prevent the Spread of AIDS. *Morbidity and Mortality Weekly Report (MMWR)* 1988; 37 (Jan 29): 1-14S.

JOURNALS/NEWSLETTERS

AIDS Alert, The Monthly Update for Health Professionals. American Health Consultants, Inc., 3525 Peidmont Rd, Building Six, Suite 400, Atlanta, GA 30306; 1-800-688-2421.

AIDS Education and Prevention, An Interdisciplinary Journal. Guilford Publications, Inc., 72 Spring St, New York, NY 10012.

Focus, A Guide to AIDS Research and Counseling, UCSF AIDS Health Project, Box 0884, San Francisco, CA 94143-0884; 415/476-6430.

MMWR (*Morbidity and Mortality Weekly Report*) (Subscribe through the Massachusetts Medical Society, CSPO Box 9120, Waltham, MA 02254-9120; $48 for third class mail, $58 for first class mail).

Pediatric AIDS and HIV Infection, Fetus to Adolescent. [periodical] Mary Ann Leibert, Inc., Publishers, 1651 Third Ave, New York, NY 10128; 212-289-2300.

SIECUS Report, Sex Information and Education Council of the United States, 130 W 42nd St, Suite 250, New York, NY; 212-819-9770.

PAMPHLETS

Caring for Someone with AIDS, Information for Friends, Relatives, Household Members, and Others Who Care for a Person with AIDS at Home. US Public Health Service, Centers for Disease Control, American Responds to AIDS, c. 1990.

Infectious Disease (AIDS/HIV, Hepatitis-B) in the School Setting. Merced, CA: Classroom Connections, revised 1992. (Classroom Connections, PO Box 2208, Merced, CA 95344; 202-383-1008).

It's Up to You—Building A Safer Approach to Universal Hygiene. (poster/video) American Federation of Teachers, no copyright date. (AFT AIDS Education Project, 1-800-238-1133 x4490).

Voluntary HIV Counseling and Testing: Facts, Issues and Answers, 1990. US Public Health Service, Centers for Disease Control; call the National AIDS Hotline 1-800-342-AIDS.

When Someone Close Has AIDS. National Institute of Mental Health, (DHHS Publication No. [ADM] 89-1515).

ORGANIZATIONS/AGENCIES

American Foundation for AIDS Research (AmFAR)
1515 Broadway, 36th Floor, New York, NY 10036; 212-333-3118

American Red Cross National Headquarters (or local Red Cross Chapter)
  AIDS Education Program
17th & "D" Streets NW, Washington, DC 20036; 202-639-3223

American School Health Association
PO Box 708/7363 State Route 43, Kent, OH 44240; 216-678-1601

Association for the Care of Children's Health
7910 Woodmont Ave, Suite 300, Bethesda, MD 20314; 301-654-6549

Council of Chief State School Officers (CCSSO)
HIV/School Health Project Suite 379, 400 North Capitol St NW, Washington, DC 20001;
202/393-8159 *HIV Bulletin Board* —twice-monthly updates of news and activities;
  1-800-927-3000
Accessible through GTE-ES Bulletin Boards; available to subscribers of *Ed-Line*

Centers for Disease Control (US DHHS, PHS)
National Center for Chronic Disease Prevention and Health Promotion

> Division of Adolescent and School Health (DASH) 1600 Clifton Rd NE; Rhodes
> Bldg, MS K-31, Atlanta, GA 30333; 404-488-5354

> Technical Information Services Branch
> 1600 Clifton Rd, Rhodes Bldg, Mailstop K-13, Atlanta, GA 30333;404-488-5080
> New resource: CDP (Chronic Disease Prevention) File—collection of 5 databases of
> information about health promotion and disease prevention on CD-ROM

> CHID (Combined Health Information Database)—computerized database of 21
> subfiles ($80 annual fee; hourly rates of $10-45 to access data. Check with local li-
> braries first because several have a contract with BRS. Available through Maxwill
> Online, BRS Information Technical Division, 8000 Westpark Dr, McLean, VA
> 22102; 1-800-289-4277

>> AIDS Education Subfile
>> National AIDS Information/Education Program, CDC
>> 1600 Clifton Rd, Mailstop E-25, Atlanta, GA 30333 404-639-2928

>> AIDS School Health Education Database Subfile
>> National Center for Chronic Disease Prevention and Health Promotion, CDC
>> 1600 Clifton Rd, Mailstop K-13, Atlanta, GA 30333; 404-488-5080

>> Health Promotion and Education Database Subfile
>> National Center for Chronic Disease Prevention and Health Promotion, CDC
>> 1600 Clifton Rd, Rhodes Bldg, Room 1112 MS-K-13, Atlanta, GA 30333; 404-
>> 488-5080

> National AIDS Information Clearinghouse, CDC
> PO Box 60033, Rockville, MD 20849-6003; 1-800-458-5231 (print resources, net-
> work to organizations, new computer access—NAC ONLINE)

Center for Population Options
1025 Vermont Ave. NW, Suite 210, Washington, DC 20005; 202-347-5700

Education Development Center, Inc.
(for curricula- Growing Healthy, Teenage Health Teaching Modules, training)
55 Chapel St, Newton, MA 02160; 617-969-7100

ETR Associates, Network Publications
(clearinghouse of AIDS/HIV, sexuality and drug prevention resources)
PO Box 1830, Santa Cruz, CA 95061-1830; 408-4060; 1-800-321-4407

Foundation for Children with AIDS, Inc.
77B Warren St, Brighton, MA 02135; 617-783-7300 (Newsletter: *Children with AIDS*)

National Association of People with AIDS (NAPWA)
PO Box 18345, Washington, DC 20036; 202-898-0414

National Association of School Nurses
Box 1300, Scarborough, ME 04074; 207-883-2117

National Association of State Boards of Education
1012 Cameron St, Alexandria, VA 22314; 703-684-4000

National Center for Health Education, NEA
72 Spring Street, Suite 208, New York, NY 10012; 212-334-9470

National Childhood Grief Institute
3300 Edinborough Way, Suite 512, Minneapolis, MN 55436; 612-832-9286

National Clearinghouse for Alcohol and Drug Information
PO Box 2345, Rockville, MD 20852; 310-468-2600

National Pediatric HIV Resource Center, School Nurse Program
Children's Hospital AIDS Program (CHAP)
Children's Hospital of New Jersey, Newark, NJ; 201-268-8273

The National PTA
700 North Rush St, Chicago, IL 60611; 312-787-0977

National School Boards Association
1680 Duke St, Alexandria, VA 22314; 703-838-6756

The Pediatric AIDS Foundation
1311 Colorado Ave, Santa Monica, CA 90404; 310-395-9051

Contact your state/local AIDS/HIV hotline/helpline for resources.

11 | IHP: Juvenile Rheumatoid Arthritis

Susan I. Simandl Will

INTRODUCTION

Juvenile rheumatoid arthritis is a childhood acquired, autoimmune inflammatory disease which presents a challenge in management for the child, family, school, and physician. This disease, with other rheumatic childhood illness, is believed to affect about 1 in 1,000 children below 16 years of age[1] or up to 250,000 children in the United States.[2] An estimated 5,000 new cases of juvenile rheumatoid arthritis are diagnosed each year making it a fairly common childhood issue.[3] It is important to remember that this disease is a systemic illness and not limited to just the apparent involved joints.

Because of the unpredictable, intermittent nature of severe acute exacerbations, alternating with sudden remissions, the disease can be confusing and unsettling and a management challenge for the child, family, physician, and school. In addition, the disease may take the form of multijoint involvement or involvement of just a few joints, or be an active systemic disease. School program flexibility is essential in planning a successful academic career for a child who may experience multiple absences, then enjoy lengthy periods relatively disease-free, and then perhaps be physically limited for variable periods of time. All these changes are possible within any given school year making the child's individual needs great and variable.

The school nurse as advocate and resource for the child who has juvenile rheumatoid arthritis is an essential key to successful school experiences. Attention must be given to federal legislation which may be useful in planning the child's school career. Public Law 94-142 prohibits exclusion from public education because of a disability, and through this law, special education services can be provided to assist the child's school success.

Pathophysiology

Disease Prevention

The etiology of juvenile rheumatoid arthritis (JRA) remains undetermined. However, much data exist to define the course of the disease and the ways it varies in presentation. The onset of JRA can take one of three basis forms: systemic onset, multijoint onset (polyarticular JRA), or onset in one to four joints (pauciarticular JRA).

Systemic onset is characterized by high fever (104 + degrees) spikes with falls to near normal or normal. A small macular rash gelling into larger lesions may present itself for several hours and then recede. In addition, these children may exhibit the additional symptoms of mild liver dysfunction, enlarged spleen, pericarditis, pleurisy, anemia. Children with systemic onset may or may not experience joint pain. Laboratory tests usually include complete blood count (elevated neutrophils and platelets are typical), erythrocyte sedimentation rate (usually elevated), and rheumatoid factor (RF—measuring anti-IGG antibody). Diagnosis is made through ruling out other rheumatic diseases. Children presenting with systemic onset typically convert into one of the two other onset groups: polyarticular JRA or pauciarticular JRA. Polyarticular JRA is characterized by symmetrical multijoint involvement including the small hand and foot joints as well as the knee, elbow, shoulder, and ankle. Some children demonstrate a positive RF and are more likely to develop adult, chronic arthritis. With negative RF, the child may experience complete remissions. Pauciarticular JRA is characterized by asymmetrical involvement of just one to four joints, usually the large joints: knee, wrist, elbow, or shoulder. Pauciarticular JRA is further subdivided into those who exhibit minimal problems or complete remission and those who develop chronic joint involvement.

Disease Course

In any of the types of JRA, remissions of several months to several years are possible. Permanent remission in late adolescence or young adulthood is possible. Triggers for exacerbations are undetermined. During the acute inflamatory exacerbations the child may experience pain and limited range of motion. In addition, the child may experience fatigue and stiffness. Stiffness occurs especially following periods of immobility, such as sitting in a class, and can create hourly variations in the limits for activity tolerance and activity ability. With limited motion in some or many joints, the child's ability to perform normal activities of daily living can be compromised minimally or extensively. The child may need assistance with dressing, eating, carrying objects (books, cafeteria trays), stair climbing, walking, writing, toileting, opening doors, and boarding and exiting busses.

Treatment

The medical treatment focus of JRA consists of medication and occasionally use of splints and braces to support involved joints as well as to prevent contractures. Passive and active range of motion exercises are also used to facilitate mobility and prevent contractures. In addition, physical therapy and occupational therapy may be useful. Continuing education about the disease, treatment, and self-care involvement at age-appropriate levels is vital. And for the adolescent who appears to be entering adulthood with continuing involvement, vocational counselling will be necessary.

Medication management is based on minimizing inflammation with anti-inflammatory drugs as well as drug relief of pain and swelling. The severity of involvement will determine the type and dosage of drug prescribed. Initially nonsteroidal, anti-inflammatory drugs (NSAIDs) such as aspirin, ibuprofen, and indomethacin are prescribed. With these medications the child must be monitored for stomach problems, bleeding, tinnitus, and liver problems. The physician may be monitoring blood levels of the medication to assure desired dosage levels and response. For children who need additional medication the slow-acting antirheumatic drugs (SAARDs) can be initiated next. These are typically monitored by a rheumatoid specialist. Corticosteriods are the next level of medication management followed by cytotoxic drugs.

INDIVIDUALIZED HEALTHCARE PLAN

Assessment

History

- History of arthritis, onset and course
- History of involved joints

Disease Management

- Student's description and definition of arthritis
- Student's current medication
- Changes in medication which are to be implemented if condition changes
- Student's description of medication plan
- Student's understanding of arthritis
- Is student in an acute phase of condition right now?
- Is student in a non-acute phase of condition right now?
- What are the differences in treatment between acute and non-acute phases?
- What splints, braces, stabilizers does student use? When?
- Current joints involved:
  stiffness
  swelling
  tenderness
  pain with touch or painless
  warmth in joint area
  amount of joint mobility loss
  morning stiffness
  afternoon stiffness (amount of joint mobility gained as day progresses)
  stiffness after sitting for extended periods (class hour)
- Fever and fever pattern (spikes to 104 degrees F not unusual in acute phases)
- Systemic involvement (malaise, lethargy, rash, pericarditis, peritoneal involvement, anemia, pulmonary involvement)

Psychosocial

- Age and developmental level
- Student's feelings about having arthritis
- Student's perception of what family members think and feel about his/her having arthritis
- Student's perception of what friends think and feel about his/her having arthritis
- School club or athletic activities past and present
- Community and church activities past and present
- Depression or despondency
- Student's support systems: family, friends, other

Academic

- Review of academic or cumulative school record for patterns of academic performance
- Assessment of teachers' perception of student's performance and classroom adjustment
- Comparison of student's behavior, social skills, academic performance to peer norms
- School absence pattern
- Need for special education (P.L. 94-142) services to adequately educate the student (transportation, classroom adaptations, tutoring, occupational therapy, physical therapy, vocational guidance)

Self-Care

- Activities student states are limited by arthritis
- What does student find useful to manage successfully in school?
- Need for learning support systems (special education, computer aids, tutors, adaptive physical education)
- What treatments, medications can student manage on own?

Nursing Diagnoses (N.D.)

N.D. 1   Alteration in comfort: Pain (NANDA 9.1.1)* related to inflamatory joint process and/or pain related to inflammation of affected joints.

N.D. 2   Alteration in activities of daily living (NANDA 6.1.1.2)—personal, recreational, educational: hygiene, toileting, eating, writing, running, walking, stair-climbing, manipulating objects with fingers.

N.D. 3   Impaired physical mobility (NANDA 6.1.1.1) related to discomfort and/or inflammation.

N.D. 4   Alterations in self-care (NANDA 6.5.1, 2, 3 or 4) related to discomfort and/or inflammation.

N.D. 5   Knowledge deficit (NANDA 8.1.1) related to arthritis pathophysiology or medications.

Goals

Management of pain. (N.D. 1)

Student will acquire adaptations necessary to experience as normal a lifestyle as possible in the school setting. (N.D. 2-4)

Student will be able to perform activities of daily living within his/her physical limits without excessive fatigue or development of pain.(N.D. 2-4)

Student will be involved in management of arthritis and improve self-management skills. (N.D. 2-4)

Student will increase understanding of pathophysiology of arthritis and develop or improve skills to manage arthritis. (N.D. 5)

---

* (See Chapter 2, page 38 for explanation of the NANDA approved numerical system.)
See Chapter 6 for additional mental health and psychosocial nursing diagnoses relevant to children with chronic disease.

Nursing Interventions

Teacher/School Interventions

Assist teachers in development of alternative educational activities compatible with mobility abilities. (N.D. 1-4)

Arrange for anti-inflammatory medication at school as appropriate and in accordance with school district policy and procedure. (N.D. 1-4)

Arrange for mid-class walk time if sitting for full class hour stiffens joints. (N.D. 1)

Provide appropriate nursing supervision to all personnel assisting the student with any cares. (N.D. 2, 3)

Establish plan for regular communication between school and family. (N.D. 1-3, 5)

Assist teachers in development of alternative educational activities if writing impaired: (N.D. 1-4)

> verbal reporting
> computer use
> use of large grip writing tools instead of standard pen or pencil
> student or teacher tutors

Arrange for assistance as necessary for daily school activities (N.D. 2-4)

> —book carrying
> —opening food and beverage cartons
> —opening doors
> —toileting
> —getting on and off bus
> —carrying food tray
> —extra time for passing between class
> —transportation to/from school

Arrange for appropriate physical education activities and instruct physical education teachers in appropriate large motor expectations when leg or arm joints involved. (N.D. 1-4)

Refer for special education (P.L. 94-142) evaluation for occupational therapy, physical therapy, tutoring, learning aids, transportation, vocational counseling. (N.D. 1-4)

Provide access to physically handicapped bathrooms, entrances, elevators as appropriate. (N.D. 1-4)

Student Interventions

Monitor activity tolerance and observe for signs of inability to manage the demands of school activity. (N.D 1-4)

Monitor for complications of medication. (N.D 1)

Assist student with braces, splints as needed. (N.D. 2-4)

Monitor limbs with braces, splints for fit, rubbing, or circulation impairment.(N.D. 2-4)

Perform or assist student in performance of passive or active range of motion exercises. (N.D. 2-4)

Instruct student in pathophysiology of arthritis at level appropriate to age and developmental level. (N.D. 5)

Instruct student in medication actions and appropriate medication administration. (N.D. 5)

Monitor student medication compliance. (N.D. 5)

Provide opportunity for student to assist in planning and providing self-care. (N.D. 4, 5)

Expected Student Outcomes

Student will have pain managed during school attendance. (N.D 1)

Student will be involved in activities that do not enhance pain. (N.D 1)

Student will be permitted to perform activities to minimize pain during school day. (N.D. 1)

Student will be able to perform as many activities in the educational setting as possible. (N.D. 2-4)

Student will receive assistance for those activities which s/he requires assistance on a regular or intermittent basis, as the disease condition demands. (N.D. 2-4)

Student will be successful in managing mobility to and around school. (N.D. 2-4)

Student will be able to physically attend all classes. (N.D. 2-4)

Student will not be excessively fatigued or develop pain from the activities of school attendance. (N.D. 2-4)

Student will describe arthritis at level appropriate to age and development. (N.D. 5)

Student will describe medication actions and administration requirements. (N.D. 5)

REFERENCES

1. Hollister J. Rheumatic disease in childhood. *Pediatrician.* 1988;15: 65-72 (1988).
2. Simmons B, Nutting J. Juvenile rheumatoid arthritis. *Hand Clinics.* 1989; 5(2): 157-168.
3. Chaney J., Peterson L. Family variables and disease management in juvenile rheumatoid arthritis. *J Pediatr Psychology* 1989; 14 (3) 389-403.

BIBLIOGRAPHY

Ciaran M, Laxer R, Silverman E. Drug therapy for juvenile arthritis. *Compr Therapy* 1989; 14 (10): 48-59.

Gallo A. Family adaptation in childhood chronic illness: a case report. *J Pediatr Health Care* 1991;5(2): 78-85.

Larson G, ed. *Managing the School Age Child with a Chronic Health Condition.* Wayzata, MN: DCI Publishing, 1986 (distributed by Sunrise River Press, 11481 Kost Dam Road, North Branch, MN 55056, 612-583-3239).

Page G. Chronic pain and the child with juvenile rheumatoid arthritis. *J Pediatr Health Care* 1991; 5(1):18-23.

Rapoff M, Purviance M, Lindsley C. Educational and behavioral strategies for improving medication compliance in juvenile rheumatoid arthritis. *Arch Phys Med Rehab.* 1988; 69(6): 439-441.

Rennebohm R. Rheumatic diseases of childhood. *Pediatrics in Review.* 1988; 10(6): 183-190.

Ungerer J, Borgan B. Chaitow J, Champion GD. Psychosocial functioning in children and young adults with juvenile arthritis. *Pediatrics* 1988; 81(2): 195-202.

Varni J, Wilcox K, Hanson V. Mediating effects of family social support on child psychological adjustment in juvenile rheumatoid arthritis. *Health Psychology* 1988; 7(5): 421-431.

Whitehouse R, Shope J, Sullivan D, Chen-Lin K. Children with juvenile rheumatoid arthritis at school. *Clin Pediatrics* 1988; 28(11): 509-514.

Wong D, Whaley L. *Clinical Manual of Pediatric Nursing.* 2d ed. St. Louis: CV Mosby, 1990.

12 | IHP: Asthma

Cynthia K. Silkworth

INTRODUCTION

Asthma is a chronic health condition that affects 5 to 10 percent of the children in the United States. [1-3] Despite major therapeutic advances over the past ten years, pediatric asthma morbidity has not changed, and childhood mortality from asthma has increased in the United States.[4-6] Asthma is responsible for more hospital admissions, emergency room visits, and school absences than any other chronic disease of childhood. [2, 4] Asthma can be a serious and life-threatening condition. However, for most children, asthma can be well controlled.

Pathophysiology

Asthma is a chronic disease in which the airways (bronchioles) overreact to various stimuli or triggers. (Asthma is also called reactive airway disease for this reason.) During an asthma episode the airways become narrowed or blocked, making it difficult to breathe and causing coughing, wheezing and tightening of the chest.

The airways become narrowed or blocked in three different ways: 1) the muscles encircling the bronchioles tighten causing narrowing of the airway (bronchospasm); 2) the cells lining the bronchioles swell and narrow the airway even further; and 3) the cells lining the

bronchioles secrete mucus which can plug the already narrowed airways.

The most common triggers of asthma episodes are:

- Viral infections: upper respiratory infections such as the common cold, influenza, or sinus infection.
- Exercise: especially in cold weather.
- Allergens: most common allergens are pollen, dust mite, animal fur, or feathers.
- Environmental irritants: smoke, aerosol sprays, chalk dust, paint and varnish fumes, perfume, and air pollution.
- Emotions: if they lead to an outburst of laughing, crying, or yelling.

The same triggers do not necessarily cause episodes in all persons with asthma, and even the same person may not react every time he/she is exposed to the trigger.

Asthma Management

Asthma management usually consists of one or several interventions.[3]

- Medications—beta agonists (inhaled or oral bronchodilators), theophylline (oral bronchodilator), cromolyn, steroids, and anticholinergics.
- Immunotherapy or hyposensitization therapy—decreasing sensitization to allergens.

- Child and family education—asthma education program.
- Environmental modification—avoiding or minimizing exposure to some allergens or irritants.
- Counseling—assistance with coping, individual or family.

INDIVIDUALIZED HEALTHCARE PLAN

History

- when was the diagnosis made
- healthcare providers involved in the management of the student's asthma and regular health maintenance
- asthma management plan (past and current)—medications, immunotherapy, child and family education, environmental modifications, and/or counseling
- student's participation in the development and implementation of the asthma management plan
- compliance with asthma management plan
- effectiveness of asthma management plan—student's, parents'/guardian's, and healthcare provider's perspectives
- what the student and parents do if an asthma episode occurs at home
- involvement of support persons/systems
- experience with self-medication at home
- experience with severe asthma episodes that required an emergency room visit
- experience with asthma episodes at school
- previous school asthma management plans and their effectiveness
- past school attendance patterns, specifically the number of days missed each year due to asthma
- participation in regular classroom activities
- participation in regular physical education activities
- participation in a regular exercise program—sports or leisure, school-related or non-school-related

Assessment

- knowledge about asthma (student, parents/guardians, and teachers)
- knowledge about his/her asthma triggers
- knowledge about early warning signs of an asthma episode
- student's perception of his/her health and asthma
- parents' perception of the student's health and asthma
- student's locus of control—health, school, family, and activities of daily living
- ability to self-administer medication
- ability to do and use abdominal breathing exercises
- proper use of peak flow meter
- baseline peak flow rate
- self-care skills
- motivation to do self-care, self-medication
- barriers to self-care, self-medication
- decision-making skills

- ability to recognize early warning signs of an asthma episode
- environment—exposure to triggers

Nursing Diagnoses (N.D.)

N.D. 1 (Potential for) alteration in respiratory function. (NAN.D.A 1.5.1.3)*

N.D. 2 (Potential for) ineffective airway clearance. (NAN.D.A 1.5.1.2)

N.D. 3 (Potential for) alteration in breathing pattern/gas exchange (NAN.D.A 1.5.1.1) related to bronchospasm/inflammation of the airways/increased mucus production.

N.D. 4 (Potential for) alteration in activity tolerance related to asthma. (NAN.D.A 6.1.1.3)

N.D. 5 (Potential for) self-care deficit related to:
- knowledge deficit about asthma
- inability to correctly do self-care skills required
- poor decision-making skills
- non-participation in asthma management measures

N.D. 6 (Potential for) noncompliance (NAN.D.A 5.2.1.1) with prescribed medications related to:
- knowledge deficit
- improper administration of medication
- perceived ineffectiveness of medication
- denial of need for medication
- inability to access medication

N.D. 7 (Potential for) alteration in role performance (NAN.D.A 3.2.1) (student) related to absence from school/class due to asthma symptoms.

Goals

Attain and maintain near normal pulmonary function. (N.D. 1-3)

Prevention of asthma symptoms, such as chronic cough and difficulty breathing.(N.D. 1-3)

Prevention of recurrent asthma episodes. (N.D. 1-3)

Develop and implement asthma action plan addressing what to do if an asthma episode occurs. (N.D. 1-3)

Participation in regular school/class activities, including physical education class, with modifications made as necessary. (N.D. 4)

Increase knowledge about his/her asthma. (N.D. 1-7)

Development of asthma self-care skills. (N.D. 5)

Development of decision-making skills. (N.D. 5)

Participation in asthma management measures. (N.D. 5)

Compliance with prescribed asthma management plan. (N.D. 6)

Good school attendance pattern. (N.D. 7)

Good classroom attendance and participation. (N.D. 7)

*(See Chapter 2, page 38 for explanation of the NANDA approved numerical system.)

Nursing Interventions

Develop an asthma action plan. (N.D. 1-3)
- include student, parent/guardian, teachers, and healthcare providers in the development process
- coordinate and incorporate with asthma management plan at home and with healthcare providers
- list and describe management measures to follow if an asthma episode occurs
- special considerations for field trips
- set guidelines for seeking assistance—include when early warning signs appear, if medication was used in the past 1 to 3 hours and symptoms have not cleared or have redeveloped, and when and how to notify parents/guardians and healthcare providers, including phone numbers
- make modifications in the plan as needed

Obtain medication orders and authorization for any asthma medications needed at school (parent and healthcare provider). (N.D. 1-3)
- for regular management of asthma condition
- for asthma episodes
- for premedication prior to activities that may trigger asthma

Keep accurate records of asthma episodes. (N.D. 1-3)
- time of onset of symptoms
- time episode was reported to teacher/health office/other school personnel
- presenting symptoms—tightness in chest, cough, wheeze, shortness of breath, skin color, anxiety level, peak flow rate, breathing rate, heart rate
- medication—drug, dose and time administered
- effectiveness of medication
- other asthma management measures—belly breathing, fluids, rest
- who was notified and when they were notified

In-service teachers and other appropriate school staff. (N.D. 1-4, 7)
- what asthma is
- common triggers of an asthma episode and the individual student's known triggers
- symptoms of an asthma episode
- importance of recognizing early warning signs
- what to do if an episode occurs
- importance of prompt treatment
- medications that need to be taken during the school day and why these medications are necessary
- ways to minimize exposing students to common triggers in the classroom
- need for flexible educational programming (such as classroom and physical education adjustments, past and advance assignments, field trip modifications)

Assist physical education teachers to modify physical education requirements, if necessary, (e.g., walking the specified distance instead of running that distance will be given the same amount of credit toward their grade). (N.D. 1-4, 7)

Assist parents/guardians, teachers, and healthcare providers in understanding the student's need to participate in regular classroom activities and discuss: (N.D. 4,7)
- classroom modifications that may be needed
- premedicating prior to activities that may trigger an asthma episode

Assist parents/guardians to talk with their child's teachers about their child's asthma. (N.D. 1-4, 7)
- known triggers
- symptoms the child has when he/she is having problems with asthma
- asthma management plan—home and school
- how to manage an asthma episode
- school/classroom/field trip modifications (modification to environment or in activities which may need to be done to prevent triggering an asthma episode, e.g., no flowering plants, feathers, animals, paint fumes, etc.; staying inside on extremely cold days (below 10 degrees F), unless his/her mouth is covered with a scarf; no long distance running activities; etc.)

Provide information to parents about when it is appropriate and not appropriate to send their child to school, based on specific symptoms (see Supplement A). (N.D. 4,7)

Discuss the need for regular school and classroom attendance with the student, parents/guardians, and healthcare providers. (N.D. 4,7)

Assist the student to administer prescribed medications (dependent on the student's knowledge and skills).(N.D. 1-6)
- medications are easily accessible at all times
- self-medication program
- premedication, as prescribed, before classes or activities that expose the student to known triggers
- with the least amount of classroom disruption necessary

Monitor medication administration and reinforce proper technique as needed. (N.D. 1-6)

Discuss with the student: (N.D. 1-7)
- importance of participating in classroom and physical education activities
- activities that may be a trigger for him/her in the classroom or in physical education
- pre-medicating prior to activities that may trigger an asthma episode to occur
- signs and symptoms that indicate the student should stop the activity he/she is doing
- importance of telling his/her teacher(s) if signs and symptoms of an asthma episode are present
- what to do if an asthma episode occurs

Provide health education opportunities—individual or group instruction regarding: (N.D. 1-7)
- what asthma is
- identification of his/her asthma triggers
- early warning signs of an asthma episode
- what to do if an episode occurs
- identification of asthma medications and how they work
- proper technique for administering asthma medications (oral, metered dose inhaler, nebulizer)
- proper technique for abdominal breathing exercises
- proper use of a peak flow meter
- how to get help, if needed

Assist the student to identify motivators and barriers to participating in self-care. (N.D. 5)

Choose and implement motivators to participating in self-care. (N.D. 5)

Remove as many barriers to participating in self-care as possible. (N.D. 5)

Assist the student to develop self-care skills. (N.D. 5)
- demonstrate proper technique for administering asthma medications, require a repeat demonstration using placebo medications and his/her medications
- demonstrate proper abdominal breathing technique, require a repeat demonstration
- demonstrate proper use of a peak flow meter, require a repeat demonstration
- discuss how to recognize early warning signs of an asthma episode and what to do if any of those signs occur
- monitor self-care skills—reinforce with practice of skills, as needed, and acknowledge demonstration of good self-care skills

Assist the student to develop appropriate decision-making skills. (N.D. 5)

Assist the student to participate in his/her asthma management measures. (N.D. 5, 6)
- allow the student to have control over designated measures or parts of the measures (dependent on knowledge, self-care, and decision-making skills
- increase the amount of participation and control the student has, dependent on an increase in knowledge and skills
- monitor student, parent/guardian, and teacher perceptions and responses to student participation in the asthma management measures
- make modifications in the asthma management measures as needed, in consultation with the student, parents/guardians, teachers and healthcare provider

Discuss with the student: (N.D. 6)
- need to take medications as prescribed, (on time, at designated intervals, in proper dose, using the proper method)
- importance of his/her participation in medication administration
- benefits of compliance
- consequences of noncompliance
- motivators and barriers to compliance

Assist the student to choose and implement motivators to compliance. (N.D. 6)

Remove as many barriers to compliance, as possible. (N.D. 6)

Monitor student's medication compliance. (N.D. 6)

Monitor classroom and physical education activity tolerance. (N.D. 1-7)

Assist the teacher to adjust activity participation based on activity tolerance and endurance. (N.D. 7)

Monitor attendance patterns and reasons for absences. (N.D. 7)

Monitor academic performance—referral to child study team as needed. (N.D. 7)

Expected Student Outcomes

The student will:
- participate in regular classroom activities, with modifications made when necessary. (N.D. 1-7)
- participate in regular physical education activities, with modifications made when necessary. (N.D. 1-7)

- define what asthma is (at a developmentally appropriate level). (N.D. 1-7)
- identify his/her asthma triggers. (N.D. 1-7)
- premedicate prior to activities that may trigger an asthma episode (as prescribed). (N.D. 1-7)
- list the early warning signs of an asthma episode. (N.D. 1-5)
- recognize early warning signs of an asthma episode and stop his/her activity. (N.D. 1-5)
- describe what to do if an asthma episode occurs. (N.D. 1-5)
- inform his/her teacher (and/or other school personnel) when he/she is having an asthma episode. (N.D. 1-5)
- initiate and follow his/her prescribed asthma action plan. (N.D. 1-6)
- name the medications he/she uses for management of his/her asthma. (N.D. 5,6)
- state why he/she needs to take the medications. (N.D. 5,6)
- describe how his/her asthma medications work. (N.D. 5,6)
- demonstrate proper administration of his/her medication as prescribed (dose, interval, time, and technique). (N.D. 1-6)
- demonstrate proper use of a peak flow meter. (N.D. 1-5)
- read and state his/her peak flow rate accurately. (N.D. 5)
- describe how he/she participates in his/her asthma management. (N.D. 5)
- participate in his/her asthma management measures (dependent on demonstrated knowledge and skills). (N.D. 5)
- describe the benefits of taking medications as prescribed. (N.D. 6)
- describe the consequences of not taking medications as prescribed. (N.D. 6)
- list motivators and barriers to compliance with taking asthma medications. (N.D. 6)
- demonstrate compliance with his/her asthma management plan (maintenance and emergency). (N.D. 6)
- have a good school attendance pattern (absent less than ten days per year). (N.D. 7)
- have a good classroom attendance pattern. (N.D. 7)
- have (minimal) disruptions in his/her educational program due to asthma. (N.D. 7)

REFERENCES

1. Evans R, Mallally DI, Wilson RW, Gergen PJ, Rosenberg HM, Grauman JS, Chevarley FM, Feinleib M. National trends in morbidity and mortality of asthma in the US prevelance, hospitalization, and death from asthma over two decades: 1965-1984. *Chest* 1987; 91:65S-74S.
2. Plaut T. *Children with Asthma: A Manual for Parents*. Amherst, MA: Pedipress, Inc., 1988.
3. Traver GA. Martinez M. Asthma update. Part I: Mechanisms, pathology and diagnosis. *J Pediatr Health Care*. 1988; 2(5):221-226; Asthma update. Part II: Treatment. *J Pediatr Health Care*. 1988; 2(5):227-233.
4. Hen J. An overview of pediatric asthma. *Pediatric Annals* 1986; 15(2):92-96.
5. Stempel DA, Mellon M. Management of acute severe asthma. *Pediatr Clin North Am*. 1984; 31:879-891.
6. Woolcock AJ. Worldwide differences in asthma prevalence and mortality, why is asthma mortality so low in the USA. *Chest* 1986; 90:40S-45S.

BIBLIOGRAPHY

American Lung Association. *Asthma: A Matter of Control*. New York American Lung Association, 1990.

American Lung Association. *The Efficacy of Asthma Education: Selected Abstracts*. New York: American Lung Association 1989.

Blue CL. Exercise-induced asthma: the silent asthma. *J Pediatric Health Care* 1988; 2(4):167-174.

Cropp GJ. Special features of asthma in children. *Chest* 1985; 87(1):55S-62S.

Freudenberg N, Feldman CH, Clark NM, Millman EJ, Valle I, Wasilewski Y. The impact of bronchial asthma on school attendance and performance. *J School Health* 1987; 50(9):522-526.

Garcia MK. Asthma: old problems and new strategies. *School Nurse* 1989; (Oct): 25-36.

Leffert F. Asthma. In: Hobbs N, Perrin J, eds. *Issues in the care of children with chronic illness*. San Francisco: Josey-Bass Publishers, 1985.

Mendoza G, Garcia MK, Collins MA. *Asthma in the School: Improving Control with Peak Flow Monitoring*. California: HealthScan, 1989.

Minnesota Department of Health. *Guidelines of Care for Children with Special Health Care Needs: Asthma*. Minneapolis, MN: Minnesota Dept of Health, Services for Children with Handicaps, 1991.

National Asthma Education Program. *Guidelines for the Diagnoses and Management of Asthma*.Bethesda, MD: National Institutes of Health, August 1991. (NIH publication No. 91-3042).

National Asthma Education Program. *Managing Asthma: A Guide for Schools*. Rockville, MD: US Dept of Health and Human Services and Dept of Education, September 1991 (NIH publication No. 91-2650).

SUPPLEMENT A.

School Attendance

Asthma and School Attendance: Checklist For Deciding About School Attendance

Clues for Sending Child to School:

1. Stuffy nose but no wheezing.

2. Mild wheezing which clears after medicine.

3. Good exercise tolerance (able to participate in usual daily activities).

4. No extra effort needed with breathing pattern.

Clues for Keeping Child at Home:

1. Evidence of infection-red/sore throat, or swollen glands.

2. Fever over 100 degrees (hot and flushed).

3. Wheezing which continues to increase one hour after medicine is taken.

4. Child is too weak or tired to take part in routine daily activities.

5. Breathing pattern is labored, irregular, rapid (more than 25 breaths per minute at rest).

Each child is different and follows his/her own special pattern during an asthma episode. Therefore, it is best to observe your child closely and learn his/her particular body signs which serve as a guide to his/her state of health.

SUPPLEMENT B.

MEDICATION PROCEDURE THAT ALLOWS SELF-MEDICATION—*SAMPLE*

Medication Procedure

The purpose of administering medications in school is to assist students who require medication during school hours to maintain an optimal state of health and, therefore, enhance their educational program.

The intent of this procedure is to assure safe administration of medications in school for those students who require them. This procedure applies to both prescription and over-the-counter medications.

Long-Term Medications: Prescribed for more than two weeks.

1. A written statement shall be required *annually*.

   a. From the physician, who will indicate the name of the medication, the route, the dosage, frequency and time of administration, the reason the medication needs to be given (diagnosis), possible side effects, and termination date.

   b. From the parent, who will request and authorize the school to give the medication in the dosage prescribed by the physician.

2. Parents/guardians are required to supply the medication in the original container labeled by the pharmacy or physician. The container will be labeled with the student's name, name of medication, dose to be given, frequency and time it is to be given, the name of the prescribing physician, and the date the medication was obtained.

Short-Term Medications: Over-the-counter or prescribed for less than two weeks.

1. A written statement will be required from the parent/guardian giving permission to give the medication in school. The statement must include: the name of the medication, the reason for the medication, the route, the dosage, and the time and date the medication is to be given.

2. Parents/guardians are required to supply the medication in the original container labeled by the pharmacy or physician. The container will be labeled with the student's name, name of the medication, dose to be given, frequency and time it is to be given, the name of the prescribing physician, and the date the medication was obtained.

Supervision

Medication will be given by or under the direction of the school nurse (during school hours).

Storage of Medication

Medications will be stored in a locked drawer or cabinet.
Medications requiring refrigeration will be refrigerated in a secure area.
(Exceptions as listed in *Self-Administration of Medications*.)

Self-Administration of Medications

The objective of some medication programs includes facilitating self-responsibility for medication. Prior to any self-medication program, the student needs to be knowledgeable about his/her specific health condition and the medications used to manage his/her condition.

After health counseling with his/her physician and the school nurse, self-administration of medication may be considered as an option.

If the student can demonstrate proper administration of the medication *and* if the student, his/her parent/guardian, physician, and school nurse agree it is appropriate for the student to self-administer the medication, the student will be allowed to carry and self-administer medication.

Record of Administration of Medications

Each dose of medication will be documented on the medication record. Documentation will include: the name of the student, name of the medication, dosage, date, time, route, and the initials of the person administering the medication or monitoring the student self-administering their medication.

Unauthorized Use of Medication

Students observed by school personnel self-administering unauthorized medications will be reported to their parents/guardian and the school administrator.

SUPPLEMENT C.
MEDICATION AUTHORIZATION FORM—*SAMPLE FORM*

Medication Authorization Form

School Year _____

School _____

Physician's Order

Name of Child: _____

Name of Medication: _____

     Dosage: _____

     Time/Frequency:_____

Reason for Medication: _____

Possible Side Effects: _____

Estimated Termination Date: _____

(All authorizations expire at the end of the school year.)

☐   Child is knowledgeable about this medication and how to administer it.

☐   Child may self-administer medication.

Date _____

Physician's
Signature _____

Address _____

_____

Telephone Number _____

- -

I request this medication be given to my child _____
_____as prescribed by my child's physician.

☐   My child may self-administer his/her medication.

Date _____ Signature _____
                                  Parent/Guardian

SUPPLEMENT D. *SAMPLE* PARENT QUESTIONNAIRE

Questionnaire for Parents of Child with Asthma

PARENT INTERVIEW

Student's Name _____ School Year _____

School _____ Grade _____ Teacher _____

Parent's Name(s) _____ Telephone (home) _____ (work) _____

Name of Child's Doctor (for asthma) _____ Telephone _____

The following information is helpful to your child's school nurse and school staff in determining any special needs for your child. Please answer the questions to the best of your ability. If you desire a conference with the school nurse, please call for an appointment.

Nurse's Name _____ Telephone Number _____

1. How long has your child had asthma? _____

2. Please rate the severity of his/her asthma. (circle)

   (Not Severe)   0   1   2   3   4   5   6   7   8   9   10   (Severe)

3. How many days would you estimate he/she missed school last year due to asthma? _____

4. What triggers your child's asthma attacks? (Please check any that apply.)

   ____ Illness   ____ Emotions   ____ Medications   ____ Foods
   ____ Weather   ____ Exercise   ____ Cigarette or   ____ Chemical odors
                                                  other smoke   ____ Fatigue

   Allergies (please list) _____

   Other (please list) _____

5. What does your child do at home to relieve wheezing during an asthma attack? (Please check any that apply.)

   ____ Breathing exercises   Takes medication: ____ Inhaler
   ____ Rest/relaxation   ____ Nebulizer
   ____ Drinks liquids   ____ Oral medication

               Other (please describe) _____

6. Please list the medications your child takes for asthma (everyday and as needed).

	Name of Medication	Dose	Frequency
(In School)			
(At Home)			

If medications are to be given during school, a medication permission slip needs to be filled out yearly. Medications must be in the original labeled container. (When you get prescriptions filled you can ask the pharmacist to put them into two containers so you'll have one for school and one for home use.)

7. If your child does not respond to medication, what action do you advise school personnel to take?_____

_____

8. What, if any, side effects does your child have from his/her medications?

_____

9. Has your child been taught how to use an extension tube, pulmonary aid, inspirease kit or other device with his/her inhaler?   Yes   No

10. How many times has your child been hospitalized overnight or longer for asthma in the past year?

_____

11. How many times has your child been treated in the emergency room for asthma in the past year? _____

12. How often does your child see his/her doctor for routine asthma evaluations?

_____

13. Does your child need any special considerations related to his/her asthma while at school? (Check any that apply and describe briefly.)

    Modified gym class _____

    Modified recess outside _____

    No animal pets in classroom _____

    Avoiding certain foods _____

    Emotional or behavior concerns _____

    Special consideration while on field trips _____

    Special transportation to and from school _____

    Observation for side effects from medication _____

    Other _____

14. Do you know what your child's baseline peak flow rate is?

    Yes   No   Rate _____

15. Do you think your child holds him/herself back from participating in all activities at school because of his/her asthma? If so, please describe.

_____

16. Have you ever attended an asthma education class?   Yes   No

    Has your child had asthma education?   Yes   No

**Thank you for your time and assistance in assessing
your child's special needs in school.**

SUPPLEMENT E. *SAMPLE* STUDENT INTERVIEW

ASSESSING THE STUDENT'S KNOWLEDGE OF AND RESPONSIBILITY FOR CONTROL OF HIS/HER ASTHMA

STUDENT INTERVIEW

Student's Name _____ Grade _____

School _____ Classroom _____

SUBJECTIVE ASSESSMENT

1. What medications do you take? Name, dose, how often and what does it do?

    _____

    _____

    ☐ Knows well   ☐ Knows some   ☐ Knows nothing

2. Who is responsible for your medications at home? (Do you remember on your own or does someone need to remind you or actually give it to you?)

    _____

    _____

    ☐ Totally self-responsible   ☐ Needs reminding   ☐ Not responsible

3. How do you feel when your asthma is acting up? (Include symptoms just before and during an episode.) _____

    _____

4. What are your triggers—things that make you wheeze? (List)

    _____

    _____

5. What, besides taking medication, do you do to help control your asthma?

    _____

    _____

6. What do you think is happening inside your lungs during a wheezing episode?

    _____

    _____

    ☐ Understands physiology well   ☐ Understands physiology some
    ☐ Doesn't understand physiology

7. Can you demonstrate breathing exercises?   ☐ Yes   ☐ No

8. What, if any, special problems do you have in school that are related to your asthma? (phy-ed, recess, foods, teasing, other)

_____

_____

OBJECTIVE PHYSICAL ASSESSMENT

1. Observation of normal lung sounds. (Comments)

_____

_____

2. Ability to do breathing exercises. (Comments)

_____

_____

3. Peak flow reading (not during bronchospasm).

_____

_____

4. Metered dose inhaler, rotahaler, nebulization technique.

_____

_____

5. Other

_____

_____

ASSESSMENT

List out the problems in order of priority (i.e., increased absenteeism), the special needs in school setting, the severity of child's asthma, how responsible the child is in self-care for his/her asthma, etc. This assessment should include all information from parent questionnaire, student interview and physical assessment.

PLAN

The plan should address the items under assessment.

13 | IHP: Attention Deficit Hyperactivity Disorder

Susan I. Simandl Will

INTRODUCTION

Attention-Deficit Hyperactivity Disorder (ADHD) is a medical diagnosis (DSM-III-R) which includes attention deficit and hyperactive behavior as well as attention deficit without hyperactive behavior. The disorder is believed to affect 2 to 4 percent of the school-age population.[1]

The DSM-III-R lists fourteen behaviors characteristic of inattention or impulsivity. These include the inability to orient, organize, or focus; excessive talking; fidgeting; distractability; and non-goal-directed activity. Typically eight of the fourteen behaviors should be documented prior to establishing a medical diagnosis of ADHD.

Children with ADHD can have significant difficulty in the learning environment. They can have problems following directions, demonstrate inconsistent performance, skill deficiencies and underachievement, as well as have difficulty with active and passive language processing. In addition, the features of hyperactivity cause them to be very noticeable in the classroom, frequently interjecting with interruptive and disruptive behavior. These symptoms can persist, complicating academic success, contributing to low self-esteem, delinquent behavior, and poor social development. In adolescence the hyperactive behavior may recede but the inattentive and cognitive disturbances can remain. Current belief is that children with attention deficit disorder can remain disordered in adolescence and adulthood, continuing to show disorganization, impulsivity, mood swings, emotional instability, or antisocial behavior.[2]

Pathophysiology

The etiology of ADHD is unknown. The most accepted theory is that of organic disturbances in brain neurotransmitter function.[3] Allergies can be a contributing or exacerbating factor for some children,[3] and, at least, for some children, there is a probable inherited factor active in the development of ADHD symptoms.[4] Most recently the study by Zametkin and associates[4] demonstrated that adults with ADHD display a significant decrease in cerebral glucose metabolism. These findings raise thoughts of impaired cerebral glucose metabolism as an etiologic or at least contributing factor to ADHD development.

The assessment for ADHD is best done by a multiprofessional team of at least a pediatrician, neurologist, social worker, and school nurse. Chemical use/abuse should be ruled out as well as learning disabilities or sensory input acuity deficiencies. Other physiological or emotional disorders should also be ruled out.

Treatment of ADHD remains varied and controversial. Some children are helped with medications, including methylphenidate (Ritalin), dextroamphetamine (Dexedrine), pemoline (Cylert), and/or antidepressants (imipramine hydrochloride). Although the pharmacological management of ADHD remains controversial, and the results are highly variable from child to child, medication is not an uncommon management approach. Medication effectiveness should be monitored with a standardized ADHD assessment tool such as the "ACTeRS Rating Form and ACTeRS Profile Form" (see Supplement to this chapter) on a regular basis in the school. Most children do not continue the medication when school is not in session. Most medications used for ADHD are controlled substances and require proper protocol for safe administration and locked storage.

A multimodal treatment approach is often successfully implemented, and can include counseling, support group sessions, and training in impulse control techniques, biofeedback, relaxation techniques, as well as medication. The school nurse needs to be active in the planning and management of the treatment for children with ADHD.

INDIVIDUALIZED HEALTHCARE PLAN

Assessment

History

- Review of academic or cumulative school record for patterns of academic performance
- Review any previous special education assessment or interventions
- Any history of previous or current illness?
- Any history of previous injury?
- Infancy and early childhood reports of attention or hyperactivity issues
- History from family:

    Significant recent life changes: move, death, financial issues, physical illness, mental illness, social or job issues
    Any other family members with attention or behavior problems?
    Does child display attention deficit or hyperactivity at home?
    Methods family has used to manage attention deficit or hyperactivity issues: Behavior management style, counseling, medication, diet, other
    Which have been successful? Which unsuccessful?

Current Status

- Standardized assessment tool such as the "ACTeRS rating form" and ACTeRS profile form." (See Supplement)
- Learning disability assessment by special education team
- Psychological assessment by special education team
- Passive and receptive language processing assessment by special education team.

- Interview teacher(s).
- Vision and hearing assessment.
- Student's self-description.
- Student's comparison to peers, in behavior and performance.
- Student's perception of family's feelings toward him/her.
- Chemical use/abuse.
- Physical exam to rule out other physiological problems.

Nursing Diagnoses (N.D.)

N.D. 1 Impaired thought processes (NANDA 8.3)* related to:
- inability to consistently conceptually process input
- learning disability
- shortened attention span
- decreased ability to exert mental effort
- decreased ability to selectively focus, concentrate

N.D. 2 Self-esteem alteration (NANDA 7.1.2) due to:
- behaviors: impulsivity, aggressiveness, inability to self-control
- inadequate peer relationships or preference for delinquent/abusing peer groups
- internalization of negative feedback from parents, teachers, other authority figures
- school failure or academic delays
- self-perception that s/he is more tense, restless than peers
- stigma of feeling "different" or singled out

N.D. 3 Ineffective coping skills (NANDA 5.1.1.1) related to:
- decreased ability to plan
- decreased ability to self-limit behaviors (self-control)
- decreased ability to anticipate consequences of actions
- decreased ability to generate several options of possible response to a stimulus
- increased risk-taking behavior: ethical, legal, sexual, chemical
- depressive or suicidal feelings

N.D. 4 Sensory-perception alteration (NANDA 7.2) related to:
- decreased visual or auditory acuity
- decreased ability to sort for relevant data
- decreased ability to focus on the appropriate data
- decreased ability to control sensory input
- decreased ability to choose which sensory data to consider relevant (filter for relevance)
- decreased rate of processing of sensory inputs
- incomplete processing of sensory inputs
- alteration in visual or verbal memory processing

---

*(See Chapter 2, page 38 for explanation of the NANDA approved numerical system).

Goals

Student will demonstrate ability to utilize intellectual capacities (thinking, focusing, concentrating) to the best of his/her ability. (N.D. 1)

Student will demonstrate increased acceptance of self and experience fewer negative encounters in school environment as measured by teacher comments, number of dismissals/suspensions from class and/or school. (N.D. 2)

Student will begin or progress in demonstrating more successful social and emotional coping patterns. (N.D. 3)

Student will demonstrate ability to use (or improve use of) appropriate sensory input. (N.D. 4)

Nursing Interventions

Teacher/School Interventions

Refer to special education team for assessment if not already involved. (N.D. 1-4)

Provide suggestions to classroom teacher: consistent structure, minimize distractions, provide separate study area, provide clear tasks and be willing to repeat instructions, suggestions to redirect student. (N.D. 1)

Obtain medical orders for medication (if used) and establish dispensing protocol in accordance with district policy and appropriate to proper management of controlled substance. (N.D. __)

Establish medication (if prescribed) protocol, as appropriate for this student, which encourages self-care. (N.D. 1-3)

Provide medical care provider with regular school evaluation data. (N.D. 1-4)

Assist faculty in establishing clear, consistent, reviewed consequences for inappropriate behaviors. (N.D. 3)

Student/Family Interventions

Encourage student to express feelings s/he has related to school: isolated, singled out, picked on, incapable, too difficult, no fun, and so on. (N.D. 2, 3)

Determine if student experiences secondary gain from behaviors. (N.D. 2, 3)

Teach or refer for impulse control techniques such as visual imagery, building a bank of options for typically difficult situations, self-talk techniques. (N.D. 2, 3)

Refer to group of students with similar issues. (N.D. 2, 3)

Suggest teachers notice and comment on appropriate behaviors. (N.D. 2, 3)

Provide support and encouragement to student (N.D. 2, 3)

Develop trusting, communicative relationship with child. (N.D. 2, 3)

Assist student in identifying resource people in school (nurse, counselor, social worker, other) who can respond with empathy and appropriate interventions when student is in behavior crisis at school. (N.D. 2, 3)

Provide opportunities for student to identify and verbalize or share feelings of frustration, anger, hostility or depression. (N.D. 2, 3)

Refer for ophthalmologic or audiologic evaluation if acuity decreased on screening results. (N.D. 4)

Establish regular communication method with parent(s) to facilitate information on medication protocol, progress in academic, social and emotional areas. (ND ___)

Refer family to appropriate resource for counseling, if indicated. (ND ____)

Expected Student Outcomes

The student and family will follow through on medical management of ADHD, including medication if prescribed. (N.D. 1)

The student will attend to learning tasks lasting ____minutes. (N.D. 1)

The student will have increased optimum situations to utilize his/her concentrating capacities with decreased surrounding distractions. (N.D. 1)

The student will receive assistance from special education teachers for learning disability if appropriate to assessment. (N.D. 1)

Student will take medication (if prescribed) with ___% reliability. (N.D. 1)

The student will (begin, progress in) demonstrating adaptation to having ADHD by: (N.D. 2, 3)

- acknowledging that s/he must use some additional techniques to maintain behavior control.
- verbalizing positive feelings about self.
- identifying several individual strengths
- describing goal(s) for current academic year and strategy(ies) to help achieve them
- being able to review a behaviorially inappropriate encounter and suggest other options for self-management.

Student will (begin, progress in) ability to articulate alternative behavior options. (N.D. 2, 3)

Student will (begin, progress in) ability to select behavior responses to stimuli. (N.D. 2, 3)

Student will decrease risk-taking behavior (ethical, legal, sexual, chemical). (N.D. 2, 3)

Student will articulate feelings. (N.D. 2, 3)

Student will identify resources in school for times when frustrations or feelings are overwhelming. (N.D. 2, 3)

Student will acquire and wear glasses if required. (N.D. 4)

Student will pursue treatment for physiologic hearing conditions if indicated. (N.D. 4)

Student will demonstrate improved ability to focus and process appropriate data as reported by teacher. (N.D. 4)

Student will demonstrate improved ability to choose relevant sensory data as reported by teacher. (N.D. 4)

REFERENCES

1. Barkley RA. *Hyperactive Children: A Handbook for Diagnosis and Treatment.* New York: Guiford Press, 1981.
2. Thorley G. Adolescent outcome for hyperactive children. *Arch Dis Childhood* 1988; 63:1181.
3. Marshall P. Attention deficit disorder and allergy: a neurochemical model of the relation between the illnesses. *Psychological Bulletin* 1989; 106(3): 434-446.
4. Zametkin A, et al. Cerebral glucose metabolism in adults with hyperactivity of childhood onset. *N Engl J Med* 1990; 323(20): 1361-1366.

BIBLIOGRAPHY

Connors CK. A teacher rating scale for use in drug studies with children. *Am J Psychiatry* 1969; 126 (6): 884-888.

Demma CM. School nursing management of attention deficit disorder. *School Nurse* 1989; (Oct): 8-16.

Herrly L. *Roles and Practices of Minnesota Elementary School Nurses in the Identification and Management of Children with Attention Deficit Hyperactivity Disorder, thesis.* University of Minnesota School of Public Health, Maternal and Child Health, 1989.

Levine MD. Attention and memory: progression and variation during the elementary school years. *Pediatric Annals* 1989; 18(6): 366-8, 370-2.

Levine MD, McCarthy ER. *Early Adolescent Transitions.* Lexington, MA: Lexington Books, 1988.

Myers DA, Claman L, Oldham DG, Waller DA, Crumley FE, Hebeler JR, Pearson GT, Shadid LG. The hyperactive child: an update. *Texas Med* 1989; 85 (3): 25-31.

Munoz-Millan R, Casteel CR. Attention-deficit hyperactivity disorder: recent literature. *Hosp Community Psychiatry* 1989; 40(7): 699-707.

National Association of School Nurses. *Guidelines for Identification and Program Management for Students with Attention Deficit Hyperactivity Disorder.* Scarborough, ME: National Association of School Nurses.

Norbert R, Barr MA. Diagnosing attention-deficit hyperactivity disorder and learning disabilities with chemically dependent adolescents. *J Psychoactive Drugs* 1989; 21(2): 203-15.

Stephenson PS. The hyperkinetic child: some misleading assumptions. *Can Med Assoc J*, 1975; 113(8): 764, 767-9.

Ullmann RK, Sleator EK, Sprague RL. *ADD-H Comprehensive Teacher's Rating Scale.* Champaign, IL: MetriTech, 1991 (MetriTech, Inc., 111 N. Market St., Champaign, IL 61820, 217-398-4868).

SUPPLEMENT A

2nd Edition

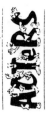

Rina K. Ullmann, M.Ed.
Esther K. Sleator, M.D.
Robert L. Sprague, Ph.D.

Below are descriptions of behavior. Please read each item and compare the child's behavior with that of his or her classmates. Circle the number that most closely corresponds with your evaluation. Transfer the total raw score for each of the four sections to the profile sheet to determine normative percentile scores.

Child's Name: CHRIS STUDENT
Rater: MRS ANDERSON
ID #: 71245
Date: 5/1/92

ATTENTION

	Almost Never				Almost Always
1. Works well independently	1	②	3	4	5
2. Persists with task for reasonable amount of time	①	2	3	4	5
3. Completes assigned task satisfactorily with little additional assistance	1	②	3	4	5
4. Follows simple directions accurately	1	2	③	4	5
5. Follows a sequence of instructions	1	②	3	4	5
6. Functions well in the classroom	1	②	3	4	5

ADD ITEMS 1-6 AND PLACE TOTAL HERE 12

HYPERACTIVITY

	Almost Never				Almost Always
7. Extremely overactive (out of seat, "on the go")	1	2	3	④	5
8. Overreacts	1	②	3	4	5
9. Fidgety (hands always busy)	1	2	③	4	5
10. Impulsive (acts or talks without thinking)	1	②	3	4	5
11. Restless (squirms in seat)	1	2	3	④	5

ADD ITEMS 7-11 AND PLACE TOTAL HERE 15

SOCIAL SKILLS

	Almost Never				Almost Always
12. Behaves positively with peers/classmates	1	2	③	4	5
13. Verbal communication clear and "connected"	1	2	3	④	5
14. Nonverbal communication accurate	1	2	3	④	5
15. Follows group norms and social rules	1	②	3	4	5
16. Cites general rule when criticizing ("We aren't supposed to do that")	1	2	3	④	5
17. Skillful at making new friends	1	②	3	4	5
18. Approaches situations confidently	1	2	3	4	⑤

ADD ITEMS 12-18 AND PLACE TOTAL HERE 24

OPPOSITIONAL

	Almost Never				Almost Always
19. Tries to get others into trouble	1	②	3	4	5
20. Starts fights over nothing	①	2	3	4	5
21. Makes malicious fun of people	1	②	3	4	5
22. Defies authority	1	②	3	4	5
23. Picks on others	1	②	3	4	5
24. Mean and cruel to other children	1	②	3	4	5

ADD ITEMS 19-24 AND PLACE TOTAL HERE 11

MetriTech, Inc.

ACTeRS Rating Form and ACTeRS Profile Form are copyright © 1986, 1988, 1991 by MetriTech, Inc., 111 North Market Street, Champaign, IL. (217) 398-4868. Reproduced by permission of the copyright holder.

SUPPLEMENT B

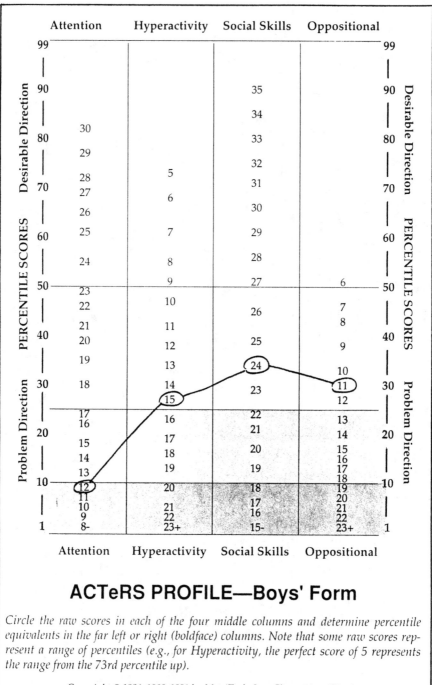

ACTeRS PROFILE—Boys' Form

Circle the raw scores in each of the four middle columns and determine percentile equivalents in the far left or right (boldface) columns. Note that some raw scores represent a range of percentiles (e.g., for Hyperactivity, the perfect score of 5 represents the range from the 73rd percentile up).

Copyright © 1986, 1988, 1991 by MetriTech, Inc., Champaign, Illinois

14 | IHP: Brain Injury, Acquired Traumatic

Mary J. Villars Gerber

INTRODUCTION

Acquired brain injuries are those occurring after birth. They should be differentiated from congenital brain injuries that produce other types of impairments and resultant intervention and treatment.

According to the National Head Injury Foundation,[1] causes of acquired brain injury include:

1. Traumas from accidents, falls, assaults, and surgical procedures.
2. Infections such as meningitis or encephalitis.
3. Stroke and other vascular accidents.
4. Anoxic injuries resulting from anesthetic accidents, hanging, choking, near drowning and severe blood loss.
5. Tumors of the brain.
6. Metabolic disorders such as insulin shock, liver and kidney disease.
7. Toxic products taken into the body through inhalation or ingestion.

Traumatic brain injuries are the most common form of acquired brain injury in young adults. Those who have suffered serious traumatic brain injuries rarely achieve preinjury levels of functioning.

A wide range of deficits have been noted following traumatic brain injuries and are seen in the following areas: psychomotor, sensory/perceptual, cognitive, psychosocial, and communication. The nature of the impairment depends on the location and severity of the injury, in addition to the individual's preinjury functioning. Brain injuries can result in a varied and complex range of deficits that require assessment and services offered by a wide range of professionals.

Impairments of motor function result in limitations in locomotion or motor functioning and/or physiological dysfunction of a body part or system. These include paralysis or weakness of one side of the body or both, muscle spasticity, muscle coordination, involuntary movement disorders, and problems sequencing goal-directed motor acts (apraxias).

Sensory impairments include deficits with smell and taste, as well as visual and auditory problems. Vision problems may include damage to the eye itself, the optic nerve, the nuclei and related cranial nerves which control eye muscles, and primary and secondary visual areas of the brain. Loss of vision may be complete or partial, affecting all or part of one visual field. Visual pathways may be intact but interpretation of visual information may be altered and responded to as though it were complete. Double vision and disturbed visual tracking may result from injury to the nerve supply of the muscles.

Partial hearing loss is frequently seen. It is most commonly sensorineural and the highest frequency ranges are most affected. Conductive losses occur as a result of damage to the structure of the ear. Dizziness and ataxia are caused by brain injury to areas controlling balance and orientation in space. Routine testing of smell, vision, hearing, and vestibular function should be conducted in all cases of traumatic brain injury.

Impairments caused by brain injury are usually nonprogressive, but in some cases may occur months or years after the injury. Epilepsy is the most common delayed complication, and has been reported up to ten years following injury.

Hydrocephalus, a dilation of the ventricles of the brain, may occur with or without increased intracranial pressure. Symptoms may include gait disturbances, urinary incontinence, and progressive intellectual deterioration. A surgical procedure to place a shunt may be necessary.

Other long-term consequences of brain injury are side effects produced by medications used to control physical and behavioral manifestations. Drugs used to control impulsive and/or aggressive behavior, muscle spasticity, and seizures depress cognitive functioning. Major tranquilizers may cause tardive dyskinesia.

Cognitive impairments may include loss of memory, attention, concentration, judgement, and problem-solving abilities; mental flexibility; organizational thinking skills; spatial orientation; and information retention.

Psychosocial impairments include behaviors that may interfere with interpersonal relationships and coping behaviors. These difficulties may be organic in origin or a natural response to the injury. Some of these difficulties include withdrawal or depression, frustration, irritability, restlessness, impulsiveness, lability of mood, poor social judgement, disinhibition, fatigue, and apathy. Goal setting, planning, and working toward a goal may also be difficult.

Communication functions that may be affected include speaking; writing; listening; comprehension of written or spoken material, especially in stressful situations; interrupting; and speaking loudly or rudely.

The school nurse will be a team member involved in assisting the student to reintegrate into the school setting. Other members will include special education teacher, classroom teachers, parents, healthcare personnel, school counselor, school psychologist, speech and language clinician, occupational therapist, physical therapist, vocational rehabilitation counselor, neuropsychologist, and neuroeducators.

INDIVIDUALIZED HEALTHCARE PLAN

History

What was the student's preinjury level of functioning?
What is the nature of the injury and medical diagnosis?

Assessment

Because the concerns and individual needs of each student are so complex following an acquired brain injury, a great number of professionals will be involved in assessment and service provision for the student. Those areas identified for nursing assessment may be somewhat limited due to the complexity of the assessment required. It will be essential to identify a case manager to coordinate services. Service needs must be addressed in conjunction with each other. This is a role that the school nurse may also assume.

- Review of healthcare records. It will be necessary for the school nurse to gather medical and other healthcare records for review by the educational team.

- Safety. Observe student for ability to function safely in the school environments where they will be present.

- Vision. Assess for vision loss in all or part of a visual field. Observe for double vision. Observe for tracking ability.

- Hearing. Screen for hearing acuity. Both sensorineural and conductive losses are seen.

- Seizures. If seizures occur as a result of brain injury, a full assessment will need to be conducted. (See also Chapter 41—Seizures.)

- Hydrocephalus. If the student has developed hydrocephalus and a shunt has been placed, a full assessment will need to be conducted. (See also Chapter 46—Ventriculo-Peritoneal Shunts.)

- Medications. Identify current medications taken, actions, current and potential side effects.

- Self-care. Abilities in the area may be affected due to cognitive, sensory-perceptual, and motor involvement.

- Family's understanding of the needs their child may have, and their ability to provide the care and support needed. Assessment of family processes: family members' response to condition, behavior toward student, family communication and roles, access and use of healthcare, use of community resources. Family functioning and support for the child will influence student's adjustment at home/school.

Nursing Diagnoses (N.D.)

N.D. 1   Potential for injury (NANDA 1.6.1)* related to inability to control movements, neuromuscular impairment, perceptual and cognitive impairment. (Specify)

N.D. 2   Potential for injury (NANDA 1.6.1) related to visual impairment.

N.D. 3   Sensory perceptual alteration: visual. (NANDA 7.2)

N.D. 4   Potential for injury (NANDA 1.6.1) related to uncontrolled movements of seizure activity. (See chapter on seizures.)

N.D. 5   Diagnosis related to hydrocephalus/shunt placement if present. (See chapter on ventriculo-peritoneal shunts.)

N.D. 6   Potential self-care deficit (NANDA 6.5.1, 2, 3, 4) related to visual impairment.

N.D. 7   Self-care deficit (NANDA 6.5.1, 2, 3, 4) related to (specify).

N.D. 8   Alterations in family processes (NANDA 3.2.2) related to difficulty adjusting to family member with acquired brain injury.

N.D. 9   Sensory perceptual alteration: visual. (NANDA 7.2)

N.D. 10   Impaired communication (NANDA 2.1.1.1) related to hearing loss.

---

* (See chapter 2, page 38 for explanation of the NANDA approved numercial system.)

Goals

Prevent injury related to (specify). (N.D. 1, 2, 4)

Maintain optimal visual acuity, facilitate methods for compensation of vision loss. (N.D. 2, 3, 9)

Prevent injury during seizure (see chapter on seizures). (N.D. 4)

Prevent injury related to increased intracranial pressure (see chapter on ventriculo-peritoneal shunts). (N.D. 5)

Maximum independence in self-care activities (specify). (N.D. 6, 7)

Support positive family adjustment and growth. (N.D. 8)

Maintain optimal auditory acuity, facilitate methods for compensation of hearing loss. (N.D. 10)

Nursing Interventions

Following review of medical and healthcare records, provide interpretation for educational staff as needed. (N.D. 1–5)

Attend hospital staffing, facilitate transition. Understanding medical/healthcare needs will be essential to ensure a smooth transition from a hospital or rehabilitation facility. (N.D. 1–5)

In-service staff on the nature of acquired brain injury and related student needs. (N.D. 1–5)

Provide classmates with age-appropriate information to encourage understanding and empathy. Encourage parent participation as appropriate. (N.D. 1–5)

Case management: Refer and followup for medical care if needed, coordinate service providers. (N.D. 1–5)

Provide for safe physical environment and necessary accommodations. (N.D. 1, 2, 5)

Screen for visual and auditory acuity annually and refer as appropriate. Maintenance of optimal visual and auditory acuity is essential for learning. (N.D. 2, 3, 6, 9, 10)

Nursing interventions related to seizures (see chapter on seizures). (N.D. 4)

Nursing interventions related to shunt functioning (see chapter on ventriculo-peritoneal shunts). (N.D. 5)

Administer medications as prescribed, maintain current medical orders and documentation of medication given. Observe for side effects and refer as appropriate. (N.D. 1, 4)

Utilize approaches consistent with the student's Individualized Education Plan (IEP). (N.D. 1–10)

Assist student in accommodation for vision impairment in self-care activities. (N.D. 6)

Assist student in achieving maximum independence in self-care activities. Utilize modifications as necessary. (N.D. 7)

Offer support to family, facilitate family strengths, and provide anticipatory guidance. Facilitation of understanding among family members promotes positive family response. (N.D. 8)

Assist student in accommodation for visual/auditory deficits in learning activities. (N.D. 9, 10)

Utilize alternative methods of communication. (N.D. 10)

Expected Student Outcomes

Will not experience injury. (N.D. 1, 2, 4)

Will utilize safety measures to accommodate for visual deficits. (N.D. 2, 3)

Outcomes related to presence of seizures (see chapter on seizures). (N.D. 4)

Outcomes related to increased intracranial pressure (see chapter on ventriculo-peritoneal shunts) (N.D. 5)

Accommodate for visual deficits in self-care activities. (N.D. 6)

Perform adaptive methods needed to complete activities of daily living/self-care. (N.D. 7)

Will give/receive support within the family system. (N.D. 8)

Will accommodate for visual/auditory deficits in learning activities. (N.D. 9, 10)

Utilizes alternative forms of communication. (N.D. 10)

Collaborative Problems

Potential complication: seizures

Potential complication: increased intracranial pressure

Potential complication: sepsis

Potential complication: paralysis

REFERENCES

1. National Head Injury Foundation, Task Force on Special Education. *An Educator's Manual, What Educators Need To Know About Students With Traumatic Brain Injury.* 1988. National Head Injury Foundation, 333 Turnpike Rd, Southborough, MA 01772, (508) 485-9950.

RESOURCES

Carpenito LJ. *Nursing Diagnosis, Application To Clinical Practice.* Philadelphia: JB Lippincott, 1989.

National Head Injury Foundation, 333 Turnpike Rd, Southborough, MA 01772, (508) 485-9950.

The Foundation has an exceptional variety of articles, educational materials, audio cassettes, and videotapes available. Request the Catalogue of Educational Materials, December 1989, and the *Education Packet.*

15 | IHP: Cancer

Susan I. Simandl Will

INTRODUCTION

Cancer is the leading childhood disease producing mortality or morbidity. Neoplastic diseases occur in 10 per 100,000 children per year. According to the American Cancer Society, in 1987, 6,600 new cases of cancer were diagnosed, with leukemia accounting for 40 percent of the newly diagnosed cases.[1]

An impressive change has occurred over the last forty years in the outcome expectation for a child diagnosed with cancer. In 1948, only 2 percent of children with cancer survived over five months.[2] Today over 60 percent of the children with leukemia and with many solid tumors survive over five years.[3] Also today, with some confidence, it can be predicted that a child who survives over five years with cancer and has no recurrence is unlikely to have a recurrence. Consequently, cancer in children has a changed focus. Childhood cancer no longer is a terminal illness. There is an expectation of cure or at the very least an expectation of living with a chronic disease, not a fatal disease.

The optimistic cure or chronic disease approach to cancer in children has been possible through changes in diagnosis and treatment. The development of CT (computed tomography), MRI (magnetic resonance imaging), and PET (positron emission tomography) scans make early identification and accurate staging possible to more carefully plan treatment. Multimodal and aggressive treatments with chemotherapy, radiation and surgical therapy are instituted quickly by growing ranks of specialists. Radiation oncology has become a specialty field as has chemotherapy. Advances in surgical techniques are permitting less radical procedures, and development of new technology has converted rare procedures to fairly common treatments (i.e., bone marrow transplant).

Nursing care of children with cancer has changed to include the advancing medical technological therapies. Because the technological therapies can free the child from long hospital stays, children managing cancer at all stages are likely to be in school. A focus on maintaining wellness and the "normalness" of the academic and social aspects of the child's life becomes a vital role for the school nurse. In addition, the school nurse must be knowledgeable about observing for chemotherapeutic side effects and managing such treatment regimens as central venous catheters. The school nurse must, however, be comfortable with death and dying issues, since some children with cancer will be facing a terminal illness.

Pathophysiology

Acute Lymphoid Leukemia (ALL)

Leukemias account for 40 percent of all childhood cancers and acute lymphoid leukemia represents 80 percent of the leukemias.[1] Acute lymphoid leukemia is a malignant condition of the blood making bone marrow cells which results in the production of high quantities of abnormal, poorly differentiated, immature and nonfunctional lymphocytes. Metastasis to the liver, spleen, lymph nodes and CNS can occur. Etiology is unknown. It is diagnosed most often in children under ten years old and most of these are around four years of age.[4] Onset is usually rapid with symptoms related to bone marrow failure complications: anemia, fever, sepsis, bruising, bleeding, joint pain, splenomegaly, and hepatomagaly. Sixty percent of the children with ALL survive the two to three year acute episode and become long-term survivors.[3]

Hodgkin's Disease Hodgkin's disease represents 4 percent of all childhood neoplasms and 60 percent of the lymphoid neoplasms.[1] Hodgkin's is distinguished from the other lymphomas by its development; the neoplastic lymph cell histology and lineage. Etiology is unknown. Hodgkin's disease is identified most often in the teen to early adult years, affecting more males than females. Symptoms are painless enlargement of the lymph nodes, especially the cervical nodes, fever, nausea, anorexia, weight loss, and occasionally night sweats or pruritis. Treatment is based on the disease stage of development and proceeds for six to eighteen months. Survival is dependent on the stage at the time of diagnosis, with a 70 percent long-term survival rate possible when identified early.[4]

Non-Hodgkin's Lumphomas Non-Hodgkin's lymphomas represent 6 percent of childhood neoplasms.[1] These are rapid growing, solid tumors of the hematopoietic system with random and diffuse involvement of the lymphatic system.[1] Etiology is unknown. Children between five and fifteen years are most frequently affected and more males than females are affected.[5] Presenting symptoms depend on body area containing the tumor mass. Common sites for the primary mass are the abdomen, mediastinum, head, neck and peripheral lymph nodes. Metastasis to the central nervous system is possible. Treatment is multimodal and based on stage. Two-year survival rates are about 70 percent.[4]

Brain and CNS Tumors Brain tumors represent 10 percent of childhood neoplasms and are a varied group in terms of lesion site, symptoms, and survival rates.[1] Etiology is unknown.

Brain stem gliomas are buried in the brain stem and inoperable. Survival rate is poor because of the location and treatment difficulties.

Medulloblastomas are rapid growing, quickly metastasizing tumors along the cerebrospinal fluid pathways. Chemotherapy and radiation are usually used conjunctively. Survival rates approach 40 percent.[5]

Cerebellar astrocytomas are typically benign, slow-growing tumors which produce difficulty because of their infringement on brain tissue space. Symptoms vary depending on cerebellar location. Surgical removal is required with survival rates above 90 percent.[5]

Rhabdomyosarcoma Rhabdomyosarcomas represent 5 percent of all childhood cancers.[1] It is a highly malignant tumor of the soft striated muscle tissue. Etiology is unknown. Identification occurs most often in the two- to six-year-old age group with more males than females affected. Primary sites can be anywhere where there is striated tissue. Common primary lesion sites are the eye orbit, nasopharyngeal area, and neck. However, primary sites can also be the bladder, pelvis, or extremities. Symptoms depend on location of the mass, with the mass itself usually firm and nontender. Survival rate depends on the extent of metastasis and type of tumor.

Neuroblasoma Neuroblastomas account for 8 percent of childhood neoplasms.[1] This tumor arises from sympathetic nervous system cells or adrenal gland cells. Primary tumors are most frequently of the adrenal medulla or of the sympathetic ganglia of the abdomen or pelvis. However, primary lesions of the head, neck, or chest are possible. Diagnosis usually occurs before age four with more males than females affected.[5] Symptoms depend on the site of original tumor with metastatic lesions often present at diagnosis. Multimodal treatment of surgery, chemotherapy, and radiation is implemented. Survival rate approaches 80 percent.[4]

Wilms Tumor Wilms tumor (nephroblastoma) represents 6 percent of childhood cancers.[1] It is a solid tumor of the kidney and often is accompanied by congenital anomalies. Diagnosis usually occurs by age 3 or 4 with presenting symptoms of an enlarged abdomen, abdominal mass, pain, hematuria, malaise, fever, anorexia, and weight loss.[5] Multimodal treatment of surgery, chemotherapy, and radiation is typical. Metastasis occurs to the regional lymph nodes and lungs as well as liver, bone, and brain. Survival rate is 83 percent.[5]

Osteosarcoma Osteosarcoma (osteogenic sarcoma), with the other bone cancer (Ewing Sarcoma), represents 7 percent of childhood neoplasms.[1] Osteosarcoma is a solid tumor of the bone mass, most likely on the rapidly growing bone ends and most commonly seen on the femur, tibia, or humerus. Other possible primary sites are the mandible, maxilla, pelvis, and fibula. As the tumor progresses, it invades soft tissues surrounding the bone. Onset is slow with the most frequent presenting complaint being pain over the tumor area . Often the child equates the pain with some recent injury, but it is more likely that the injury draws attention to the existing tumor. It is usually diagnosed in adolescence with males affected more often than females.[5] Surgical amputation is frequent with adjunctive chemotherapy. Survival rate is 60 percent if no metastasis is present.[5]

Ewing Sarcoma Ewing sarcoma is a neoplasm of the bone tissue and with osteosarcoma represents 7 percent of the childhood neoplasms.[1] Ewing sarcoma is differentiated from osteosarcoma by its histological appearance and by its behavior. Ewing sarcoma may affect any body bone, but is less common in the long bones. It spreads longitudinally through the bone marrow, destroying the bone tissue. Metastasis is usually present at diagnosis with the lungs the most common site of metastasis. Ewing sarcoma is typically diagnosed in adolescence with more males than females affected. Symptoms at diagnosis are pain and tenderness over the bone neoplasm. Treatment is multimodal with a 75 percent survival rate after three years if no metastasis is present.[4]

INDIVIDUALIZED HEALTHCARE PLAN

Assessment

History

- When was cancer diagnosed?
- What kind of cancer does child have?
- Has any metastasis been identified?
- Have there been periods of remission? How long? When was last acute episode?
- Has student had previous hospitalizations for condition? When? Why? What happened?
- Has student had previous surgical procedures? What? When?
- Has student had chemotherapy? What medications?
- Has student had radiation therapy? When?
- What has been the degree and pattern of physical disability due to the diagnosis or its treatments?
- Are there existing growth and or developmental delays?

Current Status

- Treatment regimen: chemotherapeutic or radiation treatment plan, frequency, agents
- General appearance: posture   Comparison to age norms:
                       height
                       weight
- Temperature
- Blood pressure
- Pulse
- Respirations (rate, rhythm, quality)
- Observe for signs of side effects of chemotherapeutic agents
  - Stomatitis: gingiva, oral mucosa, tongue, teeth (stomatitis is common with certain chemotherapeutic agents: inflammation and tissue breakdown)
  - Inadequate dietary intake
  - Nausea or vomiting
  - Anorexia or weight loss
  - Constipation or diarrhea
  - Bleeding—nosebleeds, easy bruising (side effect of bone marrow suppression)
  - Infection symptoms or signs (susceptible with neutropenia as a result of chemotherapeutics)
  - Alopecia
  - Dehydration
  - Neurological complications (paresthesia, neuropathies, decreased tendon reflexes, muscle weakness)
  - Pain
- Treatment orders
    activity   medications
    diet   central venous catheter

Treatment and Self-Care

- Student's description of and definition of cancer
- Student's current medication (pain, chemotherapeutic, antiemetic)
- Student's description of medication plan
- Student's understanding of diet and adherence to diet
- Student's understanding of activity limits
- Student's understanding of treatments
- Activities student states are limited by cancer diagnosis
- What does student find useful to manage successfully in school?
- Need for learning support systems (special education, computer aids, tutors, adaptive physical education)
- What treatments, medications can student manage on own?

Psychosocial

- Age and developmental level
- Student's feelings about having cancer
- Student's perception of what family members think and feel about his/her having cancer
- Student's perception of what friends think and feel about his/her having cancer
- School club or athletic activities past and present
- Community and church activities past and present
- Depression or despondency
- Student's support systems: family, friends, other
- Grieving process

Academic

- Review of academic or cumulative school record for patterns of academic performance
- Assessment of teachers' perception of student's performance and classroom adjustment
- Comparison of student's behavior, social skills, academic performance to peer norms
- School absence pattern
- Need for special education, PL 99-457 (PL 94-142), services to adequately educate the student (transportation, classroom adaptations, tutoring, occupational therapy, physical therapy, vocational guidance)
- What are the intellectual abilities? Presence of learning disability or retardation?

Nursing Diagnoses (N.D.)

N.D. 1 Alteration in activities of daily living (personal, recreational, educational—running, walking, stair climbing, sleep or rest needs) related to:
      depressed body defenses
      side effects of chemotherapy or radiation (nausea, vomiting, anorexia, diarrhea, constipation, neuropathies, stomatitis, fever, bleeding)
      decreased mobility
      amputation or other surgical procedure
      presence of central venous catheter

N.D. 2   Impaired physical mobility (NANDA 6.1.1.1)* due to:
- side effects of chemotherapy or radiation (nausea, vomiting, anorexia, diarrhea, constipation, neuropathies, stomatitis, fever, bleeding)
- amputation or other surgical procedure
- presence of central venous catheter

N.D. 3   Alteration in activity tolerance (NANDA 6.1.1.2) due to:
- depressed body defenses
- side effects of chemotherapy or radiation (nausea, vomiting, anorexia, diarrhea, constipation, neuropathies, stomatitis, fever, bleeding)

N.D. 4   Alteration in growth and development (NANDA 6.6) due to:
- depressed body defenses
- side effects of chemotherapy or radiation (nausea, vomiting, anorexia, diarrhea, constipation, neuropathies, stomatitis, fever, bleeding)

N.D. 5   Alterations in self-care (NANDA 6.5.1, 2, 3, or 4) due to:
- depressed body defenses
- side effects of chemotherapy or radiation (nausea, vomiting, anorexia, diarrhea, constipation, neuropathies, stomatitis, fever, bleeding)

N.D. 6   Potential for infection (NANDA 1.2.1.1) due to:
- depressed body defenses
- side effects of chemotherapy or radiation (nausea, vomiting, anorexia, diarrhea, constipation, neuropathies, stomatitis, fever, bleeding)

N.D. 7   Alteration in nutritional status (NANDA 1.1.2.2) due to:
- depressed body defenses
- side effects of chemotherapy or radiation (nausea, vomiting, anorexia, diarrhea, constipation, neuropathies, stomatitis, fever, bleeding)

N.D. 8   Alteration in comfort:pain (NANDA 9.1.1) due to:
- presence of cancer lesion
- side effects of chemotherapy or radiation (nausea, vomiting, anorexia, diarrhea, constipation, neuropathies, stomatitis, fever, bleeding)

N.D. 9   Alteration in fluid volume (NANDA 1.4.1.2.2.1)
- depressed body defenses
- side effects of chemotherapy or radiation (nausea, vomiting, anorexia, diarrhea, constipation, neuropathies, stomatitis, fever, bleeding)

N.D. 10   Fear (NANDA 9.3.2) related to diagnosis and prognosis

N.D. 11   Knowledge deficit (NANDA 8.1.1) related to:
- cancer pathophysiology
- medications

---

* (See Chapter 2, page 38 for explanation of the NANDA approved numerical system.)

- chemotherapy or radiation
- nutritional adaptations (including central venous catheter)

Goals

Student will receive assistance in safely managing treatments, medication and diet needs in school setting. (N.D. 2, 3, 5-7, 9)

Student will acquire adaptations necessary to experience as normal a lifestyle as possible in the school setting. (N.D. 1-5)

Student will be able to perform activities of daily living within his/her physical limits without excessive fatigue or compromising physiological status. (N.D. 1- 6)

Student will be involved in management of condition and improve self-management skills. (N.D. 5)

Student will have early, appropriate intervention if problems develop. (N.D. 5-9)

Student will progress in adaptation to living with chronic illness. (N.D. 10)

Student will progress in grieving process. (N.D. 10)

Student will progress in discussing death and dying issues. (N.D. 10)

Student will increase understanding of pathophysiology of cancer condition and develop or improve skills to manage cancer, or its treatments and side effects. (N.D 11)

Nursing Interventions

School/Teacher Interventions

Coordinate communication between medical care provider and school community. (N.D. 6–9)

Assist classroom teacher in developing activities appropriate to activity tolerance. (N.D. 1–4)

Teach classroom teachers signs and symptoms which should be reported to nurse. (N.D. 1-3, 6-9)

- change in activity tolerance
- respiratory difficulty
- pain
- irritability
- malaise
- lethargy

Arrange for lengthened or alternate passing time between classes to prevent fatigue or injury. (N.D. 1–3, 5)

Arrange for rest periods as necessary during school day. (N.D. 1–3)

Arrange for prescribed diet at school. (N.D. 7, 8)

Assist in obtaining low acid, soft foods from cafeteria if stomatitis present. (N.D. 7–9)

Assist in obtaining snacks and non-spicy, low odor foods, or high calorie foods if needed to minimize nausea or weight loss, or to maintain intake. (N.D. 7–9)

Arrange for home-hospital instruction if school attendance impossible on an extended or intermittent basis. (N.D. 1–3)

Arrange for medication at school as appropriate and in accordance with school district policy and procedure. (N.D. 5–8)

See Chapter 6 for additional mental health and psychosocial nursing diagnoses relevant to students with chronic disease.

Arrange for assistance as necessary for daily school activities. (N.D. 1–3,5, 6)
- wheelchair use
- extra time for passing between class, or separate passing time
- transportation
- book carrying

Arrange for appropriate physical education activities and instruct physical education teachers in appropriate activity tolerance expectations. (N.D. 1–3, 5)

Refer for special education (P.L. 94–142) evaluation for occupational therapy, physical therapy, tutoring, learning aids, transportation, vocational counseling. (N.D. 1–5)

Provide access to physically handicapped bathrooms, entrances, elevators as appropriate. (N.D. 1–3)

Arrange for vocational counseling and planning (for the adolescent). (N.D. 10)

Student Interventions

Monitor for signs of side effects of chemotherapy or radiation. (N.D. 6–9)

Monitor student response to activity levels: adjust activity if necessary. (N.D. 1–3, 5–9)

Assess for pain using age and developmentally appropriate tools: line graphs, color coding smiling faces to frowning faces, scales of 1–5. (N.D. 1, 5, 8)

Assist with central venous catheter care, medications, fluids or nutrients as ordered by the medical provider (since catheter brands vary in care and management requirements, obtain specific instructions from the medical source). (N.D. 6–9)

Arrange for local anesthetics to mouth ulcerations before eating if necessary. (N.D. 7–9)

Arrange for oral hygiene following meals at school. (N.D. 8)

Notify parents if there is infectious disease outbreak in school (influenza, measles, chicken pox, mumps, other). (N.D. 6)

Observe for signs of skin breakdown, notify parents. (N.D. 6, 7, 9)

Avoid temperature extreme or sudden temperature changes (ice packs, heating pads) to skin. (N.D.6–8)

Provide for student and family referral to support groups and counseling.(N.D. 10)

Encourage and provide opportunities for student's expression of feelings about cancer, its management requirements and limits it imposes. (N.D. 10)

Provide opportunities for student to discuss thoughts and feelings about death and dying. (N.D. 10)

Assist student in grieving process. (N.D. 10)

Assist student in explaining to class and friends reasons for hair loss, facial changes due to steroid therapy, fatigue, special foods, treatments, and so on. (N.D. 10)

Assist student in expressing sexuality concerns and needs (adolescent). (N.D. 10)

Instruct student in pathophysiology of cancer at level appropriate to age and developmental level. (N.D. 5, 11)

Instruct student in medication actions, administration, and side effects. (N.D. 5, 11)

Monitor student medication compliance. (N.D. 5, 11)

Instruct student in nutritional needs. (N.D. 5, 11)

Instruct student in central venous catheter care and administration of fluids, medication or nutrition via the catheter (obtain specific instructions from medical provider since brands of catheters differ in care and techniques). (N.D. 5, 11)

Instruct student in foods more easily tolerated if stomatitis present (low acid, low odor, soft or liquid). (N.D. #5, 7, 11)

Instruct student in reasons for fatigue and malaise. (N.D. 5, 10, 11)

Have student assist in planning and implementing school activity, treatments, adaptations. (N.D. 5, 11)

Expected Student Outcomes

Student's pain is minimized or absent. (N.D. 9)

Student will adhere to medical management plan, activity, diet, medications in school setting. (N.D. 6-9)

Student will be able to perform as many activities in the educational setting as possible. (N.D. 5)

Student will receive assistance for those activities which s/he requires assistance on a regular or intermittent basis, as the condition demands. (N.D. 1-5)

Student will be successful in managing mobility to and around school. (N.D. 1-3, 5)

Student will be able to physically attend all classes. (N.D. 1-3, 5)

Student will not be excessively fatigued or develop complications from the activities of school attendance. (N.D. 1-3, 5)

Student will be able to continue educational progress. (N.D. 1, 4)

Student's infection risk will be minimized in school setting. (N.D. 6)

Student will progress in grieving process. (N.D. 10)

Student will identify activities which are possible with physiological status. (N.D. 10)

Student will be involved in one (or more) school or community activity. (N.D. 10)

Student will maintain, or increase, peer contacts. (N.D. 10)

Student will make appropriate life goal plans. (N.D. 10)

Student will describe cancer pathophysiology at level appropriate to age and development. (N.D. 11)

Student will describe medication and treatment actions, and administration requirements. (N.D. 11)

Student will know medication side effects and will notify medical provider if side effects noticed. (N.D. 11)

Student will assist in planning and managing adjustment in activities of daily living within the school setting. (N.D 11)

REFERENCES

1. Hockenberry M, Coody D, Bennett B. Childhood cancers: incidence, etiology, diagnosis, and treatment. *Pediatric Nursing*. 1990; 16 (3): 239–246.
2. Sahler OJ. Caring for the child with cancer and the family: lessons learned from children with acute leukemia. *Pediatrics in Review* 1990; 12 (1): 6-8.
3. McGuire P, Moore K. Recent advances in childhood cancer. *Nurs ClinNorth Am* 1990; 25 (2): 447–460.
4. Hathaway WE, Groothuis JR, Hay WW, Paisley JW, eds. *Current Pediatric Diagnosis and Treatment.* 10th Ed. East Norwalk, CT: Appleton & Lange, 1991.
5. Waechter E, Philips J, Holaday B. *Nursing Care of Children.* 10th ed. Philadelphia: JB Lippincott, 1985.

BIBLIOGRAPHY

Berde C, Ablin A, Glaser J, Miser A, Shapiro B, Weisman S, Zeltzer P. Report of the Subcommittee on Disease-Related Pain in Childhood Cancer. In: Report of the Consensus Conference on the Management of Pain in Childhood Cancer. *Pediatrics* (Suppl.) 1990; 86 (5 Pt 2): 818–825.

Bendorf K, Meehan J. Home parenteral nutrition for the child with cancer. *Issues in Compr Pediatri Nursing* 1989; 12 (2–3): 171–186.

Johnson S. *High-Risk Parenting: Nursing Assessment and Strategies for the Family at Risk.* Philadelphia: JB Lippincott, 1979.

Martinson IM, Colaizzo DC, Freeman M, Bossert E. Impact of childhood cancer on healthy school-age siblings. *Cancer Nursing* 1990; 13 (3): 183–190.

McGrath PJ, Beyer J, Cleeland C, Eland J, McGrath PA, Portenoy R. Report of the Subcommittee on Assessment and Methodological Issues in the Management of Pain in Childhood Cancer. In: Report of the Consensus Conference on the Management of Pain in Childhood Cancer. *Pediatrics* (Suppl.) 1990; 86 (5 Pt 2): 814–817.

Morris-Jones PH, Craft AW. Childhood cancer: cure at what cost? *Arch Disease Childhood* 1990; 65: 638–640.

Rezabek P, McCullouch P. Psychosocial issues: looking at the whole person. In: Larson G, ed. *Managing the School Age Child with a Chronic Health Condition.* Wayzata, MN: DCI Publishing, 1988; distributed by Sunrise River Press, 11481 Kost Dam Road, North Branch, MN 55056, (612) 583-3239.

Sawyer MG, Toogood I, Rice M, Haskell C, Baghurst P. School performance and psychological adjustment of children treated for leukemia: a long-term follow-up. *Am J Pediatric Hematol Oncol.* 1989; 2: 146–152.

Wong D, Whaley L. *Clinical Manual of Pediatric Nursing.* 2nd ed. St. Louis: CV Mosby, 1990.

16 | IHP: Cardiovascular Disease

Susan I. Simandl Will

INTRODUCTION

Cardiovascular conditions can be divided into two types: congenital and acquired. The congenital conditions include such medical diagnoses as: ventricular septal defects, patent ductus arteriosus, tetralogy of Fallot, pulmonary stenosis, aortic stenosis, valvular stenosis, coarctation of the aorta, and transposition of the great arteries. Acquired cardiovascular conditions include such medical diagnoses as rheumatic fever, rheumatic heart disease, endocarditis, myocarditis, pericarditis, endocarditis, and hypertension. Congestive heart failure, murmurs, fibrilations and flutters may be considered part of either acquired or congenital pathophysiology.

The congenital cardiovascular conditions affect over 1 percent of all newborns and of these less than 10 percent occur as a single anomaly.[1] Currently, newborn pediatric intensive care services are able to assist in the repair of the anomaly for many children. Congenital conditions often involve other system abnormalities and may or may not involve cyanosis. Surgical repair may be a series of corrections which can result in varying degrees of physiological normality.

The cardiovascular disorders present a complex health issue for school nurse management. Often it is not only the cardiac condition alone which requires attention, since other anomalies may be present. Also, for many children, secondary growth and developmental delays develop. In addition, the disorder can present the potential for a life-threatening episode. It is essential that a thorough assessment and history be performed and that the school nurse following a child with a cardiac condition be continuously updated on the physiological status of the child. The child at school age may have a completely corrected condition which involves no need for academic or school day adjustment. However, the school-age child may require extensive monitoring, nursing intervention, and adaptation to be safe and successful.

Pathophysiology

Aortic Stenosis This acyanotic congenital heart defect is the result of aortic constriction and obstruction of blood flow from the left ventricle at or near the aortic valve. Symptoms of the defect may be absent in early life and later result in sudden development of congestive heart failure symptoms. Occasionally, a child will not develop symptoms until late childhood. The symptoms can be a persisting history of syncope, dizziness, angina. Exercise may precipitate the symptoms. Cardiac catheterization is required to diagnose the condition and palliative surgical procedures can be performed. Children without symptoms are typically not treated surgically, but followed annually for exercise tolerance testing. Participation in full activity including physical education and competitive sports can be possible with medical monitoring. Some patients are placed on prophylactic antibiotic therapy to prevent bacterial endocarditis.

Coarctation of the Aorta Coarctation of the aorta, an acyanotic condition, accounts for approximately 6 percent of congenital cardiac defects.[2] It is actually a narrowing on the aortic arch just above the ductus arteriosus. The condition usually involves a patent ductus, ventricular septal defect, and a bicuspid aortic valve. Because the left ventricle pumps against the constricted aorta, pressure increases in the ventricle causing the cardiac, mammary and intercostal arteries to become dilated. As a result, decreased blood volume is available for systemic circulation and congestive heart failure may develop. The defect will be identified in infancy if cardiac symptoms are present; however, some patients do not present symptoms until school age or later. The symptoms are absent or diminished peripheral pulses, a lower blood pressure in the legs than in the arms, a discrepancy between the brachial and femoral pulses, and bounding arm pulses. Medical diagnosis is made with x-ray films, EEG, and cardiac catheterization. Following surgical repair, hypertension can be an ongoing problem.

Congestive Heart Failure Congestive heart failure is indicative of the heart's inability to meet the perfusion needs of the body. Both congenital and acquired cardiac diseases can result in congestive heart failure. Cardiac congenital defects which increase cardiac load or obstruct blood flow can produce congestive heart failure

(valvular insufficiencies, aortic or pulmonary stenosis, coarctation of the aorta or pulmonary artery, septal defects, tetralogy of Fallot, transposition of the great vessels). Acquired cardiac infections (rheumatic cardiac disease, myocarditis) can decrease the heart's capacity and strength, resulting in congestive heart failure. Progressive compensatory cardiac and systemic alterations attempt to compensate for the altered heart action: tachycardia, ventricular dilation, ventricular hypertrophy, pulmonary and systemic circulation congestion, impaired pulmonary gas exchange, liver engorgement, increased sodium and water retention, edema. Symptoms are irritability or lethargy, fatigue, anorexia, palor, weak peripheral pulses, hyperpnea, retractions, rales, tachycardia, and edema.

Hypertension Hypertension is the persistent elevation of either systolic or diastolic blood pressure to levels above the norms appropriate for the child's age. Essential hypertension, hypertension not related to identifiable disease, is the most common form in children. Hereditary factors and lifestyle risk factors (overweight, excessive salt intake, smoking, lack of exercise) as well as medications (oral contraceptives) can elevate the blood pressure. Regular screening for blood pressure elevations by school nurses and healthcare practitioners is becoming more routine and is helping to identify children at younger ages who are developing hypertension.

Murmurs Cardiac murmur refers to the presence of abnormal cardiac sounds. These may be loud or soft, audible with auscultation in one or more locations, and may be connected to cardiac dysfunction or may be benign. Functional murmurs occur frequently. All cardiac murmurs need physican evaluation and even though determined innocent, functional, or benign, may require continued medical surveillance. The school nurse may be helpful in interpreting medical meaning of functional murmurs to parents and school staff and may be responsible for helping with the anxiety that this diagnosis can cause.

Patent Ductus Arteriosus This acyanotic congenital defect results from the closure failure of the fetal vessel which shunts blood from the pulmonary artery to the aorta. Normally this vessel closes within the first week of life. The condition is more prevalent in premature infants and spontaneous closure by two years is possible. Surgical treatment is available for those that do not spontaneously close. A child with a large patent ductus arteriosus may have pulmonary hypertension, congestive heart failure, and frequent respiratory illness. These can result in growth and developmental delays which may need addressing during the school-age years.

Rheumatic Heart Disease This acquired heart condition is a potential residual from rheumatic carditis, a complication of rheumatic fever. Rheumatic fever is an inflammatory disease following an untreated infection of A beta-hemolytic streptococci, usually of the upper respiratory tract. It occurs most frequently in older children and adolescents at a rate of up to 2 per 1,000.[3] Major symptoms are arthritic joints, heart murmur, rash (erythema marginatum), congestive heart failure, tachycardia, shortness of breath, and exercise dyspnea. Medical treatment during the carditis is bed rest, diuretics, and possibly steroid therapy. Prolonged preventive antibiotic therapy follows the acute illness because of the possibility of recurrence.

Septal Defects Atrial or ventricular septal defects are noncyanotic congenital heart diseases. Atrial septal defect is an opening in the septum between the atria which results in the shunting of blood between the atria. This opening may spontaneously close, but generally requires surgical closure. Both surgical correction and spontaneous closure typically result in the ability to have a normal lifestyle without limitations. Undiagnosed atrial defects can produce later obstructive pulmonary vascular disease, arrhythmias, and congestive heart failure.

Ventricular septal defect is the single most common congenital heart condition. The defect can occur in the muscle or the membranous tissue of the ventricle and results in the shunting of blood between the ventricles. Up to 75 percent of the defects spontaneously close,[1] the others require surgical closure. Children with this defect will typically be acyanotic, have a murmur, and may have signs of congestive heart failure. X-rays, electrocardiography (ECG), and cardiac catheterization are diagnostic measures. Disability seldom follows early surgical intervention or spontaneous closure.

Tetralogy of Fallot This cyanotic congenital cardiac defect is usually apparent in infancy, but occasionally may not be identified until later childhood. If previously undiagnosed, it can be the cause of cyanosis in school-age children. Symptoms are sudden cyanotic spells, squatting behavior (pulling knees to chest in sitting or squatting type positions), and dyspnea spells. Tetralogy of Fallot represents several cardiac anomalies: a ventricular septal defect, pulmonary stenosis, right ventricular hypertrophy, and dextroposition of the aorta. X-rays, ECG, and cardiac catheterization are diagnostic measures. Surgical correction is performed via cardiopulmonary bypass and involves closing the ventricular septal defect and resectioning the pulmonic stenosis. Following surgical correction, children can do fairly well. If the surgical correction occurs during school-age years, arrhythmias and sudden death are possible.[2]

Transposition of the Great Arteries This cyanotic congenital condition accounts for the majority of all cardiac defects. Males are affected three times more often than females.[2] In this defect, the great vessels are reversed, the aorta rises off the right ventricle and the pulmonary artery rises off the left ventricle, placing the aorta anterior to the pulmonary artery. A ventricular septal defect may or may not accompany the transposition. Transposition is diagnosed during infancy with symptoms developing in the early months, if not noticed in the neonate. Cardiac catheterization is required to medically diagnose the condition. Surgical treatment may be delayed and performed in progressive procedures. Children with corrections typically show varying degrees of continuing cardiac dysfunction as well as growth and developmental problems.

INDIVIDUALIZED HEALTHCARE PLAN

ASSESSMENT

History

- How long has cardiovascular condition been present?
- Has student had previous hospitalizations for condition? When? Why? What happened?
- Has student had previous surgical procedures? What? When?
- What has been the degree and pattern of physical disability due to the cardiovascular condition?
- Are there developmental delays?

Current Status

- General appearance: presence of chromosomal abnormalities
      posture
      height
      weight
- Blood pressure (reading and character)
    readings
    equality of pressure between arms
    20mm Hg or lower in legs than arms
    narrow or wide pulse pressures
- Pulse (rate and quality)
    rate
    visible chest pulsations
    discrepancy between apical and radial pulses
    tachycardia
    bradycardia
    pulse quality (alternans, bounding, weak, thready, diminished)
- Respirations (rate, rhythm, quality)
    tachypnea
    hyperpnea

lung sounds (rales or ronchi)
shortness of breath
- Heart auscultation
intensity
presence of abnormal sounds: murmur, snapping, clicks
- Other physical observations:
gums and teeth (gum hypertrophy and poor dentition possible with long-term conditions)
cyanosis
clubbing of fingers, toes
engorged neck veins
chest deformities
edema
peripheral pulses (absence or presence, quality, equality, strength)
temperature
rashes (erythema marginatum)
joint pain
- Treatment orders
activity   medications
diet   pacemaker

Self-Care

- Student's description and definition of cardiovascular condition
- Student's current medication (routine and emergency)
- Student's description of medication plan
- Student's understanding of diet and adherence to diet
- Student's understanding of activity limits and adherence
- Student's understanding of treatments (pacemaker, surgeries, other)
- Activities student states are limited by cardiovascular condition
- What does student find useful to manage successfully in school?
- Need for learning support systems (special education, computer aids, tutors, adaptive physical education)
- What treatments, medications can student manage on own?

Psychosocial

- Age and developmental level
- Student's feelings about having cardiovascular condition
- Student's perception of what family members think and feel about his/her having cardiovascular condition
- Student's perception of what friends think and feel about his/her having cardiovascular condition
- School club or athletic activities past and present
- Community and church activities past and present
- Depression or despondency
- Student's support systems: family, friends, other

Academic

- Review of academic or cumulative school record for patterns of academic performance
- Assessment of teachers' perception of student's performance and classroom adjustment
- Comparison of student's behavior, social skills, academic performance to peer norms
- School absence pattern
- Need for special education (P.L. 94-142) services to adequately educate the student (transportation, classroom adaptations, tutoring, occupational therapy, physical therapy, vocational guidance)
- What are the intellectual abilities?   Presence of learning disability or retardation?

Nursing Diagnoses (N.D.)

N.D. 1   Alteration in activities of daily living (personal, recreational, educational: running, walking stair climbing, sleep or rest needs) due to:
- cardiovascular dysfunction
- cardiac structural defect
- cardiovascular infection
- inadequate tissue oxygenation and nutrition
- imbalance between tissue oxygen demand and vascular supply

N.D. 2   Impaired physical mobility (NANDA 6.1.1.1)* due to:
- cardiovascular dysfunction
- cardiovascular infection
- inadequate tissue oxygenation and nutrition
- imbalance between tissue oxygen demand and vascular supply

N.D. 3   Alteration in activity tolerance (NANDA 6.1.1.2) due to:
- cardiovascular dysfunction
- imbalance between tissue oxygen demand and vascular supply

N.D. 4   Alteration in growth and development (NANDA 6.6) due to:
- inadequate tissue oxygenation and nutrition
- imbalance between tissue oxygen demand and vascular supply

N.D. 5   Alterations in self-care (NANDA 6.5.1, 2, 3, or 4) due to:
- cardiovascular dysfunction
- inadequate tissue oxygenation and nutrition
- imbalance between tissue oxygen demand and vascular supply

N.D. 6   Alteration in tissue perfusion (NANDA 1.4.1.1) due to:
- cardiovascular dysfunction
- cardiac structural defect
- imbalance between tissue oxygen demand and vascular supply

N.D. 7   Alteration in cardiac output (NANDA 1.4.2.1) due to:
- cardiovascular dysfunction
- cardiac structural defect
- cardiovascular infection

N.D. 8   Knowledge deficit (NANDA 8.1.1) related to:
- cardiovascular pathophysiology
- medications, treatments, diet

---

* (See chapter 2, page 38 for explanation of the NANDA numerical system.)
See Chapter 6 for mental health and psychosocial nursing diagnoses relevant to students with chronic disease.

N.D. 9   Altered parental or family coping (NANDA 5.1.2.1.2) or altered family process (NANDA 3.2.2) due to having a child with a cardiovascular condition.

N.D. 10   Potential for physiological injury (NANDA 1.6.1) due to cardiac insufficiency
or inadequate tissue perfusion.

Goals

Student will improve cardiac strength. (N.D. 1–4, 6, 7)

Student will acquire adaptations necessary to experience as normal a lifestyle as possible
in the school setting. (N.D. 1–5)

Student will be able to perform activities of daily living within his/her physical limits
without excessive fatigue or compromising physiological condition. (N.D. 1–6)

Student will be involved in management of condition and improve self-management
skills. (N.D. 5)

Student will have early, appropriate intervention if problems develop. (N.D. 6, 7, 10)

Student will increase understanding of pathophysiology of cardiac condition and develop
or improve skills to manage cardiac condition. (N.D. 8)

Reduction in family anxiety and stress relative to school attendance, activity, and management. (N.D. 9)

Nursing Interventions

School/Teacher Interventions

Develop individual emergency plan for (with) student and share with faculty. (N.D. 6, 7,
10)

Coordinate communication between medical care provider and school community. (N.D.
6, 7, 9, 10)

Assist classroom teacher in developing activities appropriate to activity tolerance. (N.D.
1–3)

Instruct classroom teachers in signs and symptoms which should be reported to nurse:
(N.D. 6, 7, 10)
- change in activity tolerance
- respiratory difficulty
- cyanosis
- pain
- irritability
- malaise
- lethargy

Arrange for home-hospital instruction if school attendance impossible on an extended or
intermittent basis. (N.D. 1–3)

Arrange for medication at school as appropriate and in accordance with school district
policy and procedure. (N.D. 6, 7, 10)

Arrange for assistance as necessary for daily school activities (N.D. 1–4)
- wheelchair use
- extra time for passing between classes
- transportation
- book carrying
- rest opportunities
- class schedule adaptations

Arrange for appropriate physical education activities and instruct physical education teachers in appropriate expectations for activity tolerance. (N.D. 1–7, 10)

Refer for special education (P.L. 94-142) evaluation for occupational therapy, physical therapy, tutoring, learning aids, transportation, vocational counseling. (N.D. 1– 3, 5–7, 10)

Provide access to physically handicapped bathrooms, entrances, elevators as appropriate. (N.D. 1–3, 5)

Arrange for prescribed diet at school. (N.D. 1, 6)

Arrange for rest periods as necessary during school day. (N.D. 2, 3)

Provide appropriate supervision to any personnel involved in student's care. (N.D. 10)

Student/Family Interventions

Monitor blood pressure, pulse, respirations. (N.D. 6, 7)

Monitor student response to activity levels: adjust activity if necessary. (N.D. 1–3)

Instruct student in pathophysiology of cardiac condition at level appropriate to age and developmental level. (N.D. 8)

Instruct student in medication actions, administration, and side effects. (N.D. 5, 8)

Monitor student medication compliance. (N.D. 8)

Instruct student in dietary needs and limitations. (N.D. 5, 8)

Teach student how to plan daily diet. (N.D. 5, 8)

Instruct student in reasons for activity limits. (N.D. 5, 8)

Have student assist in planning and implementing school activity. (N.D. 5, 8)

Develop relationship with parent (family). (N.D. 9)

Support family. (N.D. 9)

Involve parents in planning school management plan. (N.D. 9)

Help family identify coping strategies and support systems. (N.D. 9)

Expected Student Outcomes

Student's heart rate, volume, and rhythm will remain within acceptable limits. (N.D. 6, 7, 10)

Student will adhere to medical management plan, activity, diet, medications in school setting. (N.D. 6, 7, 10)

Student will be able to perform as many activities in the educational setting as possible. (N.D. 1–5)

Student will receive assistance for those activities which s/he requires assistance on a regular or intermittent basis, as the condition demands. (N.D. 1–5)

Student will be successful in managing mobility to and around school. (N.D. 1–5)

Student will be able to physically attend all classes or __ % of classes. (N.D. 1–7)

Student will not be excessively fatigued or develop complications from the activities of school attendance. (N.D. 6, 7, 10)

Student will be able to continue educational progress. (N.D. 1–5)

Student will describe cardiovascular pathophysiology at level appropriate to age and development. (N.D. 5, 8)

Student will describe medication actions, and administration requirements. (N.D. 5, 8)

Student will know medication side effects and know to notify medical provider if side effects noticed. (N.D. 5, 8)

Student will assist in planning and managing adjustment in activities of daily living within the school setting. (N.D. 5, 8)

Student will have support from family in condition management. (N.D. 9)

Student and family will be able to verbalize concerns and anxieties. (N.D. 9)

Student and family will be involved in planning the school program. (N.D. 9)

REFERENCES

1. Waechter E, Philips J, Holaday B. *Nursing Care of Children.* 10th ed. Philadelphia: JB Lippincott, 1985.
2. Hathaway WE, Groothuis JR, Hay WW, Paisley JW, eds. *Current Pediatric Diagnosis and Treatment.* 10th ed. Norwalk, CT: Appelton & Lange, 1991.
3. McCance K, Huether S. *Pathophysiology - The Biological Basis for Disease in Adults and Children.* St. Louis: CV Mosby, 1990.

BIBLIOGRAPHY

Gillette, PC. Dysrhythmias. In: Adams FH, and Emmanouilides GC, eds. *Moss' Heart Disease in Infants, Children and Adolescents.* 3rd ed. Baltimore: Williams & Wilkins, 1983.

Huang SH, Kessler CA, McCulloch CD, Dasher LA. *Coronary Care Nursing.* 2nd ed. Philadelphia: WB Saunders, 1989.

Lamb JI, Carlson VR. *Handbook of Cardiovascular Nursing.* Philadelphia: JB Lippincott, 1986.

National Heart, Lung, and Blood Institute, Second Task Force on Blood Pressure Control in Children. Tabular data prepared by Dr. B. Rosner. Bethesda, MD: National Heart, Lung, and Blood Institute, 1987.

Wong D, Whaley L. *Clinical Manual of Pediatric Nursing.* 2nd ed. St. Louis: CV Mosby, 1990.

17 | IHP: Cerebral Palsy

Mary J. Villars Gerber

INTRODUCTION

Cerebral palsy is a nonspecific term applied to impaired muscle control caused by damage to the brain. The chief cause is lack of oxygen to the fetal or newborn brain. Other causes include perinatal asphyxia, congenital and perinatal infections, and congenital brain anomalies. Acquired cerebral palsy may be the result of accidents, head injury, or child abuse. The diagnosis is established based on a history that the motor disability is nonprogressive.

The three main types of cerebral palsy include: spastic, stiff and difficult movements; dyskinetic, involuntary and uncontrolled movement; and ataxic, disturbed sense of balance and depth perception. A combination of these may occur in one individual. There are six types of spastic cerebral palsy. They include hemiparesis, quadriparesis, diplegia, monoplegia, triplegia, and paraplegia.

Medications used to decrease spasticity include dantrium, baclofen, robaxin, and valium.

Orthopedic surgery is sometimes used to decrease spastic muscle imbalance. These include tendon lengthening procedures, procedures to the hip and adductor muscles to improve locomotion, release of contractures, and release of wrist flexors. A neurosurgical procedure sometimes utilized is the selective posterior rhizotomy. Surgical procedures are only employed after other more conservative methods of management are ineffective.

Devices to enhance mobilization and maintain joint alignment are often utilized. These include braces, wedges, special seating devices, wheeled carts, and wheelchairs.

INDIVIDUALIZED HEALTHCARE PLAN

History

What is the history related to prenatal and perinatal factors that predispose to fetal anoxia?
What is the student's medical diagnosis?
At what age was the diagnosis made?
What were the student's developmental milestones?
What medications have been utilized?
What is the surgical history?

Assessment

- Gross motor development. Gross motor development is universally delayed and becomes more so as the child grows.

- Fine motor development. Delays may be evidenced by poor sucking, feeding difficulties, tongue thrust, and fine motor movements.

- Alterations in muscle tone. Increased or decreased resistance to passive movements, arching of the back, general stiffness, rigid hip and knee movements when pulled to sitting.

- Activity tolerance. Lack of sufficient energy and fatigue may influence tolerance to certain activities.

- Abnormal posture. Scissoring and extension of legs in supine position. Legs and arms flexed when prone.

- Abnormal reflexes. Tonic neck reflex, Moro, plantar, and palmar grasp reflex, ankle clonus may be present.

- Nutrition. Due to involvement of facial muscles and tongue muscles, inadequate nutritional intake may be present.

- Evidence of mental retardation. This is an associated disability that may or may not be present.

- Seizures. This is an associated disability that may or may not be present.

- Hearing acuity. Athetoid cerebral palsy is often accompanied by a high-frequency hearing loss or deafness.

- Visual acuity. A conjugate upward gaze palsy is often present in children with athetoid cerebral palsy. The eyes are converged toward the midline and displaced upward.

- Medications and side effects, particularly those that will interfere with learning.

- Self-care. Deficits may be present related to involuntary muscle movements and/or mental retardation. Incontinence may be present in some individuals.

- Self-concept. The student may experience negative feelings, thoughts, or views about him/herself.

- Educational needs. There may be an individual need for further information on their medical condition, medications, educational opportunities, community services, and so on.

- Communication. Speech and communication delays are present due to involvement of facial and tongue muscles.

- Classroom needs and modifications necessary to maximize the child's participation in classroom activity.

Nursing Diagnoses (N.D.)

N.D. 1   Potential for injury (NANDA 1.6.1)* related to inability to control movements, neuromuscular impairment, perceptual and cognitive impairment.

N.D. 2   Potential altered nutrition: less than body requirements (NANDA 1.1.2.2) related to sucking difficulties (infant) and dysphagia.

N.D. 3   Potential for injury (NANDA 1.6.1) related to uncontrolled movements of seizure activity.

N.D. 4   Sensory perceptual alteration: visual. (NANDA 7.2)

N.D. 5   Impaired physical mobility (NANDA 6.1.1.1) related to limited use of limbs. (specify)

N.D. 6   Potential self-care deficit (NANDA 6.5.1, 2, 3, or 4) related to visual impairment.

N.D. 7   Potential diversional activity deficit (NANDA 6.3.1.1) related to effects of limitations on ability to participate in recreational activities.

N.D. 8   Self-care deficit (specify) (NANDA 6.5.1, 2, 3, or 4) related to sensory-motor impairment.

N.D. 9   Activity intolerance (NANDA 6.1.1.2) related to decreased energy and fatigue.

N.D. 10   Self-concept disturbance (NANDA 7.1.1, 7.1.2, 7.1.2.1) related to appearance, immobility, loss of function (specify), secondary to physical disability.

N.D. 11   Impaired verbal communication (NANDA 2.1.1.1) related to impaired ability to articulate words secondary to facial muscle involvement.

N.D. 12   Impaired communication (NANDA 2.1.1.1) related to hearing loss.

N.D. 13   Potential altered health maintenance (NANDA 6.4.2) related to insufficient knowledge of: (specify).

Goals

Prevent injury related to uncontrolled movements. (N.D. 1)

Prevent deformity. (N.D. 1)

Maintain adequate nutrition. (N.D. 2)

Prevent injury related to uncontrolled movements associated with seizure activity. (N.D. 3)

Maintain optimal visual and auditory acuity. (N.D. 4, 6, 12)

Facilitate methods for compensation of vision/hearing loss. (N.D. 4, 6, 12)

Establish/promote locomotion. (N.D. 5)

Maximum independence in self-care activities. (specify). (N.D. 6, 8)

Promote involvement in recreational activity, assist in modification as necessary. (N.D. 7)

Promote rest and relaxation. (N.D. 9)

Promote positive self-concept. (N.D. 10)

Facilitate communication, utilize alternative methods of communication. (N.D. 11, 12)

Health teaching for student/family as appropriate. (N.D. 13)

---

* (See chapter 2, page 38 for explanation of the NANDA approved numerical system.)

Nursing Interventions

Utilize splints, braces, specialized equipment as directed. (N.D. 1, 5)

Employ appropriate range of motion activities to increase limb mobility and/or prevent contractures. (N.D. 1, 5)

Perform postoperative care for student who requires corrective surgery. (N.D. 1)

Provide for safe physical environment. Padding on firm surfaces, use of sturdy equipment, and avoidance of slippery surfaces are needed to avoid injury. (N.D. 1)

Use of appropriate restraints when positioned or when in vehicles. Safety belts and other restraint devices can prevent accidental injurys. (N.D. 1)

Reduce contributing factors to feeding difficulties, promote alternative methods of food preparation. (N.D. 2)

Refer to healthcare provider for assessment of growth patterns as needed. (N.D. 2)

Nursing interventions related to seizures (see chapter on seizures). (N.D. 3)

Screen for visual and auditory acuity annually and refer as appropriate. Maintenance of optimal visual and auditory acuity is essential for learning. (N.D. 4, 6, 12)

Ensure adequate rest before attempting locomotion activity. (N.D. 5)

Administer medications as prescribed. Maintain current medical orders and documentation of medication given. (N.D. 1, 3)

Refer for occupational therapy and physical therapy, and for speech and language, audiological, adaptive physical education, and cognitive assessment as appropriate. Health assessment will often identify needs that can be further assessed by other related services employed in schools. (N.D. 1, 2, 6, 8–10)

Case management: Refer and follow up for healthcare if needed, coordinate service providers. (N.D. 1–4, 13)

Assist student in accommodation for visual impairment in self-care activities. (N.D. 6)

Identify recreational activities of interest and assist in modifications as needed. (N.D. 7)

Assist student in achieving maximum independence in self-care activities. Utilize modifications as necessary. (N.D. 8)

Promote regulated schedules allowing for adequate rest and sleep periods. Observe for evidence of fatigue which may aggrevate symptoms. (N.D. 9)

Support strengths, set realistic goals, encourage appealing appearance, and allow/encourage student to discuss feelings. (N.D. 10)

Utilize alternative methods of communication. (N.D. 11, 12)

Health teaching for student/family as needed related to areas of insufficient knowledge. (N.D. 13)

Expected Student Outcomes

Maintain adequate range of motion. (N.D. 1)

Will not experience injury. (N.D. 1, 3)

Maintain adequate growth patterns. (N.D. 2)

Accommodate for sensory perceptual visual deficits. (N.D. 4)

Acquire locomotion within capabilities (specify). (N.D. 5)

Accommodate for vision deficits in self-care activities. (N.D. 6)

Participate in recreational activities. (N.D. 7)

Demonstrate adaptive methods needed to perform activities of daily living. (N.D. 8)

Student is sufficiently rested. (N.D. 9)

Exhibit behaviors indicating positive self-concept (specify). (N.D. 10)
Is well groomed, clean, and appropriately dressed. (N.D. 10)
Is able to discuss feelings and concerns regarding self. (N.D. 10)
Utilize alternative forms of communication. (N.D. 11, 12)
Actively participate in health behaviors prescribed or desired. (N.D. 13)

Collaborative Problems

Potential complication: contractures
Potential complication: seizures

BIBLIOGRAPHY

Batshaw ML., Perret YM. *Children With Handicaps: A Medical Primer.* Baltimore: Paul H. Brookes
    Publishing, 1981.
Bleck EE. Management of the lower extremities in children who have cerebral palsy. *J Bone Joint Surg* 1990;
    72A (1): 140–144.
Carpenito LJ. *Handbook of Nursing Diagnosis.* Philadelphia: JB Lippincott, 1989.
Carpenito LJ. *Nursing Diagnosis, Application to Clinical Practice.* Philadelphia: JB Lippincott, 1989.
Russman BS, Gage JR. Cerebral palsy. In: *Current Problems in Pediatrics.* Chicago: Year Book Medical
    Publishers, 1989.
Staudt LA, Peacock WJ, Oppenheim, W. The role of selective posterior rhizotomy in the management of
    cerebral palsy. In: *Infants and Young Children.* Frederick, MD: Aspen Publishers, 1990.
Whaley LF, Wong DL. *Nursing Care of Infants and Children.* St. Louis: CV Mosby, 1987.
Wong DL, Whaley LF. *Clinical Manual of Pediatric Nursing.* St. Louis: CV Mosby, 1990.

18 | IHP: Contraceptive Counseling

Kathleen M. Kalb

INTRODUCTION

By the time adolescents reach their senior year in high school, more than half are sexually active.[1] With such a large number of students who have made the decision to become sexually active, the school nurse can help many of them make healthy choices which will minimize the negative impact that early sexual activity may have. One negative consequence of sexual activity is unwanted pregnancy. Although there are some sexually active adolescents who desire to be pregnant, the vast majority do not wish to become so.[2] This leaves a responsibility for those adults who work with adolescents to not only inform the adolescents' choices, but to help these youngsters find their way to resources and methods that will work for their individual needs.

Background

With the onset of puberty both males and females become physically capable of re-production. Pregnancy usually takes place when the ovum of the female is fertilized by the sperm of the male during vaginal/penile sexual intercourse. Contraceptive measures must be taken if pregnancy is to be avoided by the sexually active student.

The decision to become sexually active is a complex one and highly individual. It is impacted by many factors including family standards, peer influence, cultural expectations, and self-esteem.[3-5] Once the decision to be sexually active has been made, the adolescent is at risk for pregnancy, sexually transmitted disease, and AIDS. Since females may ovulate prior to menstruation, it is possible for them to become pregnant without ever having had a menstrual period. It is therefore important that all sexually active individuals have access to information and resources for contraception.

Methods

Contraceptive method depends on the individual student's needs. The most common types are listed below:

Method	Action	Usage
Abstinence	Prevents pregnancy by avoiding genital contact.	Both male and female partners agree to abstain from intercourse.
Condoms	Barrier: prevents sperm from reaching ovum.	Worn by male partner over penis during intercourse.
Spermicide	Kills sperm and other organisms.	Usually inserted into vagina as cream, jelly, foam or vaginal suppositories by female partner during intercourse. May be in lubricant used for condoms.
Combination Pill ("The Pill")	Blood levels of artificial estrogen and progesterone prevent ovulation.	Taken orally by female once daily.
Progestin-only Pill ("Mini-pill")	Prevents ovulation and creates uterine lining nonreceptive to implantation of fertilized ovum.	Taken orally by female once daily.
Progestin-only Subdermal Implants ("Norplant")	Prevents ovulation and creates uterine lining nonreceptive to implantation of fertilized ovum.	Implanted under the skin in six flexible, thin capsules. Usually implanted in upper arm.
Diaphragm	Shallow rubber cup, acts as crude barrier, holds spermicide at opening of cervix to kill sperm.	Placed against cervix in female partner. Used with spermicidal jelly or cream.
Cervical Cap	Like small version of diaphragm, is better barrier due to tighter fit around cervix.	Placed tightly over cervix, used with spermicide.

Method	Action	Usage
IUD	Small device which creates hostile environment for fertilized ovum. May contain hormone to decrease ovulation.	Placed by healthcare provider into uterus. Stays in place until removed by healthcare provider.
Sterilization	Surgical procedure which alters reproductive structures so that sperm or ova are not available to become fertilized	In females fallopian tubes are cut and tied off, therefore preventing egg from reaching sperm. In the male, vas deferens is cut and/or blocked so that sperm cannot mix with seminal fluid.
Fertility Awareness	Familiarization with fertility cycle of female to avoid intercourse during ovulatory phase	Both male and female partners abstain from sexual intercourse during female's fertile days of cycle.

Since there are pluses and minuses for each method as it relates to the individual adolescent, methods must be evaluated in light of the particular student's needs. Some of the essential considerations for each method are listed below:[6]

Method	Considerations
Abstinence	Must sometimes be legitimated for the student, since there may not be peer support to sustain this method. Safest of all methods for preventing both pregnancy and sexually transmitted disease. May be more acceptable to adolescents who are familiar with alternatives to intercourse which demonstrate affection (so called "outercourse").
Condoms	Males may be resistant to using them.[7] Adolescents who choose this as a method must be instructed in their proper use. Girls may need to rehearse how to discuss their use with a male partner.[5] They are readily available over the counter and when used with spermicide are a very effective method. This method has the added advantage of providing protection against sexually transmitted disease.
Spermicides	These are also readily available to adolescents over the counter. They are safe and may be used by females with or without their partner's knowledge. Adolescents must be counseled in their proper use. They afford some protection from sexually transmitted disease, and are very effective when used in conjunction with condoms

Diaphragm	Insertion of the diaphragm must be taught carefully. Use with spermicide must be stressed since "barrier" method is something of a misnomer, and effectiveness depends on use of spermicide concurrently. The adolescent must be a motivated contraceptor, since this method must be inserted every time sexual intercourse occurs in order to be maximally effective.
Contraceptive sponge	Similar considerations as with the diaphragm, but sponge is readily available without a prescription. Insertion should be taught so that it is not inserted improperly and therefore difficult to remove. Spermicide is activated by contact with liquid, so user should be cautioned to wet it prior to insertion.
Combination pill	This is a common choice for adolescent females. It is best used by adolescents who can be responsible for taking the pill daily and who will call with questions regarding side effects. It requires a prescription and a physical exam. This method does not protect against sexually transmitted disease.
Minipills	Although quite effective, these pills are less so than combination pills and are more likely to cause spotting. They may be a good choice where medical history precludes estrogen compounds for the adolescent.
Norplant	This is an appropriate method for adolescents who desire reliable birth control but who are not reliable pill-takers. There may be some spotting initially. Adolescents may find the cost prohibitive, but since it is intended as a 5-year method, the cost is comparable to other methods in the long run. Insertion and removal both require a minor surgical procedure using local anesthetic which must be performed by a health practitioner.
Intrauterine Device	Seldom the method of choice for an adolescent, it may cause increased likelihood of menstrual cramping, bleeding, and pelvic inflammatory disease.
Sterilization	Almost never an appropriate choice for an adolescent, since this is considered a permanent method of contraception.
Fertility awareness	This is good information to have, but in only the most reliable hands is this a truly effective method of contraception and therefore not likely to be the appropriate choice for an adolescent.

INDIVIDUALIZED HEALTHCARE PLAN

History

Update the student's history with particular emphasis on the sexual history. Taking a sexual history is a sensitive and delicate process. The nurse who wants to be effective as a contraceptive counselor needs to be comfortable with sensitive topics and aware of the adolescent's emotional boundaries.

A thorough sexual history includes gathering information that will impact the choice of contraceptive method. Suggested questions follow.

Review of Systems

(General review of systems) In addition, ask the female student considering oral contraceptive use:

Has anyone in your family had a heart attack, stroke, heart disease or high blood pressure? If yes, who was it? How were/are they treated for that condition?

Have you had high blood pressure yourself? Heart disease? Are you being treated for either of these conditions?

Do you or anyone in your family have diabetes? If yes, how is this being treated? Do you (or your family member) see a specialist for diabetes?

Are you taking any medications? Which ones? How often and in what doses? Why are you taking these medications? (Many medications interact with birth control pills and can reduce their effectiveness.)

Are you taking any over-the-counter medicines, like pain killers or diet pills?

If the student indicates regular doses of analgesic for headache, ask questions to determine whether the headaches are vascular in nature, since vascular headaches may be precursors to stroke.

- How often do you get these headaches?
- Where does it hurt? (one side, both sides, temple, occipital area, etc.)
- What makes them better?
- Do certain things seem to make them worse or cause them?
- Do any members of your family have migraine headaches?

Menstrual History (female students)

How old were you when you started your period?
How often do you have a period?
Do you ever miss periods?
Do you have cramps with your periods? (Cramping may mean ovulatory cycles.)
Have you ever been pregnant? If yes, what did you decide to do about the pregnancy?
When did your last period start? Was it a normal one?
Have you had sex since your last period? If yes, did you use any birth control?

Coital History (male and female students)

How old were you when you first had sex?
How old was your partner? Did you want to have sex?

Assessment

Current Status

Current sexual activity:
Do you ever have sex now?
How many partners have you had in the last six months?
How old were they?
Was/were your partner(s) male? Female?
What kind of sexual contact did you have with your partner(s) (Anal, vaginal, oral)?
Are you comfortable with your decision to be sexually active? If not, what can you tell me about that?
What are you using for birth control? Are you using it every time you have sex?

The nature of these questions is obviously very sensitive. The nurse should provide privacy[8] and establish a solid rapport with the student before asking questions that are sexually explicit.[9] If the student seems reluctant to answer these questions, it may help to explain that the information will help you know whether (s)he is at risk for sexually transmitted diseases and will allow you to recommend contraception that will work for that student. If there is still hesitation on the part of the student, it may be best to either postpone the appointment or refer the student to another counselor.

Physical Assessment

The sexually active student should be referred to a physician or nurse practitioner for a complete physical exam.

Psychological/Emotional Assessment

While interviewing the student and taking the history, note the student's attitude toward his/her sexuality and sexual activity. Determine whether there will be social or family support for effective contraception.
Some questions which may give you clues:

Are any of your friends sexually active? What do they use for birth control?
Are any of your friends pregnant or parents of a baby?
Did anyone in your family have a baby while still a teenager? If yes, who was it?

If the student seems ambivalent about sexual activity or pregnancy, refer to appropriate resources for decision-making counseling.

Nursing Diagnoses (N.D.)

N.D. 1   Altered sexuality patterns (NANDA 3.3)* related to initiation of sexual intercourse
N.D. 2   Potential disturbance in personal identity (NANDA 7.1.3) related to behavior inconsistent with personal values
N.D. 3   Knowledge deficit (NANDA 8.1.1) related to fertility patterns

---

* (See chapter 2, page 38 for explanation of the NANDA approved numerical system.)

Goals

The school nurse will:
1. Assess the student's need for contraception and refer for physical exam if student is sexually active.
2. Assess student's risk for sexually transmitted disease and refer as appropriate.
3. Assess the student's knowledge base regarding sexual activity, risks, and contraception in order to assist with choice of contraceptive method.

Nursing Interventions

Update history as above to provide foundation for nursing assessment and information for referral. (N.D. 1–3)

Listen carefully to the student's primary concern(s) so they may be addressed first. (N.D. 1–3)

Formulate list of resources for sexuality related services. (Ideally these providers will be particularly sensitive to issues of adolescent sexuality.) (N.D. 1)

Educate the student as indicated in regard to risk factors for sexually transmitted disease and unwanted pregnancy. (N.D. 3)

Review the minor consent laws for the state in which you are practicing, so that appropriate counseling and notifications may be made with optimal regard for confidentiality. (N.D. 1–3)

Explain all methods and risk/benefits of each. Educate student regarding proper management of contraception method chosen. Answer questions thoroughly and respectfully. (N.D. 3)

Follow up with student on a monthly or bimonthly basis to determine emotional status and risk behavior. (N.D. 1–3)

Expected Student Outcomes

The student will be comfortable with his or her current level of sexual activity as indicated by self report.

The sexually active student will avoid sexually transmitted diseases and unwanted pregnancy.

The student will demonstrate, by report, adequate knowledge of risk factors for sexually transmitted disease and unwanted pregnancy.

The student will comply with suggested follow-up activities, including suggested referrals as well as meetings with the school nurse.

REFERENCES

1. Davis S. Pregnancy in adolescents. *Pediatr Clin North Am* 1989; 36 (3): 665–80.
2. Shea JA, et al. Factors associated with adolescent use of family planning clinics. *Am J Public Health* 1984; 74 (11): 1227–30.
3. Hatcher R, et al. *Contraceptive Technology 1990-1992.* 15th rev ed. New York: Irvington Publishers, 1990.
4. Neinstein LS. Contraception. In: *Adolescent Healthcare, A Practical Guide.* Baltimore: Urban and Schwarzenberg, 1984: 399–403.
5. Spain J. *Sexual, Contraceptive, and Pregnancy Choices: Counseling Adolescents.* New York: Gardner Press, 1988.

6. Howard M, McCabe JB. Helping teenagers postpone sexual involvement. *Family Planning Perspectives* 1990; 22 (1): 21–26.
7. Freeman EW, et al. Adolescent contraceptive use: comparisons of male and female attitudes and information. *Am J Public Health* 1980; 70 (8): 790–97.
8. Worth D. Sexual decision-making and AIDS: Why condom promotion among vulnerable women is likely to fail. *Studies in Family Planning* 1989; 20 (6): 301–06.
9. Smith PB, et al. Social and affective factors associated with adolescent pregnancy. *J School Health* 1982; (Feb): 90-93.

BIBLIOGRAPHY

Croxton TA, Churchill SR, Fellin P. Counseling minors without parental consent. *Child Welfare* 1988; 67 (1): 3–14.
Gorosh VA. Predicting school nurse involvement in meeting sexuality related needs of youth in New Jersey. *Public Health Reports* 1981; 96 (4): 363–68.
Zabin LS, Clark SD. Why they delay: a study of teenage family planning clinic patients. *Family Planning Perspectives* 1981; 13 (5): 205–17.

19 | IHP: Cystic Fibrosis

Cynthia K. Silkworth

INTRODUCTION

Cystic fibrosis (CF) is a chronic health condition that affects about 1:2,000 births in the Caucasian population, 1:17,000 in the Afro-American population, and is rare in the Asian and Native American populations.[1]

The disease is usually recognized in infancy or early childhood with the exact symptoms and severity of symptoms varying from person to person. In the United States, CF affects about 30,000 people, making it the most common fatal inherited disease.[2] Fifteen years ago, few children with CF lived past the age of six. Today, because of improvements in diagnosis and medical management, many persons with CF live into their mid-twenties and older.[1]

Pathophysiology

Cystic fibrosis is an inherited autosomal recessive disorder which affects the exocrine glands of the body. In CF, the mucus-producing glands fail to produce normal free-flowing fluid. Instead, they produce thick, sticky mucus that interferes with proper functioning of body organs.

In the lungs, the sticky thick mucus causes problems by obstructing the airways and coating the cilia, which impairs normal respiration and cleansing and clearing of dust and pathogens. This leads to repeated respiratory infections and chronic lung disease. Almost every person with CF will eventually develop lung disease.

In the pancreas, the sticky, thick mucus blocks the passageways that carry enzymes into the intestine. As a result, proteins and fats cannot be properly digested, absorbed, and utilized by the body. This problem with malabsorption can cause poor weight gain and growth despite having a large appetite. It can also cause frequent, large, foul-smelling fatty stools, abdominal pain/discomfort, and excessive gas.

Cystic fibrosis also affects the sweat glands. Every person with CF loses more than the normal amount of salt in their sweat. However, this rarely causes problems since there is usually enough salt in the diet to cover the amount lost in the sweat. Persons with cystic fibrosis can be at risk for heat exhaustion and dehydration, especially during strenuous exercise, hot weather, or fevers.

The reproductive system can also be affected by CF. In males, the vas deferens may become blocked by thick mucus which does not allow the sperm to pass. In females, the mucus produced by the vaginal exocrine glands may be so thick and sticky that the sperm cannot move through to reach the egg. In addition, women with

CF may ovulate less frequently and may have more irregular menstrual cycles, especially when they are having lung problems.[1]

Cystic Fibrosis Management

Persons with CF receive treatment interventions which are based on their particular condition.[2] Interventions generally include:
- chest physical therapy—helps loosen mucus in the lungs and keep the air passages open—done manually or by machine.
- physical activity—helps loosen mucus and stimulates coughing.
- aerosol therapy—decongestants, bronchodilators, antibiotics, and mucolytics.
- antibiotic therapy—helps fight respiratory infections.
- dietary management—vitamins, pancreatic enzyme replacement, and a well-balanced diet, with nutritional supplements as needed.
- child and family education—CF education program.
- counseling—assistance with coping, individual and/or family.

INDIVIDUALIZED HEALTHCARE PLAN

History

- when the diagnosis was made
- severity of the student's CF: lungs, digestive system, and other affects
- student's prognosis
- healthcare providers involved in the management of the student's CF and regular health maintenance
- CF management plan (past and current)—chest physical therapy, physical activity, aerosol therapy, antibiotic therapy, dietary management, child and family education, counseling
- student's participation in the development and implementation of the CF management plan
- assistance needed to implement the CF management plan
- compliance with CF management plan
- effectiveness of CF management plan—student's, parents'/guardian's, and healthcare provider's perspectives
- growth pattern
- bowel elimination pattern
- past history of respiratory infections
- involvement of support persons/systems
- past experiences with hospitalizations
- past experiences with heat exhaustion and dehydration
- experience with self-care at home—medications, chest physical therapy, physical activity, dietary management
- past school attendance patterns—specifically the number of days missed due to CF
- participation in regular school activities
- participation in regular physical education activities
- participation in regular exercise program—sports or leisure, school-related or non-school-related

Assessment

- knowledge about CF—student, parents/guardians, and teachers
- student's perception of his/her health and CF
- parents'/guardian's perception of the student's health and CF
- current height and weight
- current daily nutritional intake
- daily activity schedule—including CF management measures
- student's locus of control—health, school, family, and activities of daily living
- ability to do self-care—medications, chest physical therapy, physical activity, and dietary management
- motivation to do self-care
- barriers to self-care
- decision-making skills

Nursing Diagnoses (N.D.)

N.D. 1   (Potential for) alteration in respiratory function (NANDA 1.5.1.3)* related to CF.

N.D. 2   (Potential for) ineffective airway clearance (NANDA 1.5.1.2) related to CF.

N.D. 3   (Potential for) respiratory infections (NANDA 1.2.1.1) due to CF.

N.D. 4   (Potential for) alteration in nutrition, less than body requirements, (NANDA 1.1.2.2) related to CF.

N.D. 5   (Potential for) alteration in bowel elimination pattern (NANDA 1.3.1.2) (frequent, large, foul smelling, fatty stools) related to CF.

N.D. 6   (Potential for) injury (heat exhaustion, dehydration) (NANDA 1.6.1) related to CF.

N.D. 7   (Potential for) noncompliance (NANDA 5.2.1.1) with prescribed CF management measures related to:
- knowledge deficit.
- improper administration of medication or chest physical therapy.
- denial of need for treatments.
- perceived ineffectiveness of management measures.
- inaccessibility of time and place to carry out management measures.

N.D. 8   (Potential for) alteration in student role (NANDA 3.2.1) related to:
- recurrent absences from school because of respiratory infections.
- recurrent absence from class due to need for management measures during the school day.

Goals

Maintain optimal respiratory function and airway clearance. (N.D. 1, 2)
Reduce blockage of airways. (N.D. 1, 2)
Prevent blockage of airways. (N.D. 1, 2)
Prevent respiratory infections. (N.D. 3)
Increase knowledge about how CF affects his/her lungs. (N.D. 1–3)
Increase knowledge about CF and CF management measures. (N.D. 1–8)
Maintain good nutritional management. (N.D. 4)

---

*(See chapter 2, page 38 for explanation of NANDA approved numerical system.)

Maintain adequate growth and weight gain pattern. (N.D. 4)

Maintain appropriate diet and enzyme supplements. (N.D. 4, 5)

Maintain near-normal, well-formed stools. (N.D. 5)

Prevent heat exhaustion and dehydration. (N.D. 6)

Compliance with prescribed CF management measures. (N.D. 7)

Good school attendance pattern. (N.D. 8)

Management measures are done with the least educational disruption as possible. (N.D. 8)

Nursing Interventions

Set guidelines for seeking assistance. (N.D. 1, 2)

- occurrence of symptoms of airway blockage: frequent or lingering cough, excessive sputum production, intermittent wheezing, difficulty breathing, difficulty exercising, repeated lung infections
- indications of flare-ups or worsening of lung problems: increase in cough or wheezing, increase in sputum production, decrease in exercise tolerance, increase in fatigue or feeling tired, fever, poor appetite or weight loss, decrease in lung function as measured by pulmonary function tests
- notifying parents/guardians
- notifying healthcare providers

Obtain medication and orders for specialized healthcare procedures, and authorization for any management measures that need to be done at school from healthcare providers and parents/guardians. (N.D. 1–2, 4, 5)

In-service teachers and other appropriate school staff. (N.D. 1–8)

- what CF is and how it affects the body
- the student's specific health status
- management measures that will need to be done at school
- the importance of coughing and management of the disruption that might occur in the classroom due to coughing
- symptoms that would indicate the student may have airway blockage and the need to inform you if they occur
- importance of maintaining a well-balanced diet
- need for pancreatic enzymes for meals and snacks
- allowing snacks to be eaten in the classroom and/or hallways between classes
- allowing the student to use the drinking fountain as often as he/she feels a need to
- symptoms of salt depletion and dehydration
- need for flexible educational programming (daily schedule adjustments, use of the bathroom, past and advance assignments, hospital and home tutoring, temporary classroom and physical education adjustments)
- encourage teachers to ask questions or raise concerns if they have them

Assist parents/guardians to talk with their child's teachers about their child's CF. (N.D. 1–8)

- what CF is and how it affects their child
- CF management measures needed at home and school
- presence of symptoms which indicate that parents/guardians need to be contacted
- need for flexible educational programming

Assist the parents/guardians to maintain current immunization status against childhood diseases for their child, including: measles, mumps, rubella, diptheria, tetanus, pertussis, and haemophilus influenzae. (N.D. 3)

Encourage and assist parents/guardians to provide annual influenza immunization for their child. (N.D. 3)

Avoid *unnecessary* exposure to persons who have communicable diseases, especially those that affect the respiratory system. (N.D. 3)
- regular school attendance should be encouraged
- normal, healthy interaction with other children and the surrounding world should be encouraged.
- contact with someone who actually has influenza is an example of *unnecessary* exposure.

Assist the student to administer his/her prescribed management measures. (N.D. 1–8)
- medications are easily accessible to the student when they need them
- self-medication program
- private area and assistance in doing chest physical therapy with the least classroom disruption necessary

Monitor administration of medications and other management measures and reinforce proper techniques as needed. (N.D. 1–7)

Provide health education opportunities—individual or group instruction. (N.D. 1–8)
- how the body systems work
- how CF affects the body
- importance of coughing and exercise
- need for and importance of a well-balanced diet
- need for and importance of maintaing adequate water and salt intake
- symptoms that may be caused by blockage of the airways
- indications of flare-ups or worsening of lung problems
- measures used to clear the airways of obstructions and to treat or prevent infections—what they are and how they work
- medications used to manage his/her CF and what each medication does
- proper technique for administering medications

Encourage coughing to help loosen mucus and clear airways. (N.D. 1, 2)
Encourage physical exercise. (N.D. 1, 2)
- school and non-school-related
- may need extra fluids and salt when exercising strenuously or during hot weather
Encourage good hand-washing practices and reinforce proper technique as needed. (N.D. 3)

Encourage the student to eat regular, well-balanced meals with pancreatic enzyme supplements. (N.D. 4, 5)

Assist the students to eat any snacks that are needed during the school day. (N.D. 4, 5)
- in the classroom or between classes
- extra supply in health office in case snack is forgotten at home

Assist the student, parents/guardians and healthcare providers to determine the amount of pancreatic enzyme needed for good absorption of food; for near-normal, well-formed stools; and for adequate weight gain. (N.D. 4,5)

Monitor height and weight gain at specified intervals of time (such as every three months). (N.D. 4)

Provide the student easy access to a bathroom at school where he/she can have privacy. (N.D. 5)

During periods of increased sweating (hot weather, strenuous exercise, or fever), encourage the student to drink more fluids and increase salt intake. (N.D. 6)
- allow the student to drink water as often as he/she feels the need to
- encourage the student to eat salty snacks and/or extra salt on his/her food at lunch (unless contraindicated by healthcare provider)

Monitor the student for ablility to maintain adequate fluid and salt intake. (N.D. 6)

Monitor the student for symptoms of salt depletion: fatigue, weakness, fever, muscle cramps, abdominal pain, vomiting, dehydration, heat stroke. (N.D. 6)

Discuss CF management measures with the student. (N.D. 7)

- need for prescribed treatment measures
- importance of his/her participation in implementing the measures
- how school measures fit in with management measures at home and with his/her healthcare provider
- effectiveness of prescribed management measures
- benefits of compliance
- consequences of noncompliance
- motivators and barriers to compliance

Assist the student to choose and implement motivators to compliance with prescribed management measures. (N.D. 7)

Remove as many barriers to compliance as possible. (N.D. 7)

Monitor attendance patterns and reasons for absences. (N.D. 8)

Discuss the need for regular school and classroom attendance with the student, parents/guardians, and healthcare providers. (N.D. 8)

Monitor academic performance—referral to child study team as needed. (N.D. 8)

Expected Student Outcomes

The student will:
- describe what CF is and how it affects his/her body. (N.D. 1–8)
- describe symptoms that may indicate that airways are becoming blocked. (N.D. 1, 2)
- list and describe management measures he/she uses to reduce blockage of the airways. (N.D. 1, 2)
- list ways to help prevent blockage of the airways. (N.D. 1, 2)
- list indicators of flare-ups or worsening lung problems. (N.D. 1, 2)
- use coughing as a necessary, healthy way to keep the lungs and airways clear of mucus. (N.D. 1, 2)
- participate in regular exercise/physical activities. (N.D. 1, 2)
- name ways he/she can prevent respiratory infections. (N.D. 3)
- be immunized against childhood diseases. (N.D. 3)
- receive an annual influenza immunization. (N.D. 3)

- avoid unnecessary exposure to persons with communicable diseases. (N.D. 3)
- eat well-balanced diet. (N.D. 4, 5)
- eat snacks as needed to supplement diet. (N.D. 4)
- take the prescribed amount of pancreatic enzymes and vitamins with meals and snacks. (N.D. 4, 5)
- demonstrate adequate growth and weight gain. (N.D. 4)
- have near normal, well-formed stools. (N.D. 5)
- increase intake of water and salt during periods of increased sweating (hot weather, strenuous excerise, or fever). (N.D. 6)
- list the medications he/she is taking. (N.D. 1–4, 7)
- describe how his/her medication works. (N.D. 1–4, 7)
- take his/her medications as prescribed. (N.D. 1–4, 7)
- demonstrate proper technique for administering medications. (N.D. 1–4, 7)
- perform or assist in performing his/her chest physical therapy correctly. (N.D. 1, 2, 7)
- describe benefits of complying with his/her CF management measures. (N.D. 7)
- describe consequences of not complying with his/her CF management measures. (N.D. 7)
- list motivators and barriers to compliance with his/her CF management measures. (N.D. 7)
- participate in developing and implementing the CF management measures at school. (N.D. 7)
- have a normal school attendance pattern. (N.D. 8)
- have a normal classroom attendance pattern. (N.D. 8)
- have minimal disruptions in his/her educational program due to CF and CF management measures. (N.D. 8)

REFERENCES

1. Cunningham JC, Taussig LM. *A Guide to Cystic Fibrosis for Parents and Children.* Bethesda, MD: Cystic Fibrosis Foundation, 1989.
2. Cystic Fibrosis Foundation. *The Genetics of Cystic Fibrosis.* Bethesda, MD: Cystic Fibrosis Foundation, 1987.

BIBLIOGRAPHY

Cystic Fibrosis Foundation. *Cystic Fibrosis: A Summary of Symptoms, Diagnosis and Treatment.* Rockville, MD: Cystic Fibrosis Foundation, 1984.

Cystic Fibrosis Foundation. *An Introduction to Cystic Fibrosis.* Bethesda, MD: Cystic Fibrosis Foundation, 1987.

Cystic Fibrosis Foundation. *A Teachers' Guide to Cystic Fibrosis.* Rockville, MD: Cystic Fibrosis Foundation, 1985.

Lewiston NJ. Cystic fibrosis. In: Hobbs N, Perrin JM, eds. *Issues in the Care of Children with Chronic Health Conditions.* San Francisco: Jossey Bass Publishers, 1985: 196–213.

Minnesota Department of Health. *Guidelines of Care for Children with Special Healthcare Needs: Cystic Fibrosis.* Minneapolis, MN: Minn Dept of Health, 1990.

20 | Cytomegalovirus

Wanda R. Miller

INTRODUCTION

Cytomegalovirus (CMV) is a common virus in the herpesvirus family. Most people who are infected with CMV are unaware of the infection and have no signs of the disease. Throughout the world, CMV antibodies can be found in 40 to 100 percent of the adult population, whereas in the United States the rate is estimated to be 50 percent of adults. [1,2] Cytomegalovirus is found in the urine or saliva of only 0.5 to 2.2 percent of the newborn population, [1-3] but by six months of age 10 to 13 percent [1] and by three years of age up to 30 percent of all children in the United States have acquired CMV infections. [4] The congenital disease affects infants in utero, whose mothers have contracted CMV during the current pregnancy, the most severely. Between 30 to 40 percent of primary infections occurring in the first half of pregnancy result in congenital infection to the newborn. In 1987 an estimated 38,000 infants had congenital CMV. Of those infants who become infected, 10 to 20 percent, or one out of every 1,000 children born, will have developmental, neurologic, or audiological symptoms of CMV at birth. [3,5,6] The resulting neurologic symptoms range from unilateral hearing loss to severe mental retardation. Individuals who are immunosuppressed due to drugs for medical treatments, such as chemotherapy or organ transplants, or who have immune deficiency diseases are also at risk for developing pneumonia and retinitis infections from exposure to CMV. Cytomegalovirus antibodies have also been detected in high rates in homosexual males. [7]

The effects of severe congenital CMV are present at birth and include microcephaly, intracerebral calcifications, hepatosplenomegaly, chorioretinitis, and petechial or purpuric rash. Symptomatic infants are almost always born to mothers who acquired their primary CMV infection during the first half of their pregnancy. However, as many as 95 percent of congenitally infected infants are asymptomatic at birth. Ten to fifteen percent of these asymptomatic children will develop varying degrees of sensorineural deafness, seizure disorders, mental retardation, and learning disabilities during their preschool years. [3,8] Congenital CMV infection may occur despite substantial immunity in mothers, as a result of recurrent infection, which is most often due to reactivation of latent virus. The initial immunity of the mother provides a beneficial effect by reducing the virulence of the infection on the fetus. [6] Infection acquired at birth from maternal cervical excretion usually does not result in neurologic symptoms.

Most postnatal infections are asymptomatic. The potential exists for some of these infections to produce subtle effects, the long-term results of which have not been well documented. [6] In populations in which breastfeeding is common and a high proportion of mothers are seropositive, human milk is an important source of horizontal transmission of CMV to infants less than one year of age. [1] Intimate contact between mother and child is also conducive to the horizontal transmission of the virus. Familial exposure to young infants is another factor in horizontal transmission between women and children. Children in the home caused an increased seroconversion rate for women between pregnancies. Clearly, female teachers, nurses, and other staff are at no greater risk for acquiring CMV infection in the workplace than are young women in the community. It is doubtful that the risk of acquiring primary CMV infection in school personnel is increased sufficiently to warrant the many pressures placed on schools to design isolation procedures for infants known to be infected with the virus as a means of controlling horizontal infections. [2] Newborns and older infants who are infected with CMV excrete large quantities of virus into their urine and saliva [2] for many months and may continue to excrete the virus for many years following a primary infection. Therefore, schools must establish careful hand-washing procedures and diapering techniques for all children. Given these precautions for exposure to any child's bodily fluids, trained personnel should be able to avoid exposure to the virus. Studies have supported that there are no statistically significant differences in either prevalence of CMV antibodies or number of seroconversions among a group of nurses caring for infants when compared with a control group of women without such duties. [9]

The virus is readily transmitted in groups of young children of similar age. A potential vehicle for transmission was identified by the recovery of CMV from toys that had been mouthed by toddlers. The highest rate of infection occurred in children between one and three years of age, who have a high rate of oral shedding of CMV. [5] The infection rate was lowest in infants under 12 months of age. [1,5]

A CMV vaccine has been developed and is being tested in human subjects but this vaccine has not been released for general use. An experimental CMV immune globulin has been developed and is being used effectively for seronegative transplant patients. Immune globulin is also being investigated for use in preventing transmission by blood transfusion.

Pathophysiology

The virus is excreted in urine, saliva, cervical secretions (more frequently as pregnancy progresses), breast milk, and semen, and can be transmitted from the mother to child in utero. There is no indication that CMV is transmitted via respiratory droplet. The virus can, in fact, be isolated from the urine for many months and even years after birth. Salivary and fecal excretion of virus is also detectable, but for shorter periods. Nearly all children who excrete CMV in saliva also excrete the virus in their urine, but less than half of the urine shedders also excrete CMV in saliva. CMV has been recovered from fomites and caretakers' hands for up to 30 minutes after saliva contamination. In horizontal transmission of CMV a syndrome resembling infectious mononucleosis may occur, characterized by fever, sore throat, fatigue, and swollen glands. It is distinguishable from mononucleosis by the absence of heterophile antibodies, and is frequently misdiagnosed. In severe congenital CMV most infants have some degree of microcephaly, and jaundice, massive hepatosplenomegaly associated with CNS signs (lethargy, convulsions), and a petechial-purpuric rash are present. Some infants also demonstrate chorioretinitis and cerebral calcification. Surviving infants are usually severely mentally and physically handicapped. Anemia, thrombocytopenia, and hyperbilirubinemia are usually present.

CMV must be differentiated from other causes of jaundice, in particular toxoplasmosis (generalized calcification), herpetic neonatal infection (vesicular skin lesions), generalized coxsackievirus infection (myocarditis predominates), hemolytic disease, and bacterial sepsis. In the older child pneumonia must be differentiated from *Pneumocystis carinii* infection.

INDIVIDUALIZED HEALTHCARE PLAN

History

Since the maternal disease is asymptomatic, the history is of little value.

Assessment

Assessment is made through medical diagnosis. Virus isolation from a neonate is the best test for detecting congenital CMV infection. These tests must be performed within three weeks of age to avoid confusion between congenital and horizontal infections. However, elevated titers of immunoglobulin M antibodies detected by radioimmunoassay (RIA-IgM) and an ELISA technique CMV-specific IgM level can be of prognostic importance indicating abnormalities that may appear later in the child's life.

Nursing Diagnoses (N.D.)

N.D. 1 Alteration in physical regulation due to the potential for infection from cytomegalovirus. (NANDA 1.2.1.1.)*

N.D. 2 Alteration in cognitive learning due to CMV resulting in microcephaly and cerebral calcification.

N.D. 3 Potential for sensory alteration in hearing acuity due to CMV. (NANDA 7.2)

Goals

Reduce horizontal transmission of CMV to other students and staff. (N.D. 1)
Integrate student into the least restrictive classroom setting. (N.D. 2)
Identify any auditory loss at the earliest indication. (N.D. 3)

Nursing Interventions

Provide staff in-service in the care of bodily fluids. Identify urine, saliva, and feces as the bodily fluids that may transmit CMV in the school setting. (N.D. 1)

Provide staff in-service in safe handling of diapers. (N.D. 1)

Provide staff and student in-service in proper hand-washing techniques before eating, after toileting, and after diaper changes or toilet care. (N.D. 1)

---

* (See chapter 2, page 38 for explanation of the NANDA approved numerical system.)

Provide staff information about the ability to inactivate CMV on fomites with alcohol and 1:100 strength chlorine bleach. (N.D. 1)

Provide the classroom teacher with information about the level of neurologic sequelae based on the medical report. (N.D. 2)

Determine if the student is still shedding virus and if so from which routes. (N.D. 2)

In-service the teacher in the preventive measures of transmission and encourage the teacher to maintain the procedures with this child and all other children at all times. (N.D. 2)

Establish a baseline audiometric record of the child's hearing. (N.D. 3)

Develop a periodic monitoring schedule for the purpose of comparison with the baseline data. (N.D. 3)

If a hearing loss develops, assist the parent to obtain ENT and audiological consult to ensure the highest level of hearing acuity possible. (N.D. 3)

If amplification is needed, develop a daily system to review the effectiveness of the hearing aide and to replace batteries and obtain repairs as needed. (N.D. 3)

Expected Student Outcomes

Students and staff wash hands using a correct procedure and at appropriate time. (N.D. 1)

Horizontal transmission of CMV is controlled and reduced. (N.D. 1)

Student is included in the regular classroom. (N.D. 2)

Students hear within the normal range or have amplification. (N.D. 3)

REFERENCES

1. Pass RF, Stagno S, Dworsky ME. Excretion of cytomegalovirus in mothers: observations after delivery of congenitally infected and normal infants. *J Infect Dis* 1982; 146: 1–6.
2. Dworsky ME, Welch K, Cassady G, Stagno S. Occupational risk for primary cytomegalovirus infection among pediatric healthcare workers. *N Engl J Med* 1983; 309(16): 950–53.
3. Griffiths PD, Stagno S, Pass RF, Smith RJ, Alford CA Jr. Congential cytomegalovirus infection: diagnostic and prognostic significance of the detection of specific immunoglobulin M antibodies in cord serum. *Pediatrics* 1982; 69(5): 544–49.
4. Alford CA, Stagno S, Pass RF, Huang ES. Epidemiology of cytomegalovirus. In: Nahmias AJ, ed. *The Human Herpesviruses: An Interdisciplinary Perspective.* New York: Elsevier, 1981: 159–71.
5. Adler SP. Cytomegalovirus transmission among children in day care, their mothers and caretakers. *Pediatr Infect Dis J* 1988; 7 (4): 279–85.
6. Stagno S, Pass RF, Dworsky ME, Henderson RE, Moore EG, Walton PD, Alford CA. Congenital cytomegalovirus infection: the relative importance of primary and recurrent maternal infection. *N Engl J Med* 1982; 306 (16): 945–49.
7. Drew WL, Mintz L, Miner RC, et al. Prevalence of cytomegalovirus infection in homosexual men. *J Infect Dis* 1981; 143: 188–92.
8. Whaley L, Wong D. *Nursing Care of Infants and Children.* St. Louis: CV Mosby, 1983: 408–09.
9. Ahlfors K, Ivarsson SA, Johnsson T, Renmarker K. Risk of cytomegalovirus infection in nurses and congenital infection in their offspring. *Acta Paediatr Scand* 1981; 70: 819–23.

IHP: Depression/Suicide

Susan I. Simandl Will

INTRODUCTION

Depression, suicide attempts, and suicide completions are increasing in child and adolescent populations. The social, educational, and life-endangering aspects of depression and suicide are causing school personnel to become more aware of students at risk and develop strategies to identify and intervene with these students. As a healthcare provider in the school setting, the school nurse has a significant role with students experiencing depression or suicidal behaviors. This role includes both the identification and referral for students at risk as well as ongoing case management. In addition, a significant role exists for the nurse to participate in school-wide prevention strategies of education about depression, stress, stress management, and self-esteem.

Depression

Depression is one of several mood disorders (affective disorders), which can affect infants, children, and adolescents.[1, 2] Since 1970 DSM III-R criteria have been used for classification of depression as a psychiatric illness and require at least five of the following symptoms: 1) depressed mood, 2) loss of interest or pleasure, 3) significant weight loss or gain (more than 5 percent of body weight in one month or

failure to thrive), 4) insomnia or hypersomnia, 5) psychomotor agitation or retardation, 6) fatigue or loss of energy, 7) feelings of worthlessness, excessive or inappropriate guilt, 8) diminished concentration, or 9) recurrent thoughts of death, suicidal ideation, plan for suicide or a suicide attempt. The symptoms need to be present over time, a minimum of two weeks. In addition, possible organic disorders which can mimic depressive symptoms (brain tumors, brain disorders) as well as the possibility of abuse or neglect or chemical abuse or personality disorder need to be ruled out.[1, 3]

Incidence of depression in the preschool population is less than 1 percent.[1] In school-age children the rate is 2 to 5 percent.[2] The adolescent years show an increase in the rate to 5 to 7 percent, giving adolescents a rate experienced by the adult population (7 percent).[1, 3]

The probability of a student having a diagnosis of an affective disorder increases when the child or adolescent has a family member with an affective disorder. Affective disorders exist in 20 to 37 percent of the population who are related to an adult with an affective disorder.[3] Seldom, however, does the adolescent's disorder present in the same ways as that of the adult relative.[3]

Depression affects the student's ability to participate in their educational program. Untreated depression can impair social skills, disrupt the acquisition of age-appropriate competencies and slow down cognitive development.[2] Because depression can impair academic progress and success, exploring the possibility of special education (PL 94–142) assistance will be necessary.

Contemporary treatment of child and adolescent depressive disorders includes a variety of psychotherapy approaches, and may include medication. Psychotherapy can be a combination of crisis management, cognitive therapy, behavior therapy, family therapy, social skill training, and family education. Medications (tricyclic antidepressants, monoamine oxidase inhibitors, lithium carbonate, and others) may be used in conjunction with psychotherapy. Tricyclic antidepressants are not approved by the FDA for treating children under 12 years old. Data from pharmacologic research regarding the effects of antidepressant medication in young children is controversial and has not yielded clear recommendations. Often because of overdose concerns, potentially effective dosages are frequently not prescribed.[1,2] Yet, a large number of children recover from their depression when treated with antidepressants and, paradoxically, children seem to be responsive to placebos.[2] Medication is more likely to be prescribed for depressed adolescents than for preadolescent children.

Treatment of severely depressed youth may include hospital management. Electroconvulsive therapy is rarely used.

Outcomes for children and adolescents with a depressive disorder can vary. Some can show residual impairment in social functioning and learning for an indefinite time.[2] Of the children and adolescents treated for depression 60 percent will have another major episode before the end of

adolescence.[2] Up to 20 percent of children with depression will develop bipolar disorder (manic-depressive disorder).[2]

Suicide

Until the 1960s, adolescent suicides were rare events (2 percent of all completed suicides); now adolescent suicide represents 15 percent of all completed suicides.[4] Suicide is the second leading cause of death (after accidents) in adolescents.[4] Between 1961 and 1975, the completed suicide rate in adolescents increased 124 percent.[5] Between 1970 and 1980, the rate increased 40 percent.[6] The rate for males increased by 50 percent during this time period and the female rate increased 2 percent.[6]

Suicide is attempted at least thirty to fifty times more often than it is completed.[5] Many attempts by high school age students are silent or hidden by apparent accidental causes. No one may suspect suicide unless or until the injury is severe and then the student may hide the suicidal nature of the injury with deception. Among high school students there are almost 350 attempts for every completed suicide and 3 percent of high school students attempt suicide each month.[7] Ten percent of suicide attempters will eventually succeed.[8]

Epidemiology research has identified characteristics and patterns of adolescent suicides that identify some trends as to when, how, and to some degree why suicide occurs. A seasonal pattern shows the rate is highest in the fall and winter and lowest in the spring and summer. The months from September to February show a 25 to 40 percent higher rate of suicide than March to August.[5] Familiar surroundings become the site for 70 percent of suicides.[5]

In suicide completions among the 15- to 24-year-old age group, firearms represent the most frequent method (55 percent), hanging is the second method (16 to

19 percent) and overdose (poisoning) the third most frequent method (14 percent). In the 10- to 14-year-old age group, firearms represent 47 percent, hanging 45 percent, and overdose (poisoning) 5 percent.[5] Between 1970 and 1980 the use of firearms in suicide increased for both males and females, and there was a decreased proportion of suicide by poisoning by both males and females.[6] More males than females complete suicide, at a ratio of almost 5 to 1.[6] Most adolescent male suicide completers are white, 89.5 percent.[6] Suicide attempts will often be in connection with a birthday, holiday, anniversary, or national event.[8]

Depression is the clearest link to suicide and is a major predictor of suicidal behavior.[9] However, not all students who attempt or complete suicide are depressed. For some students the act is impulsive and unpredicted but related to significant stressors.[10] Adolescents interviewed after suicide attempts identified significant psychosocial stress prior to the attempt. Within six months prior to the attempt, these adolescents reported more than twice the number of stressors in their lives than did nondepressed or nonsuicidal adolescents.[11] The ten stressors most reported by adolescent attempters of suicide are: 1) breaking up of a romantic relationship, 2) trouble with brother or sister, 3) change in parent's financial status, 4) parental divorce, 5) losing a close friend, 6) trouble with a teacher, 7) changing to a new school, 8) personal injury or illness, 9) failing grades, and 10) increased arguments with parents.[11]

Cluster suicide is a phenomenon particular to adolescent suicide.[12] This concept refers to several or multiple suicide attempts or completions in one geographic area and related to a prior suicide. It is not understood why adolescents are susceptible to imitative suicidal behavior, but it is clear from reports of such events that suicides occurring later in that cluster are affected by the earlier suicides.[13] Theories suggest that media and television exposure of completed suicides, especially adolescent suicides or celebrity suicides, affect certain individuals and foster the vulnerability for a similar act.[13]

INDIVIDUALIZED HEALTHCARE PLAN

Assessment

History

- Previous history of affective disorder (depression, manic-depressive disorder, adjustment disorder), either as chronic condition or as acute episode(s)
- Loss of parent before adolescence
- Family history of depression or suicide attempts or suicide completions
- Alcohol or chemical use/abuse
- Previous suicide attempts, ideations, threats
- History of physical, sexual, or emotional abuse and/or neglect
- History from family
  - significant recent life changes: move, death, financial issues, physical illness, mental illness, social or job issues
  - any behavior problems or depressive, suicidal behaviors at home?

Developmental/Academic/Social

- Student's age and developmental level
- What are student's support systems: family, friends, church, school groups, other?
- What are patterns of academic performance as indicated by review of academic or cumulative school records?
  Recent changes?
- What is school absence pattern: Current? Previous?
- Is there a need for special education (P.L. 94–142) services to adequately educate the student?

Current Status

3 to 5 Years: DEPRESSION (adapted, with permission, from Lucas)[14]

- Somatic disorders (headaches, abdominal pain, asthma episodes)
- Encopresis, enuresis
- Erratic sleeping and eating patterns
- Excessive irritability and tantrums
- Withdrawal, noticeably different in socialization skills from peers
- Excesses in activity or lethargy
- Separation problems, unable to comfort
- Aggressive or passive-aggressive behavior
- Self-induced injury or self-endangering behavior (accident prone, head banging), or morbid play

6 to 10 Years: DEPRESSION (adapted, with permission, from Lucas)[14]

- Prolonged unhappiness, moodiness, irritability, tearfulness, sad or somber affect
- Increased and excessive irritability, anger, or frustration
- Feelings of shame indicated by low self-esteem, self-derogatory comments
- Feelings of guilt indicated by inner sense of evil or badness and evident in play or art
- Tells of frightening dreams or fantasies
- Somatic disorders (abdominal pain, headaches, nausea for which organic cause is ruled out)
- Encopresis, enuresis
- Appetite or weight changes
- Aggressive behavior, lying, stealing
- Self-endangering or self-injuring behaviors
- Morbid preoccupations
- Excessive activity or lethargy
- Withdrawal from peers (slow or sudden)
- Decrease in school performance
- Withdrawal from previously enjoyed activities

Preadolescent and adolescent: DEPRESSION (adapted, with permission, from Lucas)[14]

- Appearance of sadness, apathy
- Statements of helplessness, hopelessness
- Increased expressions of anger (verbal and physical acting out)
- Low frustration tolerance

- Sexual identity issues
- Current alcohol and chemical use/abuse
- Increased hostility to self or others
- Expressions of guilt, shame, worthlessness
- Relates frightening dreams or fantasies
- Sleep changes: insomnia, waking early, excessive sleeping
- Eating or appetite changes, weight changes
- Somatic complaints
- Withdrawal from activities previously enjoyed: sports, clubs, church groups, community groups
- Change in friends or withdrawing from friends
- Self-injuring behavior (cigarette burns, skin carvings, drug abuse, alcohol abuse)
- Decrease in school performance and attitude: work level, work accomplishment, concentration, motivation
- Legal encounters: shoplifting, stealing, drugs, violence, traffic violations
- Emotional lability, unpredictable mood fluctuations
- Depressive, despondent, worthlessness themes in written, art or verbal academic work.

Suicide Risk Assessment

- Threat or talk of suicide.
- Death themes in spoken, written or artistic schoolwork.
- Appears numb, joyless, and painless.
- Previous attempts.
- Wishes for death.
- Marked behavior changes (including sudden positive behavior after marked depression).
- Making final arrangements
  - Note
  - Giving away belongings, especially prized possessions
  - Saying goodbyes
  - Last will or testament.
- On a scale of 0 to 10, how do you feel right now about doing something to end your life?
- Specific plan for suicide (Tell me how you would do it).

Nursing Diagnoses (N.D.)

N.D. 1 Alteration in self-perception or self-concept (NANDA 7.1.2, 7.1.2.1, 7.1.2.2)*
related to anxiety, depression, and/or self-esteem disturbance.

N.D. 2 Alteration in emotional integrity (emotional pain) (NANDA 9.3.1, 9.3.2, 9.2.3, 9.2.3.1, 9.2.1.1) related to:
feelings of anxiety, despondency, and/or hopelessness
post-trauma response (loss, rape, abuse)
dysfunctional grieving

---

* (See chapter 2, page 38 for explanation of the NANDA approved numerical system.)

N.D. 3 Alteration in through processes (NANDA 8.3) related to emotional pain and/or confusion.

N.D. 4 Alteration in socialization (NANDA 3.1.1, 3.1.2) related to depression and/or anxiety.

N.D. 5 Alteration in coping pattern (NANDA 5.1.1.1) due to emotional pain, altered thought processes and/or altered self-concept.

N.D. 6 Potential for or actual self-injury (NANDA 1.6.1) related to depression and/or feelings of hopelessness.

N.D. 7 Potential for violence (NANDA 9.2.2) related to emotional pain, depression, and/or altered thought processes.

Goals

Establish relationship with student which conveys sincere interest and caring, and transfers belief that help is possible. (N.D. 1–3, 5)

Determine the type of psychosocial stressor the student is experiencing. (N.D. 1, 2, 4, 5)

Identify what further help the person is willing to accept to stop suicidal thoughts or behavior. (N.D. 6)

Provide student with options to prevent suicide or suicide attempt. (N.D. 6)

Establish support network within the school. (N.D. 4)

Arrange for referral and follow-up care for the student. (N.D. 1–7)

Establish prevention/education system for school-wide implementation. (N.D. 3–6)

Establish school crisis team to respond to individuals in distress or emergency situations. (N.D. 2, 5, 6, 7)

NURSING INTERVENTIONS

School-Wide Interventions

Crisis Interventions (suicide attempt at school or completed suicide by student)
Adapted, with permission, from Phi Delta Kappa International.[7]

First Hour: Protect privacy of family, verify death and suicide, notify principal (superintendent): Instruct student (or adult) who reports death to maintain confidentiality until it is verified. Stress that the family has experienced a terrible loss and this must be handled with respect for their needs first. (N.D. 2, 5)

Convene School Crisis Team (N.D. 2, 5)
  Prepare formal announcement of death to students and staff
  Prepare announcement for media
  Principal notify faculty of meeting to implement crisis plan
  Plan crisis room access
  Identify other students who are at "high risk," establish monitoring plan
Direct media to principal (N.D. 2, 5)

Second Hour: Announce death to students and faculty (N.D. 2, 5)

Initiate crisis center with small groups for students to access support staff (N.D. 2, 5)

Third Hour: Contact community resources: get additional support personnel from other schools, district offices, or agencies who are part of the School Crisis Team. (N.D. 2, 5)

Fourth Hour: Hold faculty meeting to establish school-wide awareness of plan, and share accurate facts about the death. Provide teachers with guidelines for handling distressed students in classroom. Identify students the faculty is concerned may be at risk for additional suicidal actions. (N.D. 2, 5, 6)

Day Two: Continue crisis center with small-group discussions for student grieving (N.D. 2, 5)

Keep media directed to single source for information. (N.D. 2, 5)

Provide meeting for teachers and crisis team at end of day to review events and obtain support. (N.D. 2, 5)

Avoid glorifying a suicide in any way: (N.D. 2, 5, 6)

Do not fly the flag at half-mast.

Do not observe a moment of silence in the school.

Do not have a memorial service.

Non-Crisis Interventions (Prevention and Proaction)

Establish a School Crisis Team (Student Services Team). (N.D. 5–7)

Establish a school-wide mechanism for referral of a student at risk for depressive behavior or suicide to the School Crisis Team. (N.D. 1–7)

Assist in the development of curriculum for instruction on self-awareness/self-esteem concepts. (N.D. 1, 3, 5)

Assist in the development of curriculum which promotes self-identification of depression and self-destructive feelings and builds skills for when and where to seek help for these feelings. (N.D. 3, 5)

Assist in the development of curriculum which instructs on topics of stress, stress management, depression, communication skills, feeling identification, and drug education. (N.D. 3, 5)

Perform a planned periodic record review of all students to identify depressive students (recurrent headaches, abdominal pains, other somatic complaints associated with depression). (N.D. 1, 3, 5)

Provide faculty with ongoing in-service on symptoms and management of depression and suicide. (N.D. 1–7)

Arrange for school library to have adequate resources available for faculty and students on depression and suicide. (N.D. 1–7)

Plan and provide parent information events (newsletter articles, evening information hour, pamphlets) on issues of child/adolescent depression, suicide, self-esteem, stress and stress management. (N.D. 3, 4, 7)

Establish peer counseling program. (N.D. 1–5)

Student/Family Interventions

Crisis Interventions: Physical Crisis Intervention (Suicide Attempt)

First Aid: Assess injuries and institute appropriate immediate care. (N.D. 6)

> **A**irway, **B**reathing, **C**irculation
>
> Call for ambulance, police
>
> For overdose of drugs or alcohol consult with Poison Control Center
>
> Control bleeding
>
> Monitor blood pressure, pulse, respirations

Document all treatment provided and observations of conditions of student. (N.D. 6)

Notify parents. (N.D. 6)

If student is awake and responsive, provide reassuring, caring and empathic comments.

> Keep student informed of what you are doing and why, but be clear that you are in charge of the student's physical safety and will take care of him/her now. Do not allow student to negotiate out of a transfer to the emergency room after an active suicide attempt by any method. (N.D. 6)

Emotional Crisis Interventions (Suicide Threat)

Make psychological contact: (N.D. 2, 5)

> Provide supportive, empathic, reflective, clarifying listening.
>
> Encourage sharing of feelings: despondence, isolation, sadness, hopelessness.
>
> Physically hold or touch.
>
> Support and encourage emotional release: verbalizing, crying.
>
> Provide emotional warmth and caring.
>
> Convey that something can and will be done to help with these overwhelming feelings and confusion.

Explore dimensions of the problem: (N.D. 3, 5)

> Inquire about event precipitating the crisis:
>
> > immediate past events
> >
> > pre-crisis functioning (strengths, weaknesses).
>
> Determine why coping skills from previous crisis situations are not functional now.
>
> Identify current strengths and weaknesses (family, social, church, friends, personal).
>
> Identify potential for handling the immediate future: after school, tonight, tomorrow.
>
> Assess for probability of imminent suicidal action. Talk frankly about how suicidal student feels.

Examine possible solutions: (N.D. 3, 5)

> Explore what student has done to solve the problems(s) thus far.
>
> Explore what student could try to do now (brainstorm).
>
> Propose other alternatives (new behaviors, redefine the problem, additional assistance, environment change).

Assist student in taking concrete action: (N.D. 3, 5)

> Inform student that confidentiality of conversation will be maintained unless there is a concern that the student is at risk for injuring self or others. Tell student that if you have to talk to others (parents, referral agencies), he or she will know when you are going to do this and can be there while you talk to them.

Facilitate perspective that "We talk, you act" for student capable of acting on own:

> Contract for action
>
>> no self-harm
>> parental notification
>> additional assessment and counseling

If student not capable of acting on own facilitate stance: "We talk, I may take action on your behalf, but you will know what I am going to do and you can be with me when I do it."

Notify parents of student's condition (with student present if student wishes).

Arrange (and/or help parents arrange) for immediate assessment by mental health center or emergency healthcare facility.

Stay with student until in the direct care of parents or healthcare facility. (N.D. 6, 7)

Allow good friend to be with student if desirable and possible. (N.D. 5)

Seek collaboration from professional colleagues or school crisis team. (N.D. 6, 7)

Non-Crisis Interventions (Depression)

Provide supportive, empathic, reflective, clarifying listening. (N.D. 2)

Help student explore the dimensions of all that is troubling. (N.D. 3)

Help student select aspects of concern that s/he can do something about. (N.D. 3,5)

Help student focus on a specific problem, create a manageable perspective: (N.D. 3,5)

> What is the hardest thing for you right now?
> What makes this so difficult right now?
> What have you tried to do with this problem?

Help student explore possible solutions: (N.D. 3, 5)

> What ideas can we come up with that might be worth a try (brainstorm)?
> Is there someone else you want to talk to about this?
> What have you done in similar situations?

Strengthen and mobilize existing coping skills: (N.D. 5)

> When you had a problem before, you handled it. I'll bet there are things you can think of that you can do for this problem.

Make a list of five, ten, or twenty things you've done before when you're upset.
Write, walk, talk, eat, be with friends, exercise, think about it, and so on.
Who else do you want to talk to?

Assist student in gaining comfort with a process to handle the discomfort: assure them that a quick fix may not be the best in the long run. (N.D. 2, 3, 5)

Provide perspective: "I understand this hurts real bad right now, but it won't feel this bad even tomorrow and even better in a few days."

Identify strengths: (N.D. 1,4,5)

Make a list with student of the five, ten, twenty great things about him/her.
Identify family, friends who can be brought into situation.
Identify clubs, organizations, churches which student belongs to and could be brought in to support student.

Arrange for involvement in school-based counseling and/or support groups. (N.D. 1–5)

Build a support network for the student of other school professionals who can be contacted for support, counseling and crisis intervention. (N.D. 1–5)

Give student a list of community agencies who can be called upon in an emergency: crisis units, hot lines. (N.D. 5)

Refer for ongoing counseling. (N.D. 1–3, 5)

Assist family in obtaining ongoing counseling. (N.D. 1–3, 5)

Provide follow up: (N.D. 1, 2, 5)

Set time for regular contacts with student.
Find student if s/he does not show up for appointment.
Collaborate with other agency(ies), professionals involved with student.
Maintain supportive contact with family.
Monitor any medication prescribed for student. Arrange for medical orders and establish dispensing system in accordance with district policy.

Expected Student Outcomes

Student feels heard, understood, accepted, and supported. (N.D. 1, 2, 5–7)

Student experiences a lessening of the intensity of the emotional distress. (N.D. 1–3, 6, 7)

Student feels there are options and that s/he has some control. (N.D. 1–5)

Student death or suicide attempt is avoided. (N.D. 6, 7)

Student and family obtain counseling. (N.D. 1–3, 5–7)

Student identifies and expands support systems within the school and the community. (N.D. 4, 5)

Student(s) will have access to competent, preplanned, appropriate, and collaborative interventions during times of crisis. (N.D. 2, 5)

REFERENCES

1. Weller E, Weller R. Pediatric management of depression. *Pediatric Annals* 1989; 18 (2): 104–13.
2. Kovacs M. Affective disorders in children and adolescents. *Am Psychologist* 1989; 44 (2): 209–15.
3. Miller D. Affective disorders and violence in adolescents. *Hosp Commun Psychiatry* 1986; 37 (6): 591–96.
4. Maris R. The adolescent suicide problem. *Suicide Life-Threatening Behavior* 1985; 15 (2): 91–109. (Available from Human Sciences Press.)
5. Garfinkel B, Golombek H. Suicidal behavior in adolescence. In: Garfinkel B, Golombek G, eds. *The Adolescent and Mood Disturbance.* Madison, CT: International Universities Press Inc., 1983.
6. Centers for Disease Control, Division of Injury Epidemiology and Control, Center for Environmental Health. Youth Suicide Surveillance Summary: 1970–1980. *MMWR* 1987; 36 (6): 87–89.
7. Phi Delta Kappa International. Responding to Student Suicide: The First 48 Hours. In: *Phi Delta Kappa International Current Issues Memo.* Bloomington, IN: Phi Delta Kappa International, Sept. 1988.
8. Phi Delta Kappa Center on Evaluation, Development, Research. *Adolescent Suicide.* Bloomington, IN: Phi Delta Kappa, 1988.
9. Hoberman H. Completed suicide in children and adolescents. *J Am Acad Child Adolescent Psychiatry* 1988; 27 (6): 689–95.
10. Garfinkel B. Major affective disorders in children and adolescents. In: Winokur G, Clayton P. *The Medical Basis of Psychiatry.* Philadelphia: WB Saunders, 1986.
11. Garfinkel B. The components of school-based suicide prevention. In: *Report of Secretary's Task Force on Youth Suicide. Volume III—Prevention and Interventions in Youth Suicide* (1989). Washington, DC: US Gov Print Off (Alcohol, Drug Abuse and Mental Health Administration), 1989.
12. Pfeffer C. Assessment of suicidal children and adolescents. *Psychiatric Clin North Am* 1989; 12 (4): 861–72.
13. O'Carroll P, Mercy J, Steward J. CDC recommendations for a community plan for the prevention and containment of suicide clusters. *MMWR* 1988; 37 (8–6): 1–11.
14. Lucas JC. *Childhood and Youth Suicide Resource Sheet, Workshop Materials.* J. Chapman Lucas, Educational Psychologist, 515 Farmers Lane, Santa Rosa, CA 95405.

BIBLIOGRAPHY

American Academy of Pediatrics. The potentially suicidal student in the school setting. *Pediatrics* 1990; 86 (3): 481–83.

Bernhardt GR, Praeger S. Preventing child suicide: the elementary school death education puppet show. *J Counseling Development* 1985; 63: 311–12.

Garfinkel B, Crosby E, Herbert M, Matus A, Pfeifer J, Sheras P (Phi Delta Kappa Task Force on Adolescent Suicide). *Responding to Adolescent Suicide.* Bloomington, IN: Phi Delta Kappa Educational Foundation, 1988.

Garfinkel B, Froese A, Hood J. Suicide attempts in children and adolescents. *Am J Psychiatry* 1982; 139 (10): 1257–61.

Garfinkel B, Golombek H. Suicide and Depression in Childhood and Adolescence. *CMA Journal* 1974; 10 (Jun): 1278–81.

Gibbs A. Aspects of communication with people who have attempted suicide. *J Adv Nursing* 1990; 15: 1245–49.

Harrington RC. Depressive disorder in children and adolescents. *Br J Hosp Med* 1990; 43 (2): 109–11.

Minnesota Department of Education. *Policies to Address Stress, Depression, and Suicide.* St. Paul, MN: Minn Dept. of Education, Memo to Superintendents of Schools, 1986 Oct 2.

Institute for Studies of Destructive Behaviors and the Suicide Prevention Center of Los Angeles & Suicide Prevention and Crisis Center of San Mateo County. *Teacher's Guide for Secondary School Unit on Youth Suicide Prevention.* 1985.

Minneapolis Public Schools. *Responding to an Urgent Student Crisis.* Minneapolis, MN: Minneapolis Board of Education, 1986.

National Education Association. *Teenage Suicide.* Washington, DC: National Education Association.

22 | IHP: Diabetes Mellitus

Susan I. Simandl Will

INTRODUCTION

Diabetes mellitus is a metabolic chronic illness characterized by abnormal carbohydrate, fat, and protein metabolism. This metabolic abnormality is the result of decreased or absent secretion of insulin by the pancreatic beta cells. The incidence of diabetes mellitus is between 1 and 3.5 cases per 1,000 in the under-18 age population.[1]

Pathophysiology

Current etiological theory is that diabetes mellitus is a pancreatic beta cell abnormality, initiated by a viral or autoimmune disorder. The result is a deficient or total lack of insulin production by the pancreatic cells. Heredity and obesity also affect the development of the disorder.

Diabetes is a complex, multisystem disease process. It affects the metabolism of fats and proteins as well as carbohydrates. Over time, the altered metabolism frequently produces complications of the vascular and neurological systems such as neuropathies, ocular changes, circulatory deficiencies, and renal complications.

Diabetes is commonly described as **Type I (insulin-dependent)** and **Type II (noninsulin-dependent)**. For Type II diabetes, diet alone may be sufficient to regulate the glucose imbalance. However,

most children and adolescents with diabetes require insulin and are therefore characterized as having Type I diabetes.

The physiological mechanism of diabetes is a decreased or absent insulin supply prohibiting the transfer of glucose to the cell. Glucose levels then increase in the blood (hyperglycemia). The glucose-loaded blood continues to the kidneys, and when sufficiently excessive glucose levels exist, reabsorption is inadequate. Glucose then appears in the urine.

Because the glucose transfer to the cell is inadequate, the tissue cells, deprived of nutrients, begin to mobilize fat and protein for energy and fuel. In the oxidation process to create this fuel, fatty acids and amino acids are produced, leading to fatty acid and amino acid accumulation in the blood. The liver then attempts to metabolize some of these acids converting them to partially metabolized acids known as ketones, which become detectable in the bloodstream. Following passage through the kidneys, ketones become detectable in the urine. This state is termed ketosis or ketoacidosis.

Ketoacidosis (diabetic coma) is an emergency state resulting from an excess of partially metabolized fatty acid and protein products in the bloodstream (ketones).

Alterations in fluid and electrolyte balance result and initiate the development of coma. Ketoacidosis happens fairly slowly and several testings with high glucose reading should increase the vigilance for this development. Signs and symptoms include: weak, rapid pulse, nausea, vomiting, weakness, confusion, twitching, seizures, numbness, low blood pressure, decreased urine output. Development of these signs and symptoms constitutes an emergency situation.

Insulin reactions are a rapid metabolic response to excess insulin or insufficient food intake to manage the insulin dose. Insulin reactions occur when the blood sugar levels are too low and may be characterized by pallor, excessive perspiration, hunger, headache, dizziness, blurred vision, irritability, inappropriate responses, crying, confusion, inattentiveness, drowsiness, lack of coordination, trembling, abdominal pain, and nausea. These reactions occur most frequently just before meals. Insulin reactions need to be treated immediately with sugar (glucose): two large sugar cubes, 1/2 cup fruit juice or pop (non-diet), candy (equivalent of seven to eight Lifesavers), two to three glucose tabs. Some students now have injectable

glucagon at school to assist in severe insulin reactions when coma is imminent. Administration of glucagon requires careful professional assessment and monitoring. It is an emergency measure necessitating immediate medical management for stabilization. Glucagon raises blood glucose by promoting conversion of hepatic glucogen to glucose.

When the diabetes is managed with a balance of diet, oral hyperglycemic agent or insulin, and exercise, functional lifestyles are the norm. Strict adherence to the medical regimen is essential for health maintenance and prevention of secondary complications. Normal developmental stresses (adolescent growth), as well as physiologic assaults (viral episodes, injuries) complicate the diabetes and create the need to closely monitor and alter the diet, insulin, and exercise balance. Students with diabetes can attend school regularly, fully participate in all activities, including competitive sports. Students can do quite well if sufficient supports exist for them. It is essential that the faculty closest to the student be thoroughly inserviced about the disease, normal maintenance requirements, and emergency interventions.

INDIVIDUALIZED HEALTHCARE PLAN

Assessment

History

- Age onset of diabetes
- Level of control child has experienced in past
- Other illness, current or chronic
- Diabetes classes or camps attended; when
- Previous difficulties in management of diabetes
- Practices or management methods which are particularly successful

Disease Management

- Regular source of medical care and ability to obtain regular care
- Student's description and general knowledge about diabetes

> Signs and symptoms of insulin reaction: shaking, sweating, fatigue, hunger, dizziness, paleness, numbness or tingling of lips, irritability, confusion, headaches, blurred or double vision, other.

- Student's knowledge of signs of ketoacidosis: high blood glucose levels, especially over several hours/days, nausea, vomiting, abdominal pain, rapid respirations, thirst, frequent urination, fatigue.
- Glucose testing method and frequency
- Student's medication (oral hyperglycemic or insulin, glucagon)
- Prescribed diet plan
  - One week dietary intake record
- Student (parent) knowledge and practice of infection control
  - Foot care, shower or bathing routines
- Knowledge of upper respiratory infection signs and symptoms: early intervention practices (rest, fluids, monitor fever)
- Knowledge of urinary tract infection signs and symptoms: early intervention practices
- Knowledge of minor skin injury treatments
- Knowledge of infection signs which require physician intervention (fever, swelling, erythema, purulent drainage, severe pain, tenderness, urinary tract infections)
- Physical limitations which complicate any aspect of the diabetic regimen
- Difficulties student experiences in following insulin or diet or exercise requirements

Self-Care

- Student's knowledge of typical signs and symptoms of insulin reaction
- Student's knowledge of what to do when early insulin reaction symptoms begin
  - Where snack is stored
  - Whom to notify
- Student's ability to perform or assist with glucose test accurately
  - Understanding of meaning of glucose levels
  - Student's reliability for regular testing
- Student's description of insulin action
  - Student's ability to self-administer or assist with injection
- Student's understanding of diet
  - Student's ability to make appropriate exchange selections
  - Student's ability to create diet plan for one day
  - Student's exercise and activity levels
  - Student's ability to weigh self
- Student's ability to recognize early signs of infection (upper respiratory, urinary tract, and skin) and manage appropriately

Psychosocial and Developmental

- Age and developmental level
- Student's feelings about having diabetes
- Perception of what family and friends think of him/her because of diabetes
- Self-perception: I can do . . . , I can't do . . . , I am. . . .
- Relationships with peers: good friends (best friends): How long?
  - Acquaintances
  - Feelings about new situations

- – Which friends know about diabetes
- – Which friends can be counted on to help if needed
- School club or athletic activities past and present
- Community/church activities past and present
- Support systems: family, friends, other
- Depression or despondency
- Family issues
  - – Who is primary caregiver?
  - – Knowledge and perceptions about diabetes
  - – Management routines in the home
- Family's resources
  - – Social
  - – Emotional
  - – Financial
  - – Knowledge
  - – Community
  - – Medical
- Knowledge, equipment, family issues, support, financial limits which may impact ability to follow regimen

Academic

- Review of academic or cumulative school record for patterns of academic performance
- Assessment of teachers' perception of student's performance and classroom adjustment
- Comparison of student's behavior, social skills, academic performance to peer norms
- School absence pattern
- Need for special education (PL 94–142) services to adequately educate the student (tutors, special education assistance)

Nursing Diagnoses (N.D.)

N.D. 1 Physiological injury (NANDA 1.6.1)* due to development of acute complications related to hypoglycemia (insulin shock) or ketoacidosis

N.D. 2 Knowledge deficit (NANDA 8.1.1) related to:
- oral hyperglycemic medication
- insulin administration
- dietary regimen
- exercise requirements
- blood sugar monitoring
- balance of insulin, diet, and exercise

N.D. 3 Self-care alteration due to:
- difficulty integrating management requirements into lifestyle
- knowledge deficit
- developmental level
- insufficient resources
- dysfunctional grieving

---

* (See chapter 2, page 38 for explanation of the NANDA approved numerical system.)

N.D. 4 Self-esteem disturbance (NANDA 7.1.2) due to:
- diabetes care requirements
- developmental level and needs
- dysfunctional grieving
- embarrassment
- stigma of having a chronic illness
- lifestyle changes demanded by diabetes and its management
- anxiety about future physiological changes related to diabetes (motor control, visual, bladder, sensory, sexual)

N.D. 5 Infection (NANDA 1.2.1.1) due to:
- high glucose levels providing bacterial or fungal growth medium
- depression of leukocyte function associated with hyperglycemia
- delayed healing associated with fluid imbalance and hyperglycemia
- knowledge deficit related to prevention
- knowledge deficit related to early intervention

See also Chapter 6 for additional mental health and psychosocial nursing diagnoses relevant to the student with chronic disease.

Goals

Student (parent) will recognize and treat early signs of insulin shock appropriately and know how to recognize and respond to early signs of ketoacidosis. (N.D. 1)

Student will increase understanding of pathophysiology of diabetes and develop or improve the skills necessary to manage diabetes. (N.D. 2)

Student will improve self-care management skills. (N.D. 3)

Student will demonstrate increased adaptation to and psychological comfort with body changes and lifestyle requirements. (N.D. 4)

Student will not experience infections and will self-treat minor illnesses and injuries appropriately. (N.D. 5)

Nursing Interventions

School/Teacher Interventions

Develop individual emergency plan for (with) student and share with faculty. Include plan for administration of glucagon if ordered. (N.D. 1)

Assess teacher(s) level of understanding of diabetes, instruct as appropriate. (N.D. 1)

Instruct teachers in what to do when early insulin reaction symptoms begin (e.g., who to contact: where to go: what snack to eat: where snack is stored). (N.D. 1)

Monitor snack supply. (N.D. 1)

Intervene with teachers, as needed, to assure student appropriate control over his/her environment and diabetes. (N.D. 4)

Establish communication and reporting system between school and home.

Arrange for medication at school as appropriate and in accordance with school district policy and procedure.

Student/Family Interventions

Interview student to determine typical insulin reaction symptoms. (N.D. 1)

Evaluate if student understands his/her reaction symptoms in early stages. (N.D. 1)

Instruct student what to do at school when early insulin reaction symptoms begin (e.g., who to contact: where to go: what snack to eat: where snack is stored). (N.D. 1)

Monitor blood glucose testing and recording, instruct and reinforce skills as needed. (N.D. 1)

Instruct student in pathophysiology of diabetes at level the student is capable of understanding (age and development appropriate). (N.D. 1–3)

Monitor insulin administration if given at school. Instruct and reinforce skills as needed. (N.D. 1–3)

Monitor diet adherence, reinforce and instruct as appropriate. (N.D. 1–3)

Instruct student in weight measurement, monitor weight regularly with student. (N.D. 1–3)

Instruct student in meaning of glucose levels, and appropriate action required at readings from 40–300. (N.D. 1–3)

Arrange space and time for student to perform self-care activities (blood glucose level monitoring, insulin injection, diet inventory, snack consumption). (N.D. 1–3)

Provide reinforcement and praise follow-through for self-management abilities. (N.D. 2, 3)

Create opportunities for student to verbalize feelings about having diabetes, management requirements, and feelings of isolation, differentness, or peer rejection. (N.D. 3, 4)

Provide opportunities for student to become increasingly self-sufficient in care provisions (private area for glucose testing or insulin injection, creation of color-coded charts to reflect blood glucose level meaning and action necessary). (N.D. 3)

Arrange dietary consult if diet incompatible with lifestyle needs and changes. (N.D. 3)

Provide referral and access to youth diabetes group. (N.D. 3, 4)

Monitor and support behaviors indicating acceptance of and positive adaptation to diabetes (regular testing, dietary adherence, verbalization of feelings). (N.D. 3, 4)

Assist student's, friend's and family's adjustment progress by active listening, communication facilitation, diabetes education. (N.D. 3, 4)

Consult physician and provide counseling referral if adjustment is nonprogressive or dysfunctional. (N.D. 4)

Clarify misconceptions about diabetes. (N.D. 4)

Instruct student in good skin care techniques. (N.D. 5)

Instruct student (parents) in signs and symptoms of upper respiratory and urinary tract infections as well as early treatment activities and need for physician evaluation. (N.D. 5)

Instruct student (parents) in early treatment of skin injuries and signs requiring physician evaluation. (N.D. 5)

Support student and family in adaptation to diabetes (referral, listening, extending support systems, teaching, regular communication). (N.D. 1–4)

Expected Student Outcomes

The student will be successful in diabetes management in the school setting. (N.D. 1-5)

The student will manage or have assistance managing insulin reactions. (N.D. 1)

The student will not experience ketoacidosis. (N.D. 1)

The student will demonstrate increasing knowledge and skill in medication management. (N.D. 2, 3)

The student will demonstrate increasing knowledge and skill in diet management. (N.D. 2, 3)

The student will perform or have assistance performing blood glucose tests. (N.D. 1–3)

The student will begin to demonstrate (beginning, progressing) adaptation to having diabetes. (N.D 3, 4)

The student will demonstrate knowledge and skill in infection prevention. (N.D. 5)

REFERENCES

1. Hathaway W, Groothuis J, Hay W, Paisley J, eds. *Pediatric Diagnosis and Treatment.* East Norwalk, CT: Appleton & Lange, 1991.

BIBLIOGRAPHY

American Diabetes Association. What the Teacher Should Know About the Student With Diabetes. New York: Am Diabetes Association, MN. Affiliate.

Balik B, Haig B. The student with diabetes. In: Larson G, ed. *Managing the School Age Child With a Chronic Health Condition.* Wayzata, MN: DCI Publishing, 1986 (distributed by Sunrise River Press, 11481 Kost Dam Rd, North Branch, MN 55056, 612-583-3239).

Dorchy H, Poortmans J. Sport and the diabetic child. *Sports Medicine* 1989; 7 (4): 248–62.

Gallo A. Family adaptation in childhood chronic illness: a case report. *J Pediatric Health Care* 1991; 5 (2): 78–85.

Smith D. Diabetes mellitus: management in the school setting. *School Nurse* 1991; 7 (1): 22–30.

Waechter E, Philips J, Holaday B. *Nursing Care of Children.* 10th ed. Philadelphia: JB Lippincott, 1985.

Wong D, Whaley L. *Clinical Manual of Pediatric Nursing.* 2nd ed. St. Louis: CV Mosby, 1990.

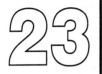

23 | IHP: Down Syndrome

Mary J. Villars Gerber

INTRODUCTION

Down syndrome, also known as trisomy 21, is one of the most common chromosomal abnormalities in humans, occurring in approximately 1:800 live births. It is characterized by varying degrees of mental retardation and associated physical defects. Heart defects occur in 40 percent of children with Down syndrome. Respiratory infections, ear infections, and conductive hearing loss are frequently seen. Low thyroid hormone levels occur in 15 to 25 percent of these children. Atlantoaxial instability is present in 10 to 20 percent of these children and is related to instability of ligaments of the upper spine. Up to 50 percent of these children experience vision problems, including nearsightedness, farsightedness, astigmatism, strabismus, and cataracts. Obesity is often a concern as the children grow older.[1]

All of these conditions associated with Down syndrome will impact a child's education in varying degrees, and will need monitoring and/or intervention in the school setting.

INDIVIDUALIZED HEALTHCARE PLAN

History

Physical growth; what are the historical height and weight measurements? Where does the student's growth fall on the Down syndrome growth chart? (See Tables 1 and 2 for growth charts for boys and girls with Down syndrome.)

Immunization status; what is the history of immunizations? Are the immunizations current?

What congenital anomalies are present and what treatment has been received?

Heart disease
Cardiac defects
Gastrointestinal abnormalities such as aganglionic megacolon, small bowel obstruction, and esophageal malformation

Is there evidence of thyroid dysfunction?

What is the history of respiratory infections, including ear infections?

Is there evidence of visual and/or auditory deficits?

What are the student's dental practices and concerns?

What delays have been present in motor development?

What delays have been present in cognitive development?

Have there been any feeding difficulties related to craniofacial skeletal differences such as short palate, underdevelopment of maxilla, and abnormal tongue size? Generalized facial and oral hypotonia may contribute to poor lip closure, poor sucking ability, and jaw instability.

Have there been any orthopedic concerns including atlantoaxial subluxation, scoliosis, slipped femoral epiphysis, knee dislocation, and foot deformities?

Assessment

- **Growth.** Height and weight charted on Down syndrome growth charts. See Tables 1 and 2 for growth charts for boys and girls with Down syndrome. Assess for obesity.

- **Current status and effects of any congenital abnormalities.** Cardiac defects may influence physical actvity tolerance or cause difficulties with feeding or poor tolerance for temperature changes. Gastrointestinal abnormalities may be present.

- **Elimination patterns.** Constipation can be a problem due to variations in autonomic patterns.

- **Current treatment for thyroid dysfunction if any.** The characteristics of low thyroid function are also those associated with Down syndrome, so thyroid function tests must be conducted to confirm a problem. Thyroid dysfunction tends to increase with age.

- **Recent respiratory infections.** Frequent, repeated, and chronic respiratory infections are common, including chronic nasal drainage.

- **Other evidence of recurrent infection.** Individuals with Down syndrome show a number of immune problems that are evidenced by a number of infections including respiratory, middle ear, hepatitis B, skin, and fungal.

- **Auditory acuity.** Individuals with Down syndrome often experience recurrent otitis media with middle ear effusion. Conductive hearing loss is common. Ear wax impaction is common and can create a hearing loss. External auditory canals are small with an increased incidence of canal narrowing. Middle ear abnormalities have been noted and are an important cause of a sensorineural hearing loss. Hearing and related speech problems must be treated. Speech and language specialists in the school system are generally involved in assessing speech and communication.

- **Visual acuity.** Abnormal eye movements and nystagmus frequently occur. This may be neuromuscular or due to significant visual deficits. Refractive error may be due to astigmatism, nearsightedness, or farsightedness. Early and periodic examination is necessary. Conjunctival inflammation is common.

- **Dental practices and concerns.** Any child with heart disease will need prophylaxis prior to any surgery, invasive procedure, or dental work. Gum inflammation is common and could lead to bone loss, tooth mobility, and eventual loss. Tooth size, eruption, shape, and enamel may all be abnormal. Malocclusion is common. More frequent dental care is usually necessary.

Table 1A. Percentiles for stature and weight of boys with Down syndrome, 1 to 36 months of age.

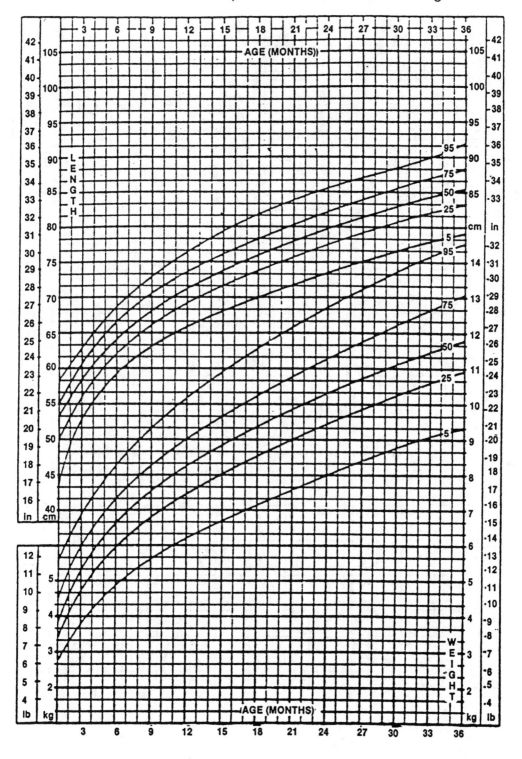

Reproduced by permission from Cronk C, Crocker A, Pueschel S, Shea A, Zackai E, Pickens G, Reed R. Growth charts for children with Down Syndrome: 1 month to 18 years of age. *Pediatric* 1988; 81(1): 107-108.

Table 1B. Percentiles for stature and weight of boys with Down syndrome, 2 to 18 years of age.

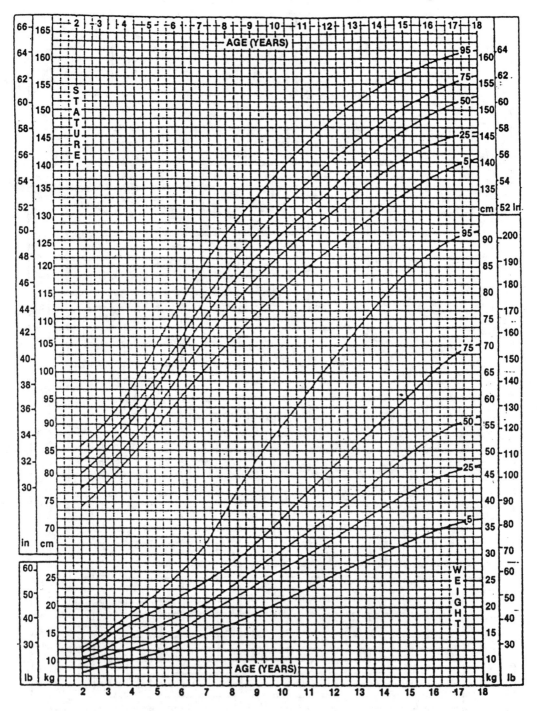

Reproduced by permission from Cronk C, Crocker A, Pueschel S, Shea A, Zackai E, Pickens G, Reed R. Growth charts for children with Down Syndrome: 1 month to 18 years of age. *Pediatric* 1988; 81(1): 107-108.

Table 2A. Percentiles for stature and weight of girls with Down syndrome, 1 to 36 months of age.

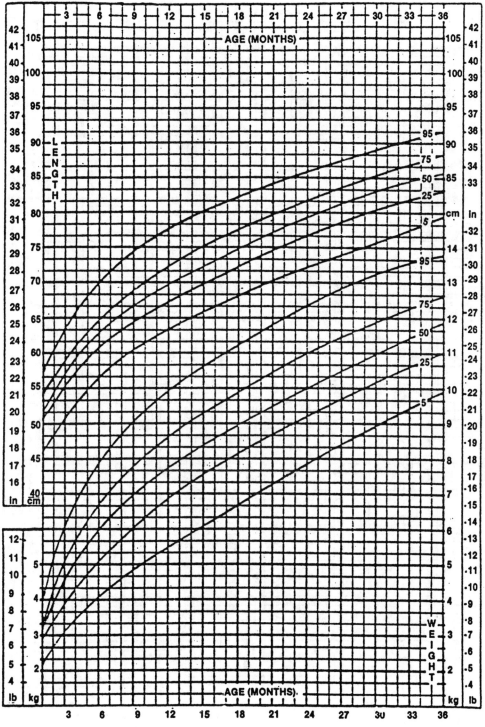

Reproduced by permission from Cronk C, Crocker A, Pueschel S, Shea A, Zackai E, Pickens G, Reed R. Growth charts for children with Down Syndrome: 1 month to 18 years of age. *Pediatric* 1988; 81(1): 107-108.

Table 2B. Percentiles for stature and weight of girls with Down syndrome, 2 to 18 years of age.

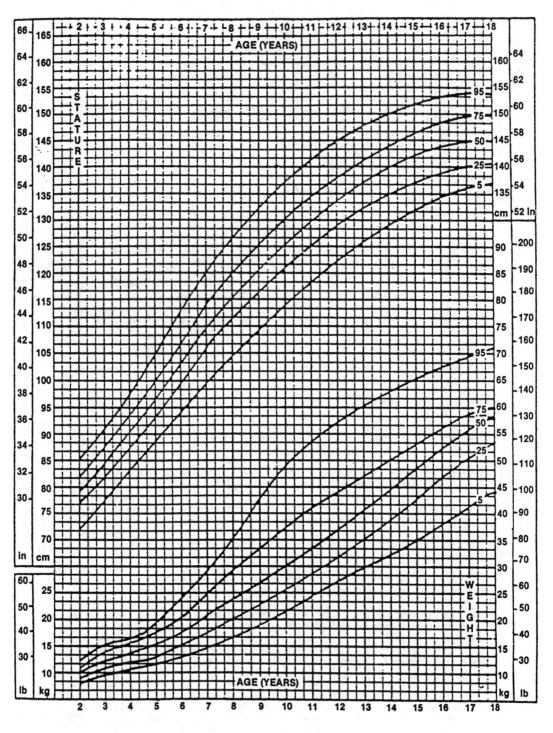

Reproduced by permission from Cronk C, Crocker A, Pueschel S, Shea A, Zackai E, Pickens G, Reed R. Growth charts for children with Down Syndrome: 1 month to 18 years of age. *Pediatric* 1988; 81(1): 107-108.

- **Motor development.** A child with Down syndrome generally follows a typical developmental progression, but at a slower rate. Low muscle tone is frequently a contributing factor. In a school setting an occupational therapist and physical therapist are commonly involved in assessing motor development.

- **Cognitive development.** There is usually some mental retardation, typically in the mild to moderate range. Teachers and psychologists are generally involved in assessing this area.

- **Nutrition and feeding concerns.** Due to the multiple craniofacial skeletal differences in children with Down syndrome, feeding difficulties are frequent but generally minor. Adequate nutrition is important. Assess for signs of obesity.

- **Orthopedic concerns.** Atlantoaxial subluxation is the instability of the space between the first two cervical vertebrae. It can result in high spinal cord compression. It occurs in 10 to 20 percent of children with Down syndrome. Only 1 to 2 percent of those individuals are symptomatic and require surgery. Symptoms include head tilt, neck pain, changes in walking gait, extremity weakness, increased tone especially in the legs, overactive reflexes, and clonus of the ankles. Periodic cervical x-rays and neurologic exams are needed. Forcible flexion of the neck may cause the vertebrae to shift and squeeze or sever the spinal cord.

  Scoliosis is also a condition seen in 50 percent of individuals with Down syndrome. These students should be carefully screened and monitored.

  Other orthopedic concerns include slipped femoral epiphysis, knee dislocation, and foot deformities including flat feet. A physical therapy referral for evaluation may be appropriate.

Nursing Diagnoses (N.D.)

N.D. 1 Altered nutrition: more than body requirements (NANDA 1.1.2.1)* related to imbalance of intake versus activity expenditures.

N.D. 2 Activity intolerance (NANDA 6.1.1.2) related to insufficient oxygenation secondary to decreased cardiac output.

N.D. 3 Potential altered body temperature. (NANDA 1.2.2.1)

N.D. 4 Potential colonic constipation (NANDA 1.3.1.1.2) related to decreased gastric motility.

N.D. 5 Potential for infection (NANDA 1.2.1.1) related to increased susceptibilty to respiratory infection secondary to hypotonia.

N.D. 6 Potential for infection (NANDA 1.2.1.1) related to susceptibility to environmental contagions secondary to compromised immune system.

N.D. 7 Potential for injury (NANDA 1.6.1) related to visual impairment.

N.D. 8 Altered growth and development (NANDA 6.6) related to (specify).

N.D. 9 Potential for injury (NANDA 1.6.1) related to forcible neck flexion.

N.D. 10 Altered oral mucous membrane (NANDA 1.6.2.1.1) related to inadequate oral hygiene or inability to perform oral hygiene.

N.D. 11 Potential self-care deficit (NANDA 6.5.1, 2, 3, or 4) related to visual impairment.

* (See chapter 2, page 38 for explanation of the NANDA approved numerical system.)

N.D. 12   Impaired communication (NANDA 2.1.1.1) related to hearing loss.

N.D. 13   Sensory perceptual alteration (NANDA 7.2): visual.

Goals

Prevent obesity. (N.D. 1)

Establish limits of activity tolerance. (N.D. 2)

Maintain normal body temperature. (N.D. 3)

Promote normal bowel elimination, prevent constipation. (N.D. 4)

Institute measures to prevent infection. (N.D. 5, 6)

Prevent vision loss, maintain optimal visual acuity. (N.D. 7, 13)

Goals related to growth and development specific to student attainment of specified developmentally appropriate skills or behavior. (N.D. 8)

Prevent injury due to forcible neck flexion. (N.D. 9)

Promote routine and periodic dental care. (N.D. 10)

Early identification and intervention of scoliosis. (Potential complication: scoliosis)

Maximum independence in self-care activities (specify). (N.D. 11)

Prevent hearing loss, maintain optimal auditory acuity. (N.D. 12)

Nursing Interventions

Update health history annually to provide current data base. (N.D. 1–13)

Counsel parents/student regarding nutrition as needed. Prevention of obesity needs to begin early. Intervention for poor nutritional intake is essential to maintain wellness. (N.D. 1)

Refer to healthcare provider for further assessment of growth patterns as appropriate. (N.D. 1, 8)

Obtain current medical orders related to cardiac condition, if present (i.e., activity tolerance/restrictions, tolerance of temperature changes). These restrictions or interventions must be carried out in the school setting. (N.D. 2, 3)

Observation of specified gastrointestinal symptoms if needed in the case of congenital anomalies. (N.D. 4)

Monitor special dietary regimen if needed for constipation, refer for further medical evaluation as appropriate. Dietary programs need to be adhered to at school as well as in the home setting. (N.D. 4)

Impedence monitoring for students with recurrent otitis media and refer for follow-up as appropriate. Many times an infection may be asymptomatic. Impedence monitoring monthly on students at high risk can be a tool to identify early infections. Visual inspections should be conducted in conjunction with this procedure. (N.D. 5)

Implement measures to prevent infection. Infection and illness that cause absence will delay learning. (N.D. 5, 6)

Screen for visual acuity annually and refer as appropriate. Prevention of visual problems and maintenance of optimal visual acuity are essential for learning. (N.D. 7, 13)

Refer for evaluation of thyroid function if problem suspected. (N.D. 8)

Provide opportunities for the student to accomplish age-related, developmentally appropriate tasks (specify). Based on assessment data, program modifications may be necessary for the student to have the opportunity to accomplish developmental tasks. (N.D. 8)

Adhere to the following activity restrictions until an evaluation to rule out atlantoaxial subluxation is completed. Injury can result in serious complications if this condition is present. (N.D. 9)

> Gymnastics
> Butterfly stroke in swimming
> Diving starts in swimming
> High jumps
> Decathalon
> Soccer
> Warm-up exercises that place pressure on the head and neck
> Contact sports
> Sommersaults
> Forward roll
> Flips
> Trampoline exercises

Monitor for periodic dental care and implement dental care as needed at school. (N.D. 10)

Screen and monitor for scoliosis annually. Refer for medical assessment as indicated. (Potential complication: scoliosis)

Refer for occupational therapy, physical therapy: speech and language, audiological, and cognitive assessment as appropriate. Health assessment will often identify needs that can be further assessed by other related services employed by schools. (N.D. 2, 5, 7–13)

Educational/emotional support for students/staff regarding the needs or care of the student with Down syndrome. (N.D. 1–13)

Case management: Refer and follow up for medical care if needed, coordinate service providers. (N.D. 1–13)

Develop healthcare plan to articulate student needs in the school setting. (N.D. 1–13)

Assist student in accommodation for visual impairment in self-care activities. (N.D. 11)

Screen for auditory acuity annually or more frequently as appropriate. Prevention of auditory problems and maintenance of optimal auditory acuity are essential for learning. (N.D. 12)

Expected Student Outcomes

The student will experience an increase in activity with weight loss. (N.D. 1)

The student will identify eating patterns that contribute to weight gain and will adhere to dietary plan. (N.D. 1)

The student will describe and perform adaptive methods needed to perform activities of daily living, and demonstrate cardiac tolerance evidenced by stable pulse, respirations, and blood pressure. (N.D. 2)

The student will adhere to specific activity limitations. (N.D. 2)

The student will utilize methods to prevent changes in temperature or adhere to directions given. The student will maintain normal body temperature. (N.D. 3)

The student will adhere to dietary and activity regimen to promote normal and less painful bowel elimination. (N.D. 4)

The student will utilize good hand-washing and personal hygiene. (N.D. 5, 6)

The student will utilize safety measures to accommodate for vision deficits. (N.D. 7)

The student will demonstrate an increase in behaviors in personal/social, language, cognition, or motor activities that are developmentally/age appropriate. (Specify the behaviors.) (N.D. 8)

The student will refrain from activities that cause forced neck flexion or will comply with directions given. (N.D. 9)

The student complies with or performs regular dental care/exams. (N.D. 10)

The student will accommodate for vision deficits in self-care routines. (N.D. 11)

The student will wear a hearing aid (if appropriate). He/she will use alternative forms of communication, and will demonstrate improved abililty to communicate. (N.D. 12)

The student will accommodate for vision deficits in learning activities. (N.D. 13)

Collaborative Problems

Potential complication: thyroid dysfunction
Potential complication: gum inflammation
Potential complication: scoliosis
Potential complication: joint dislocation

REFERENCES

1. Colwell SO. What's up in down syndrome? *Developmental Dialogue* 1990; 1 (3): 2, 8. (Available from Park Nicollet Medical Foundation, 5000 West 39th Street, Mpls., MN 55416.)

BIBLIOGRAPHY

Batshaw ML, Perret YM. *Children With Handicaps: A Medical Primer.* Baltimore: Paul H. Brookes Publishing, 1981.
Carpenito LJ. *Handbook of Nursing Diagnosis.* Philadelphia: JB Lippincott, 1989.
Carpenito LJ. *Nursing Diagnosis, Application to Clinical Practice.* Philadelphia: JB Lippincott, 1989.
Cooke RE. Atlanatoaxial instability in individuals with Down syndrome. *Adapted Physical Activity Quarterly* 1984; 1: 194–6.

Cronk C, Crocker A, Pueschel S, Shea A, Zackai E, Pickens G, Reed R. Growth charts for children with Down syndrome: 1 month to 18 years of age. *Pediatrics* 1988; 81 (1): 102–10.

National Down Syndrome Congress, 1800 Dempster St, Park Ridge, IL 60068-1146. 1-800-232-6372.

National Information Center for Children and Youth with Handicaps. General Information About Down Syndrome. Fact Sheet Number 4, 1990 (P.O. Box 1492, Washington, D.C. 20013)

Pueschel SM, Scola FH. Atlantoaxial instability in individuals with Down syndrome: epidemiologic, radiographic, and clinical studies. *Pediatrics* 1987; 80 (4): 555–59.

Springer N. *Nutrition Casebook on Developmental Disabilities.* Syracuse Un, Syracuse, NY. 1982.

Van Dyke DC. Medical problems in infants and young children with Down syndrome: implications for early services. *Infants Young Children* 1989; (Jan): 39–50.

Whaley LF, Wong DL. *Nursing Care of Infants and Children.* St. Louis: CV Mosby, 1987.

Wong DL, Whaley LF. *Clinical Manual of Pediatric Nursing.* St. Louis: CV Mosby, 1990.

24 | IHP: Dysmenorrhea (Menstrual Cramps)

Kathleen M. Kalb

INTRODUCTION

As many as two-thirds of postmenarchal adolescents experience painful menstruation, or dysmenorrhea.[1-4] It is the number one cause of repeated short-term absences from school[2] and as such is an ideal condition for school nurse intervention.

Twenty years ago this condition was considered psychogenic or some sort of rejection of a woman's "feminine role."[1] It has been well established, however, in the last two decades that this is a legitimate physiologic condition whose etiology is known and for which effective treatments are available. Unfortunately, many misconceptions remain and very few adolescents with this condition seek treatment, often assuming that it will be dismissed or blamed on the sufferer. School nurses can educate young women about this condition and oversee successful treatment, thus reducing both absenteeism of the student and any self-blame which she might have been experiencing.

Pathophysiology

Primary dysmenorrhea, that is, dysmenorrhea which is not associated with macroscopic pelvic abnormality, is caused by the release of elevated amounts of prostaglandins in the menstrual fluid. These prostaglandins are fatty acids which can cause increases in smooth muscle contractility.[2, 3, 5] The increased contractility of the uterus causes ischemia to the myometrium (decreased oxygen to the area) and thus the resultant crampy pain experienced by many women during menses. Release of these prostaglandins may also be responsible for nausea, vomiting, diarrhea, headache, and emotional changes associated with dysmenorrhea.

Since prostaglandins are released as a result of progesterone activity, dysmenorrhea is associated with ovulatory cycles. It is common for girls to have anovulatory cycles at least some of the time in the first two years following menarche; therefore, it is common for dysmenorrhea to become a problem later in the adolescent years as cycles become consistently ovulatory.[2] It is also common for this pain to be worse in the first two days of menses, since most of the prostaglandins are released during the first 48 hours.[2]

Secondary dysmenorrhea (menstrual pain associated with pelvic abnormality) may be caused by a number of conditions and should be ruled out by a healthcare practitioner before the assumption is made that the young woman has primary dysmenorrhea. Menstrual pain may be caused by sexually transmitted disease, pelvic inflammatory disease, endometriosis, congenital malformation, adhesions, cysts and other pathological conditions. Since many of these conditions have serious ramifications they must be excluded from the diagnosis before treating for primary dysmenorrhea. Table 1 outlines some of the considerations when differentiating between primary and secondary dysmenorrhea.[2]

Table 1. Differentiating Primary and Secondary Dysmenorrhea

Common Characteristics of *Primary Dysmenorrhea*	Common Characteristics of *Secondary Dysmenorrhea*
Onset within a year or two of menarche	Onset at first menses or 2-3 yrs postmenarche
Pain worst during first two days of menses	Pain not related to first day of menses. May begin prior to menses, or may not be limited to menses or increase in severity during menses
Pain pattern remains consistent during each menses	Pain increases in severity over time
May be associated with nausea, vomiting, diarrhea, headaches	May be associated with painful intercourse, abnormal bleeding, abnormal vaginal discharge

Once the diagnosis of primary dysmenorrhea has been established, there are several avenues of treatment. It is possible to treat with or without medication, with varying degrees of success. If the adolescent is willing to try more conservative measures first, she may experience relief from symptoms without drug therapy.

Nondrug Strategies

There are a number of approaches that do not rely on medication which may offer considerable relief. The young woman with menstrual cramps may try localized heat (wrapped hot water bottle, heating pad), moderate exercise, sleep, relaxation therapy, pelvic exercises, yoga, or biofeedback techniques. These measures used separately or in combination may alleviate menstrual pain.

Analgesics

If the student rejects the methods above, or wants to supplement them with analgesics, it may help to use usual doses of acetaminophen. In mild cases of dysmenorrhea, these may be sufficient.

Nonsteroidal Anti-inflammatory Drugs (NSAIDs)

These drugs act as antiprostaglandins and have been found to be very effective in managing moderate to severe menstrual pain. They must be taken at the first sign of cramping and continued through the initial two days of menses. Taken in this manner, they interfere with synthesis of prostaglandins and prevent the ischemic uterine sequelae.[1, 2] Ibuprofen (Advil, Motrin, Nuprin, Rufen) is available over the counter and may be taken in 200 mg.

doses every four to six hours throughout the first 48 hours of menses. Other NSAIDs such as naproxen sodium (Anaprox) and mefenamic acid (Ponstel) are available by prescription. If one of these medications is unsuccessful, it is advisable to try the others since one may work in persons where others are ineffective.

Some negative side effects are possible when taking NSAIDs. The most common are epigastric pain, vomiting, altered platelet function, prolonged bleeding time, headache, dizziness, blurred vision, and tinnitus.[1] These side effects are unusual, however, since the medications are used over such short duration.

It should be noted that although aspirin is also classified as a NSAID, its antiprostaglandin action is minimal and it is not recommended as an antiprostaglandin medication.

Hormonal Treatment

Oral contraceptives may also be used to treat primary dysmenorrhea. The hormones contained in these pills prevent ovulation so prostaglandins are not produced. This may be the treatment of choice in a sexually active adolescent who needs contraception in addition to relief of dysmenorrhea.

INDIVIDUALIZED HEALTHCARE PLAN

History

The history is probably the most important task the nurse will perform in designing an intervention for the student with painful menses. Update the student's history including questions about family history of dysmenorrhea. Special attention must be paid to menstrual history as well as to details of the development of menstrual pain. This information is critical in determining appropriate referral and in differentiating between primary and secondary dysmenorrhea. Following are questions addressing the most pertinent data:

- Has anyone in your family had painful periods? Your mother or sisters or any aunts? Did they ever see a doctor or nurse practitioner about it? How is or was it treated?

Menstrual History:

- How old were you (or what grade were you in) when you started having periods?
- How often do you get your period?
- Do you usually get it every month, or do you sometimes skip a month?
- How many days do you bleed?
- How much do you bleed? (Heavy, moderate, light)
- What date did your last period start? Was it a normal one?

History of Painful Periods:

- Do you have cramps with your period? If yes, how bad are they? (Severe, moderate, mild)
- When do the cramps start and how long do they last?
- Have you had cramps from your first period, or did they become more noticeable as time went on?
- Do you get any other problems with your period? If yes, what kinds of things? (Nausea, vomiting, diarrhea, headache, emotional disruption, other)
- Where does it hurt? Does it spread to any other areas?
- Do you ever miss school or work because of the pain?

- What have you tried to treat it? Does anything seem to help?
- Does anything make it worse?
- Is it generally getting better, worse or staying about the same each month?

Sexual History

- Have you started having sex yet? If yes, are you using any type of birth control?
- Have you talked to any healthcare provider about birth control or sexual activity?
- Have you had intercourse since your last period? If yes, did you use any birth control? What type?
- Have you ever had any sexual diseases? If yes, what ones?
- Have you ever been pregnant? What did you decide to do about the pregnancy (ies)?

If it seems like the appropriate opportunity, the sexual history may be completed including such information as age at first intercourse, gender and age of partners, type of sexual contact (anal, oral, vaginal), and comfort with decision to be sexually active. If, however, the student is uncomfortable or time is very short, this may be obtained at a follow-up visit. (See Chapter 18, IHP: Contraceptive Counseling.)

Assessment

Current Status

- Discuss the student's current history of painful menses. Is she having her period now, and is she in any pain.
- If she is in pain, or is just recovering from period cramping, ask her to describe the pain in terms of severity, quality, and location.
- Ascertain whether this is fairly typical, and what treatments are currently being used.

NOTE: *If the student is sexually active and experiencing severe primary or secondary dysmenorrhea following unprotected intercourse, pregnancy* must *be ruled out. She should be referred for immediate attention to a physician for assessment of pregnancy/ spontaneous abortion.*

Physical assessment

With the exception of abdominal examination, there is little physical examination which needs to be done by the school nurse. The student should be referred to a healthcare provider who is skilled in the pelvic exam, and who is knowledgeable regarding care of the adolescent. Pelvic exam is particularly important for sexually active adolescents.

Psychological/emotional assessment

- Ask the student how painful menstruation is affecting her life.
- Determine whether she has a generally positive regard for herself as a young woman, or whether dysmenorrhea is typical of negative associations with being female.
- Note the student's affect, outlook, and general attitude toward the condition.

Nursing Diagnoses (N.D.)

N.D. 1 Alteration in comfort (NANDA 9.1.1)*: Acute pain related to hormonal activity during menses.

N.D. 2 Impaired physical mobility and activity intolerance (NANDA 6.1.1.1, 6.1.1.2) secondary to pain.

N.D. 3 Alteration in self-concept: disturbance in body image and self-esteem. (NANDA 7.1.1, 7.1.2)

N.D. 4 Knowledge deficit (NANDA 8.1.1) in areas of reproductive physiology.

Goals

The school nurse will:

1. Refer appropriately for diagnosis of primary or secondary dysmenorrhea.

2. Monitor treatment plan to ensure improvement of the condition.

3. Educate student regarding normal course of treatment, typical response patterns as well as appropriate nondrug management techniques.

Nursing Interventions

Update history as above to provide foundation for nursing assessment and information for referral. (N.D. 1–3)

Educate student regarding etiology of uterine cramping and possible treatment strategies. (N.D. 4)

- Reassure student that many types of treatment are available and that if one fails others can be tried.
- Discuss nondrug treatment which may offer some relief.

Interview student to ascertain her self-concept related to this condition (N.D. 3)

Educate student regarding how media presents menstruating women, and how that may and does differ from the reality of most women. (i.e., the media presentation of menstruating women is that they are functioning at usual, optimal level. When an adolescent's reality is different from that, she may feel inadequate or abnormal and therefore have lower self-esteem.[6] Education regarding this discrepancy is often reassuring to the adolescent.) (N.D. 1, 3)

Discuss her willingness to consult a healthcare provider on this matter. (N.D. 1–4)

- Reassure her that it is a legitimate medical condition and should be medically evaluated.
- Determine whether she has a healthcare provider that she trusts and would be willing to see regarding this condition.
- If not, offer to help her find an appropriate source of healthcare.
- Refer as appropriate to diagnose primary or secondary dysmenorrhea.
- Educate her regarding what to expect at the healthcare visit (e.g., necessary history, pelvic exam, questions to ask).

---

* (See chapter 2, page 38 for explanation of the NANDA approved numerical system.)

Follow up with student on a monthly basis to determine effectiveness of treatment and student's emotional status. (N.D. 1–4)

If her response to having this condition seems inappropriately dramatic, or if her emotional status is compromised, refer for further counseling. (N.D. 3)

Expected Student Outcomes

1. The student will experience relief of dysmenorrhea as indicated by her report of lessened or absent menstrual pain.
2. The student will comply with the treatment approach outlined by her healthcare provider.
3. The student will reconcile discrepancies in self-concept and peer/media expectations as indicated by her verbalization of comfort with female role and by her acknowledgement that these expectations do not necessarily reflect her subjective reality.
4. The student will attend follow-up meetings with the nurse to monitor emotional status as well as progress and success of treatment.

REFERENCES

1. Croupy SM, Ahlstrom P. Common menstrual disorders. *Pediatr Clin North Am* 1989; 36 (Jun): 551–71.
2. Khoiny FE. Adolescent dysmenorrhea. *J Pediatr Health Care* 1988; 2 (1): 29–37.
3. Neinstein LS. Acne. *Adolesc Health Care: A Practical Guide*. Baltimore: Urban and Schwarzenberg, 1984: 221–31.
4. Wilson CA, Keye WR. A survey of adolescent dysmenorrhea and premenstrual symptom frequency. *J Adolesc Health Care* 1989; 10 (4): 317–22.
5. Barry JA. Dysmenorrhoea: periods can be a pain. *Austr Fam Phys* 1988; 17 (3): 174–75.
6. Havens B, Swenson I. Imagery associated with menstruation in advertising targeted to adolescent women. *Adolescence* 1988; 23 (89): 89–97.
7. Johnson J. Level of knowledge among adolescent girls regarding effective treatment for dysmenorrhea. *J Adolesc Health Care* 1988; 9 (5): 398–402.
8. Sigmon ST, Nelson RD. The effectiveness of activity scheduling and relaxation training in the treatment of spasmodic dysmenorrhea. *J Behav Med* 1988; 11 (5): 483–95.

25 | IHP: Eating Disorders—Anorexia, Bulimia, Morbid Obesity

Kathleen M. Kalb

INTRODUCTION

Eating disorders are an increasing problem among adolescents.[1-6] Since the age of onset for these disorders is usually between eleven and twenty-five,[2] many of the cases surface during the high school years. The school nurse may play a critical role in detecting, referring,[7] and following those students who experience disordered eating patterns.

Eating disorders have been documented as early as 1689.[2, 4] Today, they affect as many as 10 percent of adolescent females[8, 9] and are becoming more common as our cultural norm supports the notion that the ideal body for females is one that is very thin. From 80 to 95 percent of eating disordered patients are female,[8-12] therefore, the pronoun "she" will be used to refer to students who are suffering from these syndromes. Eating disorder does, however, affect males as well and should be considered in cases where there is a question of body image distortion or extreme weight control required by sports.[13, 14]

Pathophysiology

The three eating disorders that will be outlined here are anorexia nervosa, bulimia nervosa, and morbid obesity. These three conditions are distinct from one another in etiology, symptomology, and treatment,

although there are some shared and overlapping characteristics.

Anorexia Nervosa

Anorexia means loss of appetite. This is actually a misnomer for the condition, since anorexia nervosa refers to a decision to reduce body weight through calorie restriction,[15] and no actual loss of appetite occurs. This condition is marked by the determination to become as thin as possible, even in the face of life-threatening malnutrition. It has often been described in middle- to upper-middle-class white females,[2, 8, 11, 12, 16] but it is beginning to cross economic and racial lines as it becomes more widespread.[3, 17] Anorexia typically begins between the ages of 12 and 18,[2, 4, 12, 16] and has an overall incidence rate of less than 1 percent.[16, 18] The diagnosis of anorexia nervosa depends on the presence of the following characteristics:[1, 2, 6, 8, 9, 11, 12, 15, 16, 18–21]

- Inability or refusal to maintain a body weight which is normal for height.
- Loss of greater than 25 percent of original body weight.
- Disturbed body image, usually denoted by the insistence that she is "fat" even when skeletal in appearance.
- Intense fear of becoming overweight.
- Primary or secondary amenorrhea.

- Absence of organic cause for the weight loss.

Symptoms are somewhat varied and depend on how progressed the condition is. It is common for the young woman to present with a recent history of strenuous dieting and subsequent amenorrhea. Virtually all females who lose body weight to this extreme stop having menses[1, 11, 15, 16] and it may be this concern that brings the student to the school nurse. The decision to diet often follows some major change or event in the student's life, and/or a critical comment about her weight by family or peers.[4, 9, 12]

In addition to these presenting factors, other symptoms may be present in numerous combinations, among them[1, 2, 6, 9, 11, 12, 15]:

- Obsessive preoccupation with thinness.
- Food rituals, including eating only certain foods, cutting food into tiny pieces, hoarding food, eating particular foods on particular days of the week, eating only very low-calorie food, joining mealtime but not eating, and many other unusual food habits.
- Food preoccupation, participating in food-related activities but not actually eating. This might include cooking, reading cookbooks, gardening, collecting recipes, setting elaborate tables, or dreaming about food.
- Increased physical activity. In efforts to burn calories and work off agitation caused by hunger, she may jog, do sit-ups or calisthenics, climb stairs, or join a school athletic team and work tirelessly.
- Vomiting and/or laxative abuse. Since these are also seen in the bulimic patient, anorexic individuals who show symptoms of bulimia may be described as "bulimorexic."
- Indifference to emaciated status.
- Other physical symptoms include constipation, abdominal pain, cold intolerance, hypotension, bradycardia, dry

skin, lanugo, yellow skin color, edema, and cardiac abnormalities.

There are a number of personality and psychological characteristics commonly found in the anorexic individual. She is likely to have low self-esteem and experience depression, anxiety, and a general sense of ineffectiveness.[1, 3, 12, 20] She may be a "model child"[19, 21] and evidence a perfectionistic attitude as demonstrated by overachievement.[12, 22] She may, however, be quite anxious in social situations and have very little sexual interest,[12] as well as a marked need for control.[1]

The families of anorexic patients have been described as rigid, avoidant of conflict resolution, overprotective, boundary invasive, and enmeshed.[3, 12, 21, 23] As the area is researched, however, it is clear that no one type of family supports the development of anorexia nervosa, but rather several types of constellations and interactional patterns may contribute to the formation of the disorder.[17, 24] Recent work indicates that a family history of eating disorder increases the risk for eating disorder in the adolescent.[2]

Treatment of anorexia nervosa is varied and controversial. The approach which seems to hold most promise is two-staged.[3] The first stage is to return the patient to physiologic equilibrium, including weight gain to a normal weight for height and reinstating a normal nutritional status. This may be achieved by several routes, including behavior modification, education and general monitoring. Psychotherapy should be initiated during this stage in order to begin the long-term recovery and assure optimal response from the individual. Hospitalization may be required for the initial stage of intervention,[2, 18] but success has also been achieved on an outpatient basis. The second stage is the follow-up therapy which is most effective when continued for two to four years after initiation of treatment.[1] The purpose of therapy should be to assist the patient toward higher self-esteem and more generalized control over her life. It may require both individual and family sessions to be effective.[2, 3, 9, 23]

It must be kept in mind that anorexia nervosa is a serious disorder. Prognosis for morbidity and continued eating disorder is guarded, with as many as 50 percent still experiencing some symptoms at long-term follow-up.[1, 8, 11] Mortality occurs at a rate of 5 percent for treated individuals[1, 2, 4, 7, 15] and up to 20 percent in untreated populations.[2] These mortalities are usually from both the effects of malnutrition and from suicide.[23] Psychiatric disturbance including depression, anxiety, obsessive-compulsive symptoms, and affective disorder were noted in up to 45 percent of cases on follow-up.[21] The prognosis improves with early age of onset, high educational achievement, realistic body image following weight gain, initial ego strength, and supportive family.[4, 12] It worsens with late age of onset, continued body image distortion, premorbid obesity, bulimic symptoms, prolonged duration, dysfunctional family relations, marked psychopathology, and low social class.[4, 12] Clearly, the nurse can affect outcome by contributing to prompt intervention and effective, caring follow-up.

Bulimia Nervosa

"Bulimia" derives from words meaning "ox hunger" and refers to compulsive or recurrent binge eating. If it is accompanied by purging with vomiting or laxatives, it is described as a syndrome and labeled "bulimia nervosa."[1,2, 20] It typically occurs somewhat later than anorexia nervosa, usually between the ages of 17 and 25.[4, 25] Bulimic individuals tend to be of normal weight, and the disorder may go undetected for years before intervention is sought.[4, 16, 21, 25] Incidence rates seem to be in the range of 4 to 10 percent.[1, 2, 9] Diag-nosis of this disorder would include the following factors:[1, 4, 6, 15, 19, 21]:

- Recurrent episodes of "binge" eating, ingesting large quantities of food in short periods of time, usually secretively.
- Three or more of the following:
  - Binging on high calorie, easily digested food.
  - Ending binges because of abdominal pain, sleep, social interruption, or vomiting.
  - Eating secretively.
  - Approaching weight loss repeatedly through severe calorie restriction, vomiting, amphetamines, cathartics, or diuretics.
- Depression and/or very low self-esteem, especially following binge behavior.
- Absence of anorexia nervosa or medical disorder.

As with anorexia nervosa, bulimia nervosa may be precipitated by some major change in the life of the individual.[1, 4] Family dynamics seem to play a role, although what that role is is not clearly defined. Usually there is a deficit in the ability of the family to allow the bulimic patient independence or especially control over her own life. This leads to feelings of inadequacy and powerlessness.[1] Food may be the only place where the young woman feels she has any control. Ironically, in taking control of this aspect of her life, she eventually loses control over even this as her body swings into an endless cycle of binging and purging.

Bulimic individuals are even more likely than anorexics to show signs of major depression.[1, 9, 10, 25] This contributes to the mortality rate (ranging between 1 and 15 percent), which is split evenly between suicide and medical conditions leading to death.[23] Bulimia is more common than anorexia, and has an incidence rate of 4 to 19 percent.[9] The bulimic individual is more likely than peers to be chemically dependent,[9, 23] therefore chemical dependency may be explored during an evaluation for eating disorder. If there is evidence of chemical dependency, that condition must be treated prior to treating the bulimia.[9]

Additional symptoms that may be encountered in addition to those necessary for diagnosis might include: [1, 4, 6, 9, 10]

- Painless parotid enlargement
- Subconjunctival hematoma
- Erosion of teeth enamel and dental caries
- Ulcerative and/or boggy gingivae
- Tissue damage in the oral cavity
- Calluses on the dorsal aspect of the fingers
- Glossitis
- Dizziness, orthostatic hypotension
- Fluctuations of weight greater than 10 lbs. over short periods of time
- Amenorrhea
- Cardiac arrythmias
- Pretibial and ankle edema

In order to support her "habit" of binging, the bulimic individual may have had episodes of shoplifting or stealing food, or of stealing money to buy food. Sometimes families will express anger that they "can't keep any food in the house."[6] These activities can intensify the young woman's isolation and support her feelings of low self-esteem and inadequacy.[9]

Treatment of bulimia nervosa is a combination of various elements. Antidepressants have been used successfully in reducing the severity of symptoms.[2, 9, 25] These medications seem to be effective even in the absence of major depression,[26] and their mechanism of action is uncertain. Insight-oriented psychotherapy and cognitive behavioral therapy have also been effective in this disorder.[2, 4, 10, 25–27] Group and family therapy may be appro-

priate, depending on the particular characteristics of the individual. In cases of severely nutritionally compromised individuals or if there is suicidal ideation, hospitalization may be necessary to begin the process of treatment.[2, 9] Once physiologic stability has been established and the bulimic person is free of suicidal ideation, treatment may be continued on an outpatient basis.

The prognosis for bulimic individuals is not as optimistic as for those with anorexia nervosa.[23] In studies with long-term follow-up, about one third of clients were free of symptoms, one third were still experiencing symptoms during times of stress, and one third were still experiencing severe problems with their eating.[4, 18]

Much research remains to be done on the causes and treatment of this disorder. As effective treatment evolves, more will be discovered about reducing morbidity and mortality from bulimia.

Morbid Obesity

Morbid obesity is defined as body weight which is 20 percent above ideal weight as listed in weight tables, weight for height exceeding the 95th percentile, and/or triceps skinfold exceeding the 95th percentile.[12, 28] It seems to be slightly more prevalent in females, with the rate for females at 12 percent and for males at 11 percent.[12]

Many factors influence obesity in the child and adolescent, among them inherited body type, environmental effect on food intake patterns, body image, and psychological coping mechanisms.[12, 29] If a child has inherited a so-called "endomorphic" body type, which tends to retain a certain fat content, or if the family has introduced unhealthy eating patterns, the child is more likely to be obese.[12] Further, if the child has an image of him/herself as fat, and/or uses food to cope with stressors, the child is again more likely than peers to be overweight.[12, 29] As with all conditions of weight fluctuation from the norm, organic and metabolic causes must be ruled out before intervention is planned.[29] The nurse should be particularly suspicious of a metabolic cause of obesity if height is below the 50th percentile or if there is attendant mental retardation.[28, 30]

Children who indulge in binge eating are closer to the bulimic pattern discussed above, and require similar treatment strategies. Children who have more straightforward behavioral underpinnings to their obesity seem to respond more readily to behavior modification and nutritional counseling approaches. If the obese child is younger than mid-adolescence, it is imperative to involve the family in treatment since food resources and attitudes are provided at home.[12, 28, 30]

Adolescence is an opportune time for intervention. Since it is one of the periods when fat cells are added to the body (the other two being gestation and the first year of life), it is a critical period for individuals to maintain a normal weight. Otherwise, the fat cells added are permanent and can be reduced in size, but not in number.[12] In fact, 85 percent of obese adolescents will be obese adults.[12, 30] The environmental factors which increase the risk of obesity are single-parent family, greater parental age, television watching, and family eating habits.[30]

Treating obesity is important not so much because of immediate, life-threatening consequences, but because the long-term morbidity is high. Obesity is implicated in such conditions as hypertension, cerebrovascular disease, coronary heart disease, and diabetes mellitus.[12, 30] These problems occur after chronic obesity and seldom surface in childhood or adolescence. More immediate to the child are the psychological prices paid for not conforming to the cultural ideal for body type. These problems can include social isolation, poor body image, low self-esteem, and depression.[28, 30] These psychological issues often prompt the obese youngster to seek help.

Young adolescents may be unmotivated to change eating behaviors, and treatment may be postponed by the individual until later adolescence when motivation is more internalized. Treatment approaches which have met with success tend to include components of nutrition education, behavior modification, calorie restriction, exercise, and group support.[12, 28] This combination can reform food attitudes and practices, reduce body weight, and support the individual while (s)he develops a healthier body image. Often this becomes a lifelong process and requires major changes on the part of the individual in both behavior patterns and world view.

INDIVIDUALIZED HEALTHCARE PLAN

History

It is important for the nurse to realize that a nonjudgemental attitude is very important when interviewing a student regarding food issues.[25, 28] A great deal of shame may be associated with this topic and care must be taken to appreciate the natural reluctance some students will have when discussing food-related behavior. Update the student's history as appropriate. Since family history is a risk factor for these disorders,[9] note any family history of obesity, eating disorder, or chemical dependency. Following are suggestions for addressing the most pertinent data:[1, 6, 9]

Weight/Diet Information

- Diet history, including:
  - Current weight, past weight gains/losses
  - 24-hour diet recall
  - What ways have you tried to control your weight?
  - What are your favorite foods? What are some of your typical meals?
  - Have you ever eaten large amounts of foods in a single sitting?
  - What sorts of foods did you eat? How much did you eat?
  - How often does this happen?
- Do you ever have trouble with constipation, diarrhea or nausea?
- Have you ever vomited or used laxatives or diuretics to control your weight?
- Have you ever or are you now using diet pills, either over the counter or prescription types?
- On a scale of 1 to 10, with one being too skinny and ten way overweight, where would you put yourself right now? (Note how this compares to objective body size relative to weight tables.)
- Do you exercise? How often? What sorts of exercise do you do? For how long at a time?

Reproductive Information

- Menstrual history including:
  - How old were you when you started having periods?
  - Do you have (or have you ever had) regular periods?
  - How often are your periods? How many days does the bleeding last?
  - When was your last period? Was it a normal one?

Psychosocial Information

- How are things in your family right now? Do you get along with your parents pretty well? If not, how do people in your family solve these conflicts?
- Do you ever feel "down" or depressed? What do you usually do about it? Do you ever feel like hurting or killing yourself? What do you usually do about it? Do you feel that way now?
- Has anyone in your family been treated for depression? If yes, who?
- Are there any stresses in your life right now? What are they?
- Have there been any big changes in your life in the past year? If yes, what are they?
- Has anyone in your family had trouble with their weight or dieting?
- Was anyone in your family ever diagnosed with anorexia or bulimia? If yes to either of these questions, who was it? What did (do) they do about it?
- Do you use drugs or alcohol? How often?
- Is anyone in your family chemically dependent (addicted to drugs or alcohol)?

Assessment

Current Status

In assessing the status of a student who is possibly eating disordered, take into account the history as outlined above, your objective observations, and any distress the student expresses about her weight and/or eating behaviors. Be aware that anorexic individuals may try to deny or minimize the problem, and bulimic students may either deny problems or be quite distraught at their lack of control over the situation.

Physical Assessment

When doing a physical assessment, observe the student for any of the symptoms listed earlier in this section. Physical examination of a student with eating disorder may be perfectly normal, since some of the serious physical symptoms do not occur until later in the disease.

Baseline Information
- Current height.
- Current weight (Have the student weigh herself with very minimal clothing. If there are adequate provisions for privacy, take the weight with the student in underwear only. This gives the nurse an opportunity to observe the amount of body wasting which has occurred in very thin patients.) Compare this weight to both standard weight tables and to previous weights of this student if they are available.
- Blood pressure (may be lower than normal in anorexic students, higher than normal in obese students).
- Temperature (may be low in anorexic students).
- Pulse (may be elevated in anorexic or bulimic students).

Examination of the Head
- Conjunctiva may hemorrhage if there has been recent strenuous vomiting.
- Parotid glands may show painless swelling in bulimic students.
- Dental exam is important [15, 25] and should note:
  - tissue damage
  - glossitis
  - tooth erosion
  - dental caries

Examination of the Chest
- Cardiac arrythmias may indicate electrolyte imbalance, muscle weakness, or emetine (Ipecac) poisoning.
- Respiratory infection is common in obese students or may be a sign of aspiration of vomitus or generally poor immune response of a malnourished student.

Examination of the Abdomen
- Striae may be evident if weight fluctuations have been extreme.
- Either absent or hypermotile bowel sounds indicate intestinal abnormality.

Examination of the Extremities
- Calluses on dorsal aspect of fingers may indicate induced vomiting.
- Edema may be present with electrolyte imbalance or cardiac abnormality.

Examination of the Skin
- Hair loss occurs in some anorexic students.
- Dry skin or poor turgor may indicate poor nutritional status.
- Fine downy lanugo may be present on emaciated students.

Note: Be prepared to recommend hospitalization if physical exam indicates any life-threatening condition. (See "Nursing Interventions" section.)

Psychological/Emotional Assessment

While getting the student's history as outlined above, listen for signs of unrealistic body image, depression, chemical abuse, poor self-esteem, and general powerlessness. These are clues that she is at increased risk for eating disorder.[9] Determine whether family relationships are stressed to the point of dysfunction and whether the family seems unsupportive, overprotective, or otherwise inappropriate for the adolescent's stage of establishing independence.[9]

Nursing Diagnoses (N.D.)

N.D. 1   Altered nutrition: less than body requirements (actual and potential) (NANDA 1.1.2.2)*, related to self-starvation and/or vomiting.

N.D. 2   Altered nutrition: more than body requirements (actual and potential) (NANDA 1.1.2.1, 1.1.2.3), related to overeating.

N.D. 3   Altered bowel elimination (NANDA 1.3.1.1, 1.3.1.2), related to dietary intake, exercise habits, laxative use.

N.D. 4   Altered cardiac output (NANDA 1.4.2.1), related to electrolyte imbalance, drug toxicity, blood pressure abnormality.

N.D. 5   Fatigue (NANDA 6.1.1.2.1) related to metabolic rate decrease or sleep disturbance.

N.D. 6   Altered growth and development (NANDA 6.6) related to low caloric intake and/or purging.

N.D. 7   Injury (actual or potential) (NANDA 1.6.1) related to aspiration of vomitus, dental erosion, esophageal damage, malnutrition, overweight.

N.D. 8   Disturbance in self-concept : self-esteem (NANDA 7.1.2), body image (NANDA 7.1.1).

N.D. 9   Knowledge deficit (NANDA 8.1.1) in regard to healthy nutrition, appropriate eating behaviors, and treatment process.

N.D. 10   Altered thought processes (NANDA 8.3), related to effects of malnutrition, especially body image perceptions and denial of illness.

Goals

The School Nurse Will:
1. Assess student's current physical and nutritional status.
2. Work with student and other disciplines to form an optimal treatment approach.
3. Monitor student's progress in dealing with eating behaviors and nutritional health.
4. Refer student for additional services as indicated.

Nursing Interventions

It should be noted that eating disorders are chronic conditions and treatment is a long-term process. Both the nurse and student should set expectations accordingly and look for improvement over time, rather than for immediate or "quick fix" responses to interventions. Students suffering from these conditions may minimize or deny the seriousness of the disease process; they may have concrete cognitive functioning and they may

---

* (See chapter 2, page 38 for explanation of the NANDA approved numerical system.)

misperceive the actions of the nurse or "split" their loyalties, preferring one care provider and resisting another.[20] The nurse needs to continue to be helpful and nonjudgmental, recognizing these responses as part of the disordered thinking that can accompany these conditions. It is important not to be manipulated and not to personalize what may seem to be insulting or resistive behaviors.

Following are appropriate interventions for students suspected to be eating disordered [2, 7, 12, 19]:

Update history, as indicated earlier, to provide foundation for nursing assessment and information for referral. (N.D. 1–10)

Explore area resources for treatment of eating disorders in order to make informed referrals. (N.D. 1–10)

Communicate with other professionals and make appropriate referrals based on assessment and consultation. (N.D. 1–10)

Refer for immediate evaluation if her symptoms indicate cardiac involvement, suicidal ideation, electrolyte imbalance or significant. (> 25 percent of ideal) loss of body weight. (N.D. 4)

Refer to rule out pregnancy in amenorrheic students who are sexually active. (N.D. 6)

Involve student in decision-making process so that she will be invested in the outcome and more likely to be compliant with treatment. (N.D. 8–10)

Assist student in realistic goal setting and problem solving, keeping in mind the possibility that she may have difficulty with these processes if her thinking is at a concrete level. (N.D. 9, 10)

Educate the student regarding her condition, its possible consequences, usual treatment measures, and expected outcomes. (N.D. 9)

Educate the student regarding any possible side effects of medications prescribed for her. (N.D. 9)

Assist student in starting and keeping a food diary, including daily foods eaten, emotions and thoughts accompanying eating, and events precipitating eating. (N.D. 8–10)

Determine whether student seems to be coping successfully with body image concerns, including whether the student is acquiring a realistic body image. (N.D. 8)

Follow up with student on a weekly or biweekly basis to determine effectiveness of treatment and student's emotional status. (N.D. 1–10)

Note: Hospitalization is indicated if she has lost 40 percent of premorbid weight, lost more than 30 percent of premorbid weight within three months, has cardiovascular changes, decreased vital signs, is suicidal, or if she or her family continuously sabotage treatment efforts.[1, 2, 15, 23] Do not hesitate to contact appropriate professionals if any of the above occur.

Expected Student Outcomes

The student will achieve and maintain an appropriate weight for height as measured by weight tables or growth charts.

The student will experience a decrease in binge/purge symptoms and will eat a balanced, healthy diet appropriate for her age and height as demonstrated in food diary, by self-report, and by objective measurements.

The student will experience increased self-esteem as demonstrated by:

> Ability to take part comfortably in group activities.
>
> Ability to take social risks.
>
> Appropriate eye contact when interacting verbally.
>
> Affect reflecting comfort or positive emotional status.
>
> Ability to express positive opinion of self.

The student will express increased comfort with body image as demonstrated by:

> Appropriate dress and grooming as compared to peer group.
>
> Ability to verbalize acceptance of body.
>
> Lack of negative comments about body or body parts.
>
> Lack of obsessive preoccupation with thinness.
>
> Lack of denial or minimizing of symptoms.
>
> The student will demonstrate a knowledge of her condition, its consequences, and of healthy nutrition as demonstrated by verbal report of same to nurse.
>
> The student will cooperate with the treatment plan as shown by following up on referrals, attending therapy, and attending follow-up meetings with the nurse.

REFERENCES

1. Comerci GD. Eating disorders in adolescents. *Pediatrics in Review* 1988; 10 (2): 37–47.
2. Giannini AJ, Newman M. Anorexia and bulimia. *Am Family Practitioner* 1990; 41 (4): 1169–76.
3. Gilbert EH, Deblassie RR. Anorexia nervosa: adolescent starvation by choice. *Adolescence* 1984; 19 (76): 839–46.
4. Holden N. Eating disorders. *Palliere's Clinical Obstetrics and Gynaecology* 1989; 3 (4): 705–27.
5. Muuss RE. Adolescent eating disorder: bulimia. *Adolescence* 1986; 21 (82): 257–67.
6. Plehn KW. Anorexia nervosa and bulimia: incidence and diagnosis. *Nurse Practitioner* 1990; 15 (4): 22–31.
7. Mallick J. Anorexia nervosa and bulimia: questions and answers for school personnel. *J School Health* 1984; 54 (8): 299–301.
8. Barry A, Lippmann S. Anorexia nervosa in males. *Postgrad Med* 1990; 87 (8): 161–65.
9. Edelstein CK et al. Early clues to anorexia and bulimia. *Patient Care* 1989; (Aug 15): 155–75.
10. Fitzgerald BA, et al. Bulimia nervosa: uncovering a secret disorder. *Postgrad Med* 1988; 84 (2): 119–23.
11. Milman DH. When thin is not beautiful: anorexia nervosa. *Resident Staff Phys* 1981: (Jan): 47–51.
12. Neinstein LS. *Adolescent Health Care: A Practical Guide.* Baltimore: Urban and Schwarzenberg, 1984: 221–31.
13. Moore DC. Body image and eating behavior in adolescent boys. *Am J Dis Children* 1990; 144 (April): 475–79.
14. Slavin J. Eating disorders in athletes. *JOPERD* 1987; 58 (3): 33–36.
15. Brotman A, Rigotti N, Nd Herzog D. Medical complications of eating disorders: outpatient evaluation and management. *Compr Psychiatry* 1985; 26 (3): 258–72.
16. Rockwell WJ. Eating disorders: evaluation and treatment. *North Carolina Med J* 1988; 49 (10): 533–35.
17. Lachenmeyer JR, Muni-Brander P. Eating disorders in a nonclinical adolescent population: implications for treatment. *Adolescence* 1988; 23 (90): 303–12.
18. Yager J. The treatment of eating disorders. *J Clin Psychiatry* 1988; 49 (9): 18–25.
19. Jacobson K, Aughey D. What's eating our youth: overview of disordered eating. *Topics in Pediatrics* 1988; Minneapolis Children's Med. Ctr., (Winter): 11–17.
20. Muscari ME. Effective nursing strategies for adolescents with anorexia nervosa and bulimia nervosa. *Pediatric Nursing* 1988; 14 (6): 475–82.
21. Young D. Eating disorders in the adolescent. *Aust Family Phys* 1988; 17 (5): 334–36.
22. Pantanizopoulos J. "I'll be Happy When I'm Thin Enough." The Treatment of Anorexia Nervosa in Adolescent Literature. *The ALAN Review* 1989; 17 (1): 9–10.

23. Palmer TA. Anorexia nervosa, bulimia nervosa: causal theories and treatment. *Nurse Practitioner* 1990; 15 (4): 12–21.

24. Grigg DN, et al. Family patterns associated with anorexia nervosa. *Marital Family Therapy* 1989; 15 (1); 29–42.

25. Castiglia PT. Bulimia. *J Pediatric Health Care* 1989; 3 (3): 167–69.

26. Fairburn CG. Bulimia nervosa: antidepressant or cognitive therapy is effective. *Br Med J* 1990; 300 (Feb): 485–87.

27. Pyle RL, et al. Maintenance treatment and 6-month outcome for bulimic patients who respond to initial treatment. *Am J Psychiatry* 1990; 147 (7): 871–75.

28. Dietz WH. The overweight child: psychosocial effects and treatment. In: *Feelings and Their Medical Significance.* Ross Laboratories 1989; 31 (1): 1–4.

29. Basoe H, Herman CP. Nature vs. nurture in the etiology of overweight. BASH Magazine 1990; 9 (5): 140–41.

30. Griffin DW. Adolescent obesity. *Topics in Pediatrics* 1988; Minneapolis Children's Med. Ctr., (Winter): 11–17.

31. Johnson C, Connors ME. *The etiology and treatment of bulimia nervosa: a biopsychosocial perspective.* New York: Basic Books, 1988.

32. Marshall-Hoerr SL, et al. Treatment and follow-up of obesity in adolescent girls. *J Adolescent Health Care* 1988; 9 (1): 28–37.

RESOURCES

Organizations

American Anorexic and Bulimic Association
133 Cedar Lane
Teaneck, NJ 01616
(201) 836–1800

Anorexia Nervosa and Associated Disorders
P.O. Box 7
Highland Park, IL 60035
(312) 831–3438

National Anorexic Aid Society
550 S. Cleveland Ave.
Suite F
Westerville, OH 43018

Assessment Tools

Eating Disorder Screening Tool
Available from:
Healthstart, Inc.
640 Jackson St.
St. Paul, MN 55101
(612) 221–3441

Handbook of Psychotherapy for Anorexia Nervosa and Bulimia.
Garner D, Garfinkel P, eds. New York: Guilford Press, 1984.

Eating Disorders Inventory
Available from:
Psychological Assessment Resources, Inc.
P.O. Box 98
Odessa, FL 33556

Weight Control Programs

Weight Watchers
(Listed locally)

Shapedown
by Lauren Mellin
(Comprehensive weight reduction program)
Available from:
Balboa Publishing Company
583 Tenth Ave.
San Francisco, CA 94118

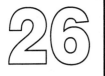

26 | IHP: Encopresis

Wanda R. Miller

INTRODUCTION

Encopresis is the persistent fecal soiling of clothing by a child who has reached 4 years of age, the age when most practitioners agree that toilet training should be accomplished. Encopresis occurs both in children who have never been toilet trained and in those who have been successfully toilet trained.[1,2] Encopresis is reported in 1.5 to 3 percent [2-4] of school-age children and is approximately four times as prevalent in boys as in girls.[5]

The cause of encopresis has not been clearly established; however, recent studies indicate faulty anal sphincter mechanics may cause constriction rather than relaxation of the sphincter when the stimuli to defecate occurs. The resulting response, or as some believe the cause,[6] is chronic constipation and may be the result of or the cause for as much as 80 to 90 percent of all cases of encopresis.[4] A small percentage of encopretic children pass stool into their clothing due to a variety of bowel diseases. Approximately 5 percent of children with encopresis do not have a history of either constipation or existing physical or bowel disease problems[6] and pass stool into their clothing due to emotional reasons. There is a great deal of discrepancy in the literature about the incidence and etiology of encopresis, therefore the percentages are only rough estimates of the incidence of encopresis and the etiology remains vague.

Anthony[1] and Levine[2] have classified encopretic children based on whether the child retains stool or not. The retentive encopretic willfully avoids defecation, while the nonretentive encopretic purposefully deposits soft, formed stool that is normal in volume. It is important to differentiate these two characteristics for the purposes of pathophysiology and intervention; however, the behavior is variable and both characteristics have been observed in the same child.[2]

Although the etiology remains inconclusive, the resulting behavior presents a serious problem to the child and to the child's family.

Pathophysiology

A variety of precipitating causes for encopresis have been studied. Many of them are associated with changes in the child's bowel routine. One of the most frequently cited causes is a simple environmental change resulting in constipation.[5] In the infant, the change can be as minor as a change from breast milk to formula, from one formula to another, or the introduction of a new food into the infant's diet. In the toddler, toilet training that requires developmental disequilibrium and change from dependence to control and autonomy has been considered by some to be a precipitating factor.[1, 7] If parental pressure is too great, the child may withhold stool, which can lead to constipation. In older children, the change can occur with stress or new situations, such as, moving to a new house, changing schools, family conflicts, loss of a parent, changing teachers, a new sibling, a sick parent, or a new bathroom facility. There is some initial information that would indicate that sexual abuse may also be a factor in the etiology of encopresis.[7] Illness associated with dehydration, diarrhea, or an anal fissure may also cause pain on defecation resulting in retention of stool. The passage of painful stool and the resulting behavior of withholding stool is believed by some to be the beginning cause of constipation.[6]

Constipation, a primary factor in encopresis, is a decrease in the passage of stool accompanied by difficulty in defecation. This decrease facilitates the absorption of water and electrolytes in the colon section of the gastrointestinal tract and results in excessively dry, hard stool which if allowed to persist contributes to an overflow of liquid incontinence from above the hard stool in the rectum and seepage out the anus.

Stool is continually moved into the descending sigmoid colon and the rectum before the urge to defecate is felt. Two sphincters at the distal end of the rectum maintain continence. The internal sphincter is controlled by the autonomic nerve system and is composed of circular muscle fibers. The sphincter is involuntarily controlled by the autonomic nerve system. The external sphincter is voluntarily controlled and contraction of this sphincter and the anal musculature maintains continence. The descending colon and the rectum are evacuated during defecation. If the external sphincter is willfully contracted, the rectum and descending colon adjust to the increased pressure.

Additional water is absorbed from the stool, progressive hardening occurs and a large mass of stool accumulates and stretches the colon. As rectal distention increases, the anal muscle relaxes and the anal canal shortens. Soft stool gathers above the mass, flows around it involuntarily and the shortened external sphincter is unable to prevent soiling. This process results in decreased rectal sensitivity, megacolon development, and a fear-pain anxiety in response to signals to defecate. What starts out as a simple constipation problem may become a habitual abnormal defecation pattern.[5]

The treatment program is dependent on the child's and parent's commitment to the program and their compliance with the medical regime. Depending on the level of constipation and the management plan of the physician, either a bowel evacuation schedule followed by an oral laxative maintenance dose is used or the oral laxative maintenance is used alone. In the more aggressive regime, Levine[8] recommends using a sodium biphosphate/phosphate (Fleets) 2 oz. enema am and pm on the first day. The same enema on the second day and a bisacodyl rectal suppository (Dulcolax) stool softener in the am and pm [dioctyl sodium sulfosuccinate (Colace) is suggested by other practitioners]. On the third day a bisacodyl oral tablet (Dulcolax) is given in the pm.

If oral laxatives are used plain mineral oil or dioctyl sodium sulfosuccinate in mineral oil (Milkinol) is given in adequate doses. If taste is a problem, flavored mineral oil (Kondremul without cascara or phenolphthalein (Agoral without phenolphthalein may be supplemented). Bulk agents such as barley malt extract (Maltsupex) are another alternative.[5]

Soothing lotions (Balneol) or local anesthetic ointments (Nupercainal, Surfacaine) may be used if there is local irritation or anal fissures.[5]

INDIVIDUALIZED HEALTHCARE PLAN

History

Update the history with particular emphasis on fecal soiling, constipation, retentive or nonretentive behavior, abdominal cramping, and pain. Consider the differentiating signs to rule out Hirschsprung's disease or other organic diseases. Hirschsprung's disease presents with constipation also; but, in contrast, exhibits failure to thrive, anemia, obstructive symptoms, and almost always has its onset with constipation in infancy. In the absence of organic causes of encopresis, following medical examination, school nurses can effectively assess, intervene, and manage the care plan for a child with encopresis.

Table 1. Guidelines for Eliciting the Encopretic History

These guidelines are intended to provide a framework for the development of a comprehensive encopretic history. All characteristics listed refer to the child under care, unless otherwise specified.

1) **Soiling Profile**
   Age at onset of soiling
   Duration of soiling
   Frequency of soiling
   Description of soiling episodes (consistency and volume of stool, time of day, activities and location when soiling occurs)

2) **Current and Past Bowel Profile: Infant, Toddler, Preschooler, School-Age)**

   Description of the stools: frequency, consistency and size of stools; presence of crying; presence of pain or blood while passing stools; positions assumed to pass a stool; frequency of stools using the toilet
   Previous evaluation and treatment approaches used to address the child's bowel problem

3) **Toilet-Training Profile**

   Age when bladder and bowel training was initiated
   Individuals responsible for training
   Techniques employed
   Age at which bladder training was completed and length of time to complete
   If bowel training was completed at any point, age at which this occurred and length of time taken to complete
   Any major family changes or significant events that occurred during bladder or bowel training

4) **Child's Response to Current Toileting and Soiling**

   Child's feelings about use of the toilet at home, in school, elsewhere
   If child tries to willfully withhold stool, describe
   Child's feelings about the soiling
   Child's ideas about the causes of his/her soiling

5) **Family's Response to Soiling**

   Parental feelings about the child's soiling
   Parental perceptions of the causes of the child's soiling

6) **Urinary Tract Profile**

   Note any history of urinary tract infections
   Establish any history of day or night wetting

7) **Dietary Profile**

   Describe the child's appetite
   Note source of dietary fiber, dairy products, protein, fluids and junk food

8) **Family Demographic and Social Profile**

Birth dates, occupations, work hours, education and marital status of parents
Child's birth order rank in family
Sibling's names and birth dates
Current household members
Current child care arrangements

9) **Behavioral Profile**

Temperament style
General behavior at home
Quality of the child's relationships with family members

10) **School-Functioning Profile**

Academic performance
Classroom behavior
Peer relationships

Reprinted, with permission, from Sprague-McRae JM, [7] p 18. Copyright, *The Nurse Practitioner: The American Journal of Primary Health Care.*

An alternative parental questionnaire is available. Developed by Levine and Barr,[10] the encopretic evaluation system focuses on the historical, demographic, and behavioral aspects of the child and families.

Assessment

An assessment of the child's classroom behavior can be obtained through classroom observation by the nurse or from reports from the teacher(s). If a more structured observation is desired, the Conners' parent and teacher rating scale may be used.[11]

On physical examination the abdomen of the encopretic child has minimal distention, and movable fecal masses are palpable. Abdominal distention suggests Hirschsprung's disease and warrants medical referral.

Problems, in addition to Hirschsprung's disease, that signal the need for referral include urinary tract infections, deep pilonidal dimples, and flat buttocks. Female encopretics should have a urinalysis to rule out urinary tract infection. Deep pilonidal dimples with hair tufts suggest spina bifida occulta, and a flat buttocks suggests sacral agenesis.[4] Nonretentive encopretics may need a psychological evaluation.

Nursing Diagnoses (N.D.)

N.D. 1 Alteration in knowledge deficit (NANDA 8.1.1)*, related to:
- developmental stages of toddlers, preschoolers, and school-age children
- the normal digestive process
- the nature of encopresis.

N.D. 2 Alteration in bowel elimination pattern, constipation and soiling, due to encopresis. (NANDA 1.3.1.1.2)

N.D. 3 Alterations in coping of the family due to ineffective and compromised behavior. (NANDA 5.1.2.1.2)

---

* (See chapter 2, page 38 for explanation of the NANDA approved numerical system.)

N.D. 4 Alteration in nutrition—mechanical—due to lack of fiber and fluids. (NANDA 1.1.2.2)

N.D. 5 Alterations in self-care: toileting. (NANDA 6.5.4.)

N.D. 6 Alterations in self-concept: disturbance in self-esteem due to fecal soiling of clothes. (NANDA 6.5.4, 7.1.2.2)

Goals

The parent (s) will increase their knowledge of the developmental stages of children. (N.D. 1)

The family and child will increase their knowledge of the pathophysiology of digestion and encopresis. (N.D. 1)

The parent (s) will develop a working knowledge of behavior modification. (N.D. 1)

The child will clear the impaction, overcome withholding behavior, and establish and maintain routine bowel evacuation. (N.D. 2)

The child will eliminate fecal soiling of clothing. (N.D. 2)

The child and family will recognize the problem. (N.D. 2)

The parents will be assured of the developmental and mechanical problems associated with constipation and relieved of feelings of guilt. (N.D. 3)

The child is supported emotionally. (N.D. 3)

The parents will emphasize responding to internal stimuli (body signals to defecate) versus external stimuli (reward system). (N.D. 3)

The parent (s) and child are informed about foods high in fiber, especially whole grain cereals and bran, raw and cooked vegetables and fruit. (N.D. 4)

The child and parent (s) will identify encopresis as a problem and work toward resolving the problem. (N.D. 5)

The guilt associated with being encopretic or having a child who is encopretic will be reduced. (N.D. 6)

Nursing Interventions

Provide the parent information in terms of Erikson's stages of development to increase their understanding of the child's normal conflict between autonomy and shame. (N.D. 1)

Provide information to the family and student to increase their knowledge of the physical aspects of digestion and encopresis. (N.D. 1)

Provide the parents a clearly defined, nonjudgmental approach to the implementation of positive and negative reinforcement and to the principles of behavior modification. (N.D. 1)

Provide the parent with information about the principles of behavior modification techniques. (N.D. 1)

Determine the need for medical management for bowel disease or psychological intervention. (N.D. 2)

The parent will keep a diary of dietary intake and bowel movements for at least two weeks. (N.D. 2)

Develop an encopresis management plan: (N.D. 2)

- Consult with the child's physician to establish medical practice.
- Engage the child and family in the treatment process.
- Include the family, student, and physician in the development of a plan.
- Assist the parent to establish a bowel evacuation protocol using enemas, stool softeners, or oral laxatives, as prescribed by the physician.
- Develop with the family and child a set of common language terms for the words bowel movement, urine, and anus.
- Explain defecation process to parent and review with child.
- Establish periods during the day when defecation is encouraged.

Maintain a supportive attitude to the child and the family through the process of gaining control of a routine bowel movement process. Support the family through the slow periods and the plateau periods when change does not occur or when positive progress is temporarily reversed. (N.D. 3)

Assist the child in identifying the internal stimuli for defecation. (N.D. 3)

Establish positive reinforcers that are currently meaningful to the child and periodically review and revise the positive reinforcer. (N.D. 3)

Establish criteria and specific monitoring times when clothing is expected to be clean. Space these in small incremental steps that allow the child to succeed. (N.D. 3)

- Determine negative consequences such as withholding privileges as a consequence for soiling. Reevaluate these negative reinforcers frequently to insure that a power struggle is not ensuing.

Identify foods that are high in fiber and assist the child in developing preference for high-fiber foods. (N.D. 4)

Develop a plan with the child and the parent for a nutritional diet. (N.D. 4)

Encourage the parent to include the child in the compiling of a shopping list and the selection of foods from the grocery store. Encourage the parent to allow the child to select fruits, vegetables, and cereal grains at the store. (N.D. 4)

Anticipatory information regarding the potential for relapse during illnesses or environmental change is given to the child and the parent. (N.D. 5)

Assist the student to develop self-care skills in the event of a soiling episode. (N.D. 5)

Promote positive self-image and student optimism to achieve freedom from constipation and soiling. (N.D. 6)

Promote social support systems at school. (N.D. 6)

Ensure psychological referral if needed. (N.D. 6)

Expected Outcomes

The student can define the digestive process and describe the mechanical process of constipation. (N.D. 1)

The student maintains routine bowel elimination and clean clothing throughout the day. (N.D. 2)

The student defines the physical sensation of the urge to defecate. (N.D. 3)

The student identifies fruits, vegetables, and cereal grains as foods high in fiber, chooses foods at the grocery store that are high in fiber. (N.D. 4)

The student comes to the school nurse's office in the event of soiling, cleans his/her body, and changes clothing independently. (N.D. 5)

The student reports to the nurse self-confidence in maintaining clean clothes. (N.D. 6)

REFERENCES

1. Anthony EJ. An experimental approach to the psychopathology of childhood: encopresis. *Br J Med Psychology* 1957; 30: 147–75.
2. Levine MD. Children with encopresis: a descriptive analysis. *Pediatrics* 1975; 56 (3): 412.
3. Bellman M. Studies on encopresis: encopretics and controls—a clientele investigation. *Acta Paediatr Scand* 1966; Suppl 170: 54–110.
4. Ellert ML. Constipation/encopresis: a nursing perspective. *J Pediatric Health Care* 1990; 4 (3): 141–6.
5. Johns C. Encopresis. *Am J Nursing* 1985; (Feb): 183–5.
6. Fitzgerald JF. Encopresis, soiling, constipation: what's to be done? *Pediatrics* 1975; 56: 348–49.
7. Spraque-McRae JM. Encopresis: developmental, behavioral and physiological considerations for treatment. *Nurse Practitioner: Am J Primary Health Care* 1990;15 (6): 8, 11–18: 21–4.
8. Levine MD. The school child with encopresis. *Pediatrics in Review* 1981; 2 (9): 285–90.
9. Levine MD. Encopresis: its potentiation, evaluation and alleviation. *Pediatr Clin North Am* 1982; 29 (2): 315–30.
10. Levine MD, Barr R. Encopretic Evaluation System. 1980. The Children's Hospital Medical Center, Division of Ambulatory Pediatrics. 300 Longwood Ave, Boston, MA 02115.
11. Conners CK. A teacher rating scale for use in drug studies with children. *Am J Psychiatry* 1969; 26 (6): 884–8.

27 | IHP: Gastrostomy

Mary J. Villars Gerber

INTRODUCTION

As greater numbers of students with physical and multiple handicaps are being mainstreamed into regular education settings, the school nurse will more likely be involved with a student who receives his/ her primary nutrition by gastrostomy feedings. The school nurse will play a primary role in management and supervision of this procedure for a student in school.

Physiology

Oral feeding is always the preferred method of nutrition whenever possible. However, in some instances, alternative methods of feeding must be considered. Students with the following conditions may be considered for gastrostomy feedings:

Central nervous system dysfunction such as cerebral palsy
Gastroesophageal reflux
Chronic gagging or vomiting
Oral hypersensitivity
Birth defects such as cleft lip/palate
Congenital anomalies of the esophagus
Inability to suck, chew, or swallow
Muscle and nerve disorder of the face or cranium
Malfunction or malformation of the stomach or intestines

Oral motor dysfunction with primitive or abnormal reflexes such as jaw thrust, lip retraction, tongue retraction, tongue thrust, and tonic bite
At risk for aspiration or choking

When all other options for oral feeding are not suitable to maintain adequate nutrition, a gastrostomy may be considered. Gastrostomy feedings are considered a longer term solution than a nasogastric feeding.

The surgery is now considered a minor procedure. A small opening is made in the wall of the abdomen. Into this opening, or stoma, a small tube is inserted. One end of this tube, known as a gastrostomy tube, opens into the stomach, and the other end can be attached to a feeding device. Recently a feeding button has also been used and functions in the same way. A plastic button is placed and it lays flat against the outer abdominal wall. It tends to be dislodged less frequently and does not need to be changed periodically, as a gastrostomy tube does. Complications of gastrostomy tube placement include obstruction of the pyloric outlet, wound dehiscence, postoperative ileus, intestinal adhesions, and peritonitis.[1]

Maintenance of optimal osmolarity is a consideration in preparing homemade tube feedings. If the formula prepared is hyperosmolar, the feeding tends to pull fluid from blood to the colon resulting in a sudden increase of volume in the colon, causing diarrhea. Commercially prepared formulas have controlled osmolarity.

Students with the condition known as gastroesophageal reflux are at frequent risk of aspiration and subsequent aspiration pneumonia, poor weight gain, and esophagitis with resultant iron deficiency anemia. Clinical evidence of aspiration includes a wet, gurgling vocal quality with feedings, coughing and sputtering, frequent respiratory illness, and weak, breathy vocalizations and cries. Medical management of this condition always precedes surgical management. The use of upright positioning, thickened foods, and medications to hasten the emptying of the stomach will be tried prior to surgical intervention. Videofluoroscopy is conducted to diagnose this condition. If a gastrostomy is chosen, a procedure known as a fundoplication will very likely be conducted in a child with gastroesophageal reflux. The Nissen technique is the most commonly used, and involves a 360 degree wrap of the upper stomach around the distal esophagus.[2] This very often prevents regurgitation, but may also prohibit normal feeding.

With the gastrostomy, it is always desirable to maintain the student's ability to eat orally, if possible, and should be done as soon as possible. Some students may continue using a combination of oral and gastrostomy feeding. The child's physician must be consulted regarding oral feeding.[3]

Certain professionals are trained to work with feeding difficulties, they include occupational therapists, nutritionists, and speech pathologists. Along with the child's physician, these people should be your first contacts in dealing with feeding difficulties.[3]

INDIVIDUALIZED HEALTHCARE PLAN

History

What is the student's history of growth and weight gain? (charted)

What were the medical history and diagnosis that resulted in placement of the gastrostomy?

At what age was the gastrostomy placement done?

To what extent have oral feedings been used?

Assessment

- Current height and weight to establish baseline.
- Current use of oral feedings, frequency and tolerance. It is possible that oral feeding may be needed during school hours.
- Type of feeding procedure used, equipment and feeding formula, and frequency of feedings. This information will be needed to develop school procedure.
- Tolerance of feeding.
- Bowel elimination patterns. Diarrhea can be a sign the feeding formula is hyperosmolar.
- Individualized instructions for feeding including positioning used. This information will be needed to establish guidelines for the individual student.

- Medical care information in the event the tube becomes dislodged, including physician and phone number, hospital, parents' names and phone numbers, insurance coverage, and procedure for tube replacement.
- Frequency of routine gastrostomy tube replacement and by whom. Old or worn tubes will function poorly or become dislodged.
- Medications administered by gastrostomy.
- Safety precautions and care of tube and stoma. To prevent accidental dislodging of the tube, it needs to be secured and can be done so in a variety of ways. Some students will need more meticulous care of the stoma to prevent skin breakdown.
- Procedures related to a Nissen fundoplication including oral feedings and nausea/vomiting. Some students cannot be fed orally because of the Nissen procedure that was done. When a child appears to be nauseated, the tube or button needs to be vented to allow stomach contents to be expelled.
- Classroom needs and modifications.

Nursing Diagnoses (N.D.)

N.D. 1 Potential for aspiration (NANDA 1.6.1.4)* related to increased intragastric pressure secondary to gastrostomy tube feeding.

N.D. 2 Impaired swallowing (NANDA 6.5.1.1) related to inability to participate in independent eating behavior secondary to decreased cognition.

N.D. 3 Altered nutrition: less than body requirements (NANDA 1.1.2.2) related to chewing or swallowing difficulties.

N.D. 4 Altered physical growth and development (NANDA 6.6) related to inability to consume adequate nutrition.

N.D. 5 Potential altered bowel elimination: diarrhea (NANDA 1.3.1.2) related to gastrostomy feedings.

Goals

Prevent aspiration during gastrostomy feedings. (N.D. 1)

Administer gastrostomy feedings as primary/supplementary form of nutrition. (N.D. 2–4)

Facilitate weight gain. (N.D. 3, 4)

Prevent diarrhea. (N.D. 5)

Nursing Interventions

To prevent aspiration, verify placement of feeding tube, aspirate for residual, position with head elevated during and after feeding, and regulate feedings to allow for stomach emptying. (N.D. 1)

Update health history. (N.D. 1–5)

Educational/emotional support for students and staff. (N.D. 1–5)

---

* (See chapter 2, page 38 for explanation of the NANDA approved numerical system.)

Supervision of staff administering feedings. In some cases it is possible that district procedure will allow properly trained and supervised staff to administer feedings, it is the school nurse's responsibility to fulfill this role. (N.D. 1–5)

Case management: Refer and follow up for medical care if needed, coordinate service providers. (N.D. 1–5)

Healthcare plan to include guidelines for residual, procedure for feeding, type and amount of feeding, time and duration of feeding, plans for action should tube become dislodged, special feeding needs, safety precautions, care of stoma, procedures related to a Nissen fundoplication, growth monitoring. (N.D. 1–5)

Refer for feeding assessment by speech and language or occupational therapist. Oral feedings can occur according to physician orders and a feeding program for the student will need to be developed. (N.D. 2, 3)

Obtain current medical orders for feedings. (N.D. 2–4)

Self-care education for the student as appropriate. (N.D. 2–4)

Provide for documentation of feedings at school. Because this is a procedure conducted by physician order, it is necessary to document it. (N.D. 2–4)

Develop procedure for administration of feedings and by whom. (N.D. 2–4)

Monitor in the case of frequent diarrhea and refer for medical/dietary assessment of feeding formula. (N.D. 5)

Expected Student Outcomes

The student will not aspirate. (N.D. 1)

The student will improve ability to swallow. (N.D. 2)

Will receive adequate nutrition by gastrostomy/orally. (N.D. 3)

Will experience improved physical growth. (N.D. 4)

Will experience infrequent diarrhea. (N.D. 5)

Collaborative Problems

Potential complication: Paralytic Ileus/Small Bowel Obstruction

Potential complication: Pneumonia

Developmental Issues

When a gastrostomy tube is placed due to a child's developmental delay related to oral motor disfunction, it is quite possible that over time the child may develop the skills to drink, chew, and swallow. In these cases it is possible that the gastrostomy tube will no longer be necessary.

REFERENCES

1. Fee MA, Charney EB, Robertson WW. Nutritional assessment of the young child with cerebral palsy. *Infants Young Children* 1988; 1 (Jul): 38.
2. Blount BW. Gastroesophageal reflux in children. *Am Family Phys* 1988; 37 (4): 201–216.
3. Larson G, ed. *Managing the School Age Child with a Chronic Health Condition: A Practical Guide for Schools, Families, and Organizations.* Wayzata, MN: DCI Publishing, 1988: 154 (Available from Sunrise River Press, 11481 Kost Dam Rd, North Branch, MN 55056, 612-583-3239.

RESOURCES

Behrman RE, Vaughan VC III. *Nelson Textbook of Pediatrics.* Philadelphia: WB Saunders, 1983.

Carpenito LJ. *Nursing Diagnosis, Application to Clinical Practice.* Philadelphia: JB Lippincott, 1989.

Colorado Department of Education, Colorado Department of Health. *Procedure Guidelines For Health Care of Special Needs Students In The School Setting.* Denver: Colorado Departments of Education and Health, 1988.

Nelson C, Hallgren R. Gastrostomies: indications, management and weaning. *Infants Young Children* 1989; 2 (Jul): 66–74.

Paarlberg J, Balint J. Gastrostomy tubes: practical guidelines for home care. *Pediatric Nursing* 1985; (Mar/Apr): 99–102.

Sondheimer JM. Gastroesophageal reflux: update on pathogenesis and diagnosis. *Pediatr Clin North Am* 1988; 35 (1): 103–116.

Springer N. *Nutrition Casebook On Developmental Disabilities.* Syracuse Un. Press, Syracuse, NY, 1982.

Supplement 1. Procedural Guidelines: Gastrostomy Tube Feedings

1. The student should have a healthcare plan outlining: how to check for residual and placement, type and amount of feeding, time and duration of feeding, and plans for action if tube becomes dislodged.

2. Written parental and physician consent for the procedure should be obtained.

3. Supplies will be sent from home.

4. Staff will not replace gastrostomy tubes if dislodged. Alternative arrangements will be specified in the healthcare plan for replacement.

5. The school nurse may provide in-services to classroom staff on gastrostomy tube feedings and supervise technical or functional concerns.

6. Wash your hands. Assemble the feeding equipment (30-60 cc syringe, stethoscope). Measure or prepare feeding.

7. Check placement of tube by pulling back on plunger of the syringe. If there is no residual present, inject a specified amount of air and listen with a stethoscope over the abdomen for gastric sounds. Delay feeding for thirty minutes if the residual is greater than specified amount.

   After that time, if residual persists, contact parent/guardian.

8. Pull back gently on the gastrostomy tube to make sure it is tight against the stomach wall.

9. Position the student as directed, generally a 45 degree angle.

10. Attach tube, syringe, or feeding bag. Fill with desired amount of feeding. Unclamp the tube, and allow feeding to flow in over specified time by gravity. Change height of feeding to vary rate or clamp with finger.

11. Monitor student during procedure. Recheck placement if student becomes distressed.

12. Flush tube with 30-60 cc water and reclamp.

13. Assess tube site and secure the tube.

14. Keep the student elevated for the prescribed number of minutes after the feeding.

15. Notify parent/guardian of any incidents or changes in feeding tolerance.

16. Document feeding on daily procedure flow sheet. Describe any problems or intolerance in progress notes. Note residual on flow sheet.

17. When using a feeding pump:

    - Follow specific manufacturer's instructions.
    - Fill bag and tubing prior to beginning feeding/unclamping tube to reduce distention.
    - Keep pump manual with pump for reference.

28

IHP: Grief—Loss—Divorce

Kathleen M. Kalb

INTRODUCTION

Sustaining a significant loss in childhood can have considerable effect on an individual. Some of these effects are short-term responses to the loss, but some may lead to lifelong pathology.[1-5] The climbing divorce rate,[6-9] means that almost half of the children born in the 1980s will experience parental divorce, with 20 percent of them experiencing a second divorce.[7,9,10] This, as well as the loss of parents through death, will mean that many children will need to grieve the loss of a parent. These children typically do not turn to school personnel for support or information during such a period of loss,[11,12] but the school nurse may be in a position to minimize the resulting trauma for both the child and family.

Background

Loss of a parent or sibling is an extreme crisis within a family system.[13] Many variables will determine how well the family can cope with the loss. These variables include ages of the children in the family, temperament of these children, what resources are available to the family, and the general quality of interpersonal relationships within the family. Responses to grief are individual and complex and generalizations about children suffering such loss

should not be made. There are, however, discernible patterns which sometimes occur in these families and the nurse's awareness of these patterns can be invaluable if she is assisting bereaved children. Many of the responses to loss are affected by the age and developmental maturity of the child.[1,5,13] For that reason, loss will be discussed in the context of age-appropriate reactions. Differences related to type of loss (i.e., death or divorce), family member lost, and coping skills of involved children will all be highlighted.

Preschool and Early-School-Age Children

Between the ages of 3 and 6 years children begin to form a concept of death.[5,7] At this age, it is usually perceived as a reversible event, explainable within the child's experience. The child may equate it with "falling asleep" or "going to heaven to be with God," and there is the sense that the person could reverse the process and join the family again.[14] If well-meaning family or friends reinforce this notion, the child may become frightened of going to sleep or may think that anyone who gets sick is in danger of going away forever to be with God. Children of this age should be told in concrete terms that the departed family member is not going to return and that people will be very sad about that for awhile. If the child has had some experience with the death of another family member or of a pet, there may be a better acceptance of the idea that the death is final. Eventual psychopathology for children who lose a parent is possible, and seems to be related to discontinuance of effective parenting and nurturance, and not to the loss per se.[10, 15] Children whose remaining family members have adequate support systems to provide for the emotional and physical needs of the young child seem to fare much better in the long run than children whose remaining parent is incapable of meeting those needs.

When a child of this age loses a sibling or a parent there is a strong tendency for the child to feel guilty. Any previous negative thoughts or death wishes that the child has had may convince the child that (s)he is responsible for the death.[5] Children must be reassured that they are in no way to blame for the death of the family member. The reason for death must be explained as clearly as possible so that the child can leave behind the feeling of responsibility for the tragedy.

A child losing a parent through divorce is also vulnerable to feeling responsible.[6, 16] Children seem to do best if they can continue to see the noncustodial parent in the period following separation,[6, 9] and if parental conflict can be minimized.[2, 6–8, 16–18] Boys seem to have more trouble adjusting to divorce in general and may begin acting out in school and at home.[2, 10, 16, 19]

Children often suffer decreased self-esteem,[8] and common responses to loss at this age are regressive behaviors, interruptions in language development and toilet training, sleep disturbance, agressive behaviors, and fear of abandonment.[6, 7, 9] Since these children may not be able to articulate their emotional state, they will act it out. Parents, teachers, and caretakers must expect a period of unusual and/or negative behaviors. It is often helpful for children of this age to have well-enforced routines to provide structure during the period of adjustment.[6]

Later School-Age Children

From the age of 5 or 6 to about 10 years, children begin to understand that death is irreversible.[5, 7] They understand it as a concrete, physical process. They may imagine that they see the deceased "breathe" while lying in state. Like the earlier school-age children, they must be reassured that they are not responsible for the death and be allowed to express any feelings of guilt, anger, or sadness that they feel. If children are not allowed to grieve effectively, they may have trouble grieving future losses.[4, 5]

In families where there is a closed system of communication, or where silence and secrecy are expected, children who lose a sibling may fall into one of three negative patterns:[5, 20] the haunted child, the bound child, or the resurrected child. Haunted children become terrified of what might happen to them and they may respond by becoming caretakers of their parents to protect their support system. They may demonstrate their stress with somatic complaints, negative school behaviors, or phobias. Bound children are overprotected by their parents, who do not want to lose another child. This may result in the child becoming angry and rebellious in order to escape their short leash. The resurrected child becomes a substitute for the lost child and may have difficulty in achieving a separate identity within the family. These three patterns are attempts to manage the pain of loss, but all of them actually interfere with appropriate grief and therefore prolong the suffering for all members of the family.

Many children of this age will develop a general fearfulness.[2, 9 14] In cases of sibling loss a child is commonly left with strong feelings of guilt for having felt normal sibling rivalry and for having ever competed with the lost sibling.[5, 20] They must be encouraged to express these feelings so adults can reassure them that all children have such feelings and that it does not mean that they were wrong or bad for having them. Even previously well-adjusted children may evidence such things as enuresis, headaches, depression, school phobia, severe separation anxiety, and abdominal pain[5] in the wake of a sibling loss.

Children of this age who experience a parent death will have an easier time if they are allowed to express their feelings.[2, 5, 13, 20, 21] They will also have more success in their grieving if their needs for parenting and nurturance can be met.[2, 21] This may mean that the remaining parent must get support to continue being available to the child, or that a close friend or relative can take over parenting responsibilities during the initial and subsequent periods when the parent is caught up in his or her own grief.[1, 18]

If the loss of a parent is through divorce, the school-age child may respond with learning problems, fearfulness, a decline in school performance, problems with peers, acting out behaviors, and/or anger toward the custodial parent.[2, 7, 9, 16] Again, boys have more difficulty with adjustment to divorce, probably due to the loss, in most cases, of the male role model.[2, 8, 10, 16] More problems occur in the acute phase of divorce, immediately following separation, because parent conflict is high, child anxiety is very high, and parent emotional availability is very low.[2] Parent availability may be further limited when income decreases and newly single parents must find work.[7, 10, 16, 17]

Children of later school age may blame one parent or the other for the divorce[9] and may act out with the custodial parent as a way of expressing this.[16] They may also experience loyalty conflicts, which are worsened when either parent has a new partner and may interfere with the child being able to connect with the new partner out of loyalty to the other parent.[6, 16] Parents need to expect these behaviors and realize they are indicative of the child's internal conflict, not a judgement about the new partner.

Adolescents

Although it may not be as evident in adolescents, it is very difficult for them to lose a sibling or parent during this period of their lives. A teenager may put up a "pseudo adult" front, giving the impression that (s)he is handling the emotional turmoil very well. In fact, the adolescent is very sensitive to the effects of a loss and may be suffering well beyond appearances.[21]

In the case of a sibling loss, the adolescent is likely to experience shock, guilt, confusion, depression, loneliness, and anger related to the death.[14] Their friends may not understand the process of grief, and may "desert" the adolescent when they are unsure how to best respond to their friend's loss.[20] This increases the adolescent's feelings of loneliness and isolation.

Adolescents have a greater understanding of the finality of death,[5, 7, 15] and are therefore at greater risk of depression and suicide.[12, 21] The possibility of suicide must always be considered when the grieving adolescent does not seem to be recovering from the loss. Safety precautions must be taken and a plan made by family members to safeguard the adolescent.[5] This not only addresses the suicide potential, but affirms the adolescent's importance in the family and demonstrates the parent's concern. Parents who are themselves recovering from the loss of a child may not be observant of the needs of their adolescent [14, 21] and may need intervention in order to be able to deal effectively with the situation. This risk of suicide is particularly high if the sibling was lost through suicide or circumstances suggesting suicide.[22]

When teenagers lose a parent through death, it has profound impact on their lives. They may be expected to grow up quickly, or to be an adult influence for younger siblings.[14] While they may appear to live up to these expectations, it postpones their identity formation and interferes with their developmental growth. They may have trouble with the separation tasks that are a part of normal adolescence, especially if they become responsible for meeting the dependency needs of the surviving parent. They may demonstrate a "learned helplessness" if they sustain many losses and feel that major events in their lives are beyond their control.[17, 21]

If the loss of the parent is through divorce, the adolescent may respond in a number of ways. It is not unusual to see many forms of acting out when parents are divorcing. In the case of an adolescent this acting out may take the form of general behavior problems,[7, 9] running away,[17] decreased academic performance,[6, 17] violence against a parent,[7] and/or sexual promiscuity.[5, 22] There are frequently feelings of loyalty conflict, anger, and depression.[2, 7, 8, 16] As with the death of a family member, there is a risk of suicide.[16] The adolescent understands circumstances more thoroughly than a younger child and may have more trouble in accepting the parents' new roles as sexual individuals when the parents begin to date or attach to another partner.[2, 16] Parental divorce may negatively impact the adolescent's socialization and expectations regarding his or her own future marriage. As with the death of a parent, there may be an impairment of the adolescent's ability to complete developmental tasks and form a healthy identity separate from the family.[8]

In Summary: Common Findings in Grief Response

- The grief process is a long one. It can, and probably will, take several years.[22] Families must understand that while the initial response may soften, it is normal to feel very strong emotions about a loss for years afterward.[5]

- Time in and of itself does not heal the hurt of a significant loss.[11, 23] If the grieving process is hampered or prevented, this unresolved grief will color the emotional life of the individual for many years.[5] The pain may be suppressed, but not diminished.[22]

- The greatest reactions to loss occur immediately following the loss.[2, 9] Therefore, children's behavior problems, inadequate parenting, depression, suicide, and other expressions of strong emotion are most likely in the first year following death or divorce.[11, 18] Parents and children should be made aware that this is the case so that additional support can be arranged for the most stressful periods.

- It is important for the grieving child (and parent) to have a forum wherein there is freedom to express all the emotions and hardships associated with the loss.[1, 13] Although parents may want to deny the situation to "protect" the child,[5, 12] all family members need the chance to tell about the loss, remember the lost family member, talk about feelings, and discuss the reactions of friends.[5, 22] The less a child is allowed to talk about the loss, the more potential there is for future problems.[5, 9]

- Very young and school-age children are likely to "act out" their strong emotional responses with negative behaviors.[8, 13, 21, 23] Adolescents are more likely to cover theirs over with a false maturity.[12, 15] Both must have an opportunity to work through the grief in an honest, productive way.

- Future psychopathology is usually related to the inadequate parenting surrounding a loss, not to the loss itself.[3, 10] Therefore, there is more risk for the child who loses a primary caregiver (usually mother) through death or divorce,[1] for children whose parents were poor or marginal performers prior to the loss,[1] and for children who remain in family situations of continuing conflict.[7-10]

- In cases of divorce, self-esteem of both boys and girls is linked with a healthy, ongoing relationship with their fathers.[8]

- People who lose a parent during childhood are vulnerable to having to renegotiate the developmental tasks of the stage in which they were when the loss occurred. This may mean regression during future stressful periods or when subsequent losses occur.[4, 5]

INDIVIDUALIZED HEALTHCARE PLAN

History

It is not uncommon for children who are grieving to experience increased somatic discomforts.[22] It may be these somatic complaints and not the divorce or death per se that bring them to the nurse's office. If the student reveals that there has been a recent death or divorce in the family, the nurse may pursue this with the following questions:

- How long ago did this take place?
- What were the circumstances surrounding the loss? (How did your dad die? Did your parents decide to separate for good or just for now? and so on.)
- Where are you living now? Is that going to change?
- Tell me how each member of your family is handling this. (What do they do to feel better when the death/divorce is upsetting them?)
- What do you do to feel better?
- Is it okay to talk at home about how you're feeling? What happens when you do?
- Who else can you talk to about all this?
- Do you see (or play with) your friends as often as before?
- How are things going at school? Are your grades about the same as they were before this happened?
- Do you seem extra tired or do you have trouble paying attention to things?
- Are you sleeping well at night? (If "no," What do you do when you can't sleep?)
- Are you eating about the same as usual? Is your weight about the same as usual?
- Do you ever feel like dying, or like hurting or killing yourself? (If "yes", do you feel like that now?)
- Have you ever been through anything like this before? (If "yes," How did that go? What seemed to help?)
- (When the loss is a death) What do you believe about death? or What do you think happens when people die?

In addition, of course, update the history in relation to the presenting physical complaint that brought the student in originally.

Assessment

Physical Assessment

Physical assessment consists of the appropriate examination for the presenting physical complaint. In addition, measure weight and vital signs and, if possible, compare to previous measurements.

Psychological/Emotional Assessment

Students may be resistant to adult interference or advice. Respect their reluctance to share sensitive information immediately following a loss event. Explain that you are interested in helping them feel better and in keeping them safe, not in prying or making their lives more difficult.

Notice whether the student looks fatigued, is labile in affect, appears sad or distressed, and whether (s)he has trouble maintaining appropriate nonverbal communication and/or attention during the conversation. Note the student's expression and general attitude when discussing the loss event.

Be aware that students with a history of addictive behavior may be vulnerable to an increase in or return to such behaviors in the wake of a significant loss. Assessment of their addictive behaviors may be necessary if there is indication that they are engaged in such activities. (See Chapter 44, IHP: Substance Abuse.)

Nursing Diagnoses (N.D.)

N.D. 1   Anxiety (NANDA 9.3.1)*, related to recent loss as evidenced by:
 Inability to concentrate
 Somatic complaints
 Negative affect or emotional overreaction to situations unrelated to loss

N.D. 2   Ineffective family coping (NANDA 5.1.2.1.2) secondary to recent loss and poor intrafamily communication as evidenced by:
 Family inability to communicate about the loss
 Frequent family conflict
 Ineffective parenting
 Inability of family to allow or express emotions

N.D. 3   Ineffective individual coping (NANDA 5.1.1.1) secondary to recent loss as evidenced by:
 Depression or suicidal feelings
 Acting out behaviors
 Regressive behaviors
 Appetite/sleep disruption
 Drop in school grades

N.D. 4   Dysfunctional grieving (NANDA 9.2.1.1), related to loss of family member(s) as evidenced by:
 Apparent recovery after very short time period
 Inability to accept loss after long period of time (greater than one year)
 Preoccupation with loss which does not diminish over time

N.D. 5   Impaired social interaction (NANDA 3.1.1), secondary to grief response

N.D. 6   Spiritual distress (NANDA 4.1.1), related to death/divorce

*(See chapter 2, page 38 for explanation of the NANDA approved numerical system.)

Goals

The school nurse will:
1. Assess student's current physical and emotional status, including coping skills.
2. Work with other disciplines to assist student in achieving healthy grief response.
3. Monitor student's process of grief and recovery.

Nursing Interventions

Update history as recommended and assess student as described. (N.D. 1–6)

Use active listening skills to allow student to express grief and process loss. Allow student to express feelings of guilt, anger, helplessness, fear, and so on. Allow student to cry. (N.D. 1–6)

Educate student regarding grief process, including: (N.D. 1–6)

- what feelings to expect and how long the process may take
- that different people handle grief differently and there are many "normal" ways to grieve
- that holidays and special events may be difficult
- that such responses as numbness, trouble concentrating, and irritability are very common

Educate the student regarding normal responses to divorce (N.D. 1–6)

- reinforce the fact that most divorces do *not* result in parental reunion
- help the student articulate what (s)he is feeling toward parents

Educate the student regarding any medical information that may be helpful in understanding a death caused by disease. (N.D. 1, 6)

Give accurate and honest information in response to student questions. (N.D. 1–6)

If possible, contact parent to express sympathy for a loss of family member. This establishes foundation for future contacts should they become necessary. (N.D. 2–4)

If friends or teachers of grieving student seem to be uncomfortable with the circumstances, meet with them to help them understand how to best support the student. (N.D. 5)

If student (or family) seems to be denying the loss or grieving inappropriately, refer student for additional counseling. (N.D. 2–4)

If student expresses suicidal ideation or depressive symptoms, refer *immediately* for mental health evaluation. Ensure that student has adequate protection to prevent suicide attempt. (N.D. 3)

Follow up with student on a weekly or biweekly basis to determine student's emotional status. (Daily follow-up may be necessary in initial stage of loss.) (N.D. 1–6)

Connect student with ongoing grief group if possible. (N.D. 1–6)

Expected Student Outcomes

1. The student will show less anxiety and more comfort as evidenced by participation in school and social activities, appropriate affect and ability to talk about loss.

2. Family will show appropriate grief response as indicated by student report.
3. Student will show appropriate grief response as evidenced by increasing comfort in discussing loss, return to usual activities, and decreased feelings of sadness, guilt, or anger related to the loss.
4. Student will find a spiritual understanding of the loss which is comfortable, evidenced by ability to articulate and agree with a perspective on the loss event which puts the event into context.

REFERENCES

1. Finkelstein H. The long-term effects of early parent death: a review. *J Clin Psychol* 1988; 44 (1): 3–9.
2. Goodyer IM. Family relationships, life events and childhood psychopathology. *J Child Psychol Psychiatry* 1990; 31 (1): 161–92.
3. Harris T, Brown GW, Bifulco A. Loss of parent in childhood and adult psychiatric disorder: the role of lack of adequate parental care. *Psychol Med* 1986; 16 (3): 641–59.
4. O'Neil MK, Lancee WJ, Freeman JJ. Loss and depression: a controversial link. *J Nerv Ment Dis* 1987; 175 (6).
5. Ross-Alaolmolki K. Coping with family loss: the death of a sibling. *Nursing Interventions for Infants and Children.* (Craft MJ and Denchy JA, eds.) Philadelphia: Saunders, 1990.
6. Dubowitz H, Newberger CM, Melnicoe LH, Newberger EH. The changing american family. *Pediatr Clin North Am* 1988; 35 (6): 1291–311.
7. Shonkoff JP, Jarman FC, Kohlenberg TM. *Curr Probl Pediatr* 1987; 17 (9).
8. Schwartzberg AZ. Divorce and children and adolescents: an overview. *Adolesc Psychiatry* 1981; 9: 119–32.
9. Weitzman M, Adair R. Divorce and children. *Pediatr Clin North Am* 1988; 35 (6): 1313–23.
10. Tennant C. Parental loss in childhood: its effect in adult life. *Arch Gen Psychiatry* 1988; 45 (11): 1045–50.
11. Balk D. How teenagers cope with sibling death: some implications for school counselors. *School Counselor* 1983; (Nov): 150–58.
12. Berman H, Cragg CE, Kuenzig L. Having a parent die of cancer: adolescents' reactions. *Oncology Nursing Forum* 1988; 15 (2): 159–63.
13. Demi AS, Gilbert CM. Relationship of parental grief to sibling grief. *Arch Psychiatric Nursing* 1987; 1 (6); 385–91.
14. Glass JC. Death, loss, and grief in high school students. *High School Journal* 1990; (Feb–Mar): 154–61.
15. Cheifetz PN, Stavrakakis G, Lester EP. Studies of the affective state in bereaved children. *Can J Psychiatry* 1989; 34 (7): 688–92.
16. Rae-Grant Q, Robson BE. Moderating the morbidity of divorce. *Can J Psychiatry* 1988; 33 (6): 443–52.
17. Brody GH, Neubaum E, Forehand R. Serial marriage: a heuristic analysis of an emerging family form. *Psychol Bulletin* 1988; 103 (2): 211–22.
18. Connell HM. Effect of family break-up and parent divorce on children. *Aust Paediatr J* 1988; 24 (4): 222–27.
19. Hetherington EM. Coping with family transitions: winners, losers and survivors. *Child Development* 1989; 60 (1): 1–14.
20. Hansen JC, Frantz TT, eds. *Death and Grief in the Family.* Rockville, MD: Aspen Systems Corp., 1984.
21. Masterman SH, Reams R. Support groups for bereaved preschool and school-age children. *Am J Orthopsychiatry* 1988; 58 (4): 562–70.
22. Gyulay J. Grief responses. *Issues in Compr Pediatr Nursing* 1989; 12: 1–31.
23. Black D, Urbanowicz MA. Family intervention with bereaved children. *J Child Psychol Psychiatry* 1987; 28 (3): 467–76.
24. Camiletti Y, Quant V. Anticipatory counseling for adolescents of divorced parents. *School Guidance Worker* 1983; 39 (1).
25. Vargas LA, Loya F, Hodde-Vargas J. Exploring the multidimensional aspects of grief reactions. *Am J Psychiatry* 1989; 146 (11): 1484–88.
26. Schonfeld DJ. Crisis intervention for bereavement support: a model of intervention in the children's school. *Clin Pediatr* 1989; 28 (1): 27–33.

IHP: Headaches

Kathleen M. Kalb

INTRODUCTION

Headache is a common complaint from school age-children and adolescents, with as many as 75 percent experiencing this condition by the age of fifteen.[1] Headaches seem to become increasingly prevalent with age,[2] and to occur more in females than males.[1, 2] Since this condition is sometimes dismissed as trivial by adults, students may be reluctant to seek help with this problem,[3] and the school nurse can be a valuable resource to help them sort out the causes and refer them for treatment.

There are several types of headache with which children typically present. Migraine or vascular, muscle contraction, psychogenic, headaches secondary to underlying organic pathology (traction, cranial inflammation, vascular malformation), and headaches secondary to disease of the head or neck structures.[1] Treatment and referral will vary depending on which type of headache the student is experiencing. Outcome of treatment is difficult to predict, with severity of the headache strongly correlated with the eventual outcome.[4] But other factors such as individual stress level and even the student's general satisfaction with the family situation[5] play a role in the success of treatment.

It should be noted that headache may be a result of head injury, and this must be ruled out before treating for more chronic causes of head pain.

Pathophysiology

Underlying etiology is quite different for each type of headache. Successful treatment, therefore, depends on determining which type of headache the child is experiencing. Following are the presumed mechanisms of pain for various types of headache[1]:

Migraine and vascular headaches are caused by the dilatation of cranial arteries, which are exquisitely pain-sensitive. Any vasoactive agent, either endogenous or introduced, may play a causative or reactive role in this type of headache. The prodromal phase is most likely the result of vasoconstriction prior to dilatation, causing initial ischemia and resultant neurological symptoms.

Muscle contraction headache, as its name implies, results from the contraction of muscles in the head and neck area. It is the most common cause of headache in both children and adults.

Traction headaches are those which involve intracranial structures. These are attributable to underlying pathology and may be seen with brain tumor, subdural hematoma, or any condition resulting in increased intracranial pressure. Suspicion of this type of headache is cause for immediate referral to a physician familiar with pediatric headache.

Inflammation of tissue is the cause of pain in meningitis or sinusitis.

The majority of headaches are of the migraine or muscle contraction types. See Table 1 for information on typical clinical presentations of the various types of headaches and possible treatment options.[1,2]

The diagnosis of headache type may be complicated by overlapping features. Students with recurrent headache must be properly diagnosed by a physician or nurse practitioner and treatment directed at the particular type of headache.

Table 1. Types of Headaches, Possible Treatment Options

Headache Type	Clinical Features	Common Treatment
Muscle Contraction	Steady, dull, "band-like" pain of gradual onset, lasting hours to days, may be precipitated by stress and/or associated with weakness or fatigue.	Conservative use of analgesics, stress reduction techniques, elimination of triggers, reassurance.
Migraine	Throbbing pain of gradual onset, lasting hours or days, may be precipitated by ingestion of alcohol, red wine, aged cheese, coffee or chocolate, or by bright lights. More common in females and may be more likely to occur in the premenstrum. Sometimes associated with neurologic prodrome, nausea, vomiting, fever, weakness, or fatigue.	Ergotamine preparation, analgesics, elimination of triggers, stress management techniques, beta-blockers (prophylactic), reassurance.
Pathological (rare, but serious)	Recent onset (gradual or acute) of dull, aching, constant pain. Tends to get worse over time and may be associated with neurological symptoms. May worsen with coughing or bending forward.	Neurologic management depending on underlying cause.
Psychogenic	May present with any of the above symptoms, alone or in combination. Marked by chronicity and nonresponse to treatment. [2]	Treatment of underlying psychological contributor and conservative use of analgesics, stress reduction techniques, reassurance. May need to involve family in treatment. [1,2,5]

(Table 1 continued)

| Sinus | Deep, full ache associated with nasal congestion, face pain. May worsen with movement of head. Usually associated with infection of sinus cavities. | Antibiotic, analgesic, and/or decongestants. |
| Cluster (rare in childhood) | Intense, boring pain. May be periodic or time-limited. May be associated with lacrimation, rhinorrhea, and conjunctival injection. Often occur suddenly in the very early morning. | Analgesic, sleep, elimination of triggers. |

INDIVIDUALIZED HEALTHCARE PLAN

History

Correct diagnosis depends on a careful and accurate history.[1] Update the student's history with particular emphasis on symptoms and on family history of headache. Following are questions addressing the most pertinent data:

Information to Rule Out Head Injury

- Do you remember hitting your head or falling recently?
- Are you playing any contact sports? Which ones?
- Have you been injured lately either accidentally or in a fight? (e.g., Automobile accident, "roughhousing" with friends, fist fight, fall on slippery surface, other)
- If so, what was done about it? Were you treated? Did you lose consciousness?

If these questions reveal a negative history for injury, go on to questions regarding more chronic headache.

How old were you when you started having these headaches?

Do they seem to happen with anything else? (Big tests, stressful family situations, relation to menstrual cycle,[6] triggers such as specific foods, bright lights, exercise, or medications.)

How long do they usually last?

Where does it hurt?

How often do you get them?

Describe the pain. (Sharp, dull, stabbing, throbbing, steady, severe, mild, other)

What time of day do you usually get them? (May wake up with migraine or cluster headaches, muscle contraction headaches tend to be later in the day.)

Does the headache interfere with your activities? Can you continue to do what you were doing, or do you have to go to bed?

Do you have any warning that you're getting one of these headaches? If yes, describe it.

Do you ever feel sick to your stomach, dizzy, feverish, confused, or have "funny" sensations with these headaches? Please describe the feeling. Do these things happen before, during, or after the headaches?

What seems to help?

Does anything make the headache worse?

Have you or your friends or family noticed that you're acting any differently lately? If yes, can you say more about that? Did this change happen before the headaches started, about the same time, or after you'd had some headaches?

Does anyone in your family have headaches like these? If yes, what have they done for them? Does it seem to work?

Does anyone in your family have seizures?

Have you ever seen a doctor or nurse practitioner for these headaches? If yes, what did they recommend?

What medications do you take? (Explore type and frequency of analgesic use, whether the student takes birth control pills, other medications, and street drugs, including anabolic steroids.)

Are you now, or have you been in the past, suffering from a long-term depression? (Psychogenic headache may accompany clinical depression.[2])

Assessment

If the student is having recurrent headaches, (s)he should see a physician or nurse practitioner for a complete physical examination as well as a thorough neurologic examination to rule out pathology.[6]

Current Status

Determine whether the student is having a headache now. If so, ask for a description. Find out whether the student would be agreeable to seeing a care provider to diagnose the headaches.

Physical Assessment

Physical assessment by the nurse can offer important information for determining the type of headaches the student is experiencing.

- Vital signs (note elevated blood pressure or temperature)
- Examination of the head
     abnormalities
     signs of infection
     facial tenderness
     otitis
     poor dentition
     vision acuity
- Examination of the neck
     muscle soreness or rigidity
     swollen glands
     pain with movement

- Neurologic signs
    mental status
    long- and short-term memory
    sensory and motor abnormalities
    cranial nerve function

Rule Out:

- Injury
  - Observe, inspect, palpate for lumps, bruises, lesions
  - Simple neuro assessment (hand squeeze, finger coordination, eye movement, pupil response to light)
  - Range of motion in neck, especially for suspected whiplash
- Intracranial Pressure
  - Mental status
  - Pain with Valsalva's maneuver
- Allergy/Sinusitis
  - Periorbital pain or tenderness
  - Fever
  - Purulent nasal discharge

Psychological/Emotional Assessment

Interview the student to determine:

- His or her general attitude toward the headaches
- Whether situational factors are affecting his/her general emotional status

Nursing Diagnoses (N.D.)

N.D. 1 Alteration in comfort (NANDA 9.1.1)* secondary to head pain.
N.D. 2 Ineffective individual coping (NANDA 5.1.1.1) with attendant recurrent headache.
N.D. 3 Knowledge deficit (NANDA 8.1.1) regarding effective treatment of recurrent headache.
N.D. 4 Sensory-perceptual alterations (NANDA 7.2) related to migraine syndrome or pathologic neurologic process.
N.D. 5 Injury (actual or potential) (NANDA 1.1.1) related to head trauma.

Goals

The school nurse will:

1. Refer appropriately for diagnosis of headache type and/or injury.
2. Monitor treatment plan to ensure improvement of the condition.
3. Educate student regarding normal course of treatment, typical response patterns as well as appropriate nondrug management techniques.

---

* (See chapter 2, page 38 for explanation of the NANDA approved numerical system.)

Nursing Interventions

Update history as above to provide foundation for nursing assessment and information for referral. (N.D. 1–5)

Refer recent injury for further evaluation. (N.D. 5)

Educate student regarding etiology of headache and possible treatment strategies. (N.D. 1–3)

- Reassure student that most headaches are benign and do not denote pathological condition.[1,2,7]
- Reassure student that many types of treatment are available and one is likely to be effective for this type of headache.
- Teach/discuss nondrug treatment which may offer some relief. (i.e., relaxation therapy, stress reduction, biofeedback, other).

Interview student to ascertain self-concept related to this condition. (e.g., self as handicapped by condition or unable to participate in normal activities with peers, etc.). (N.D. 2)

Discuss willingness to consult a healthcare provider on this matter. (N.D. 1, 3–5)

- Reassure that it is a legitimate medical condition and should be medically evaluated.
- Determine whether there is a healthcare provider that. (s)he trusts and would be willing to see regarding this condition.
- If not, offer to help find an appropriate source of healthcare.
- Refer as appropriate to diagnose headache.
- Educate regarding what to expect at the healthcare visit (e.g., necessary history, physical and neurologic exam, questions to ask).

Educate student regarding pain mechanism involved in his/her particular type of headache. (N.D. 3)

Educate student regarding stress management techniques, as these nondrug strategies have been found to be advantageous in most types of headache.[1,2,8–10] (N.D. 1, 3, 4)

Instruct student in keeping a headache diary. Instruct the student to rate headaches on a scale, from 0 to 5, 4x per day[2] for a period of one month. This information will be useful as baseline data to measure effectiveness and as historical information for referral.[10] (N.D. 1–3)

Follow up with student monthly to determine effectiveness of treatment and student's emotional status. (N.D. 1–5)

If response to having this condition seems inappropriate, or if student's emotional status is compromised, refer for further counseling. (N.D. 2)

Expected Student Outcomes

1. The student will experience relief of headache as indicated by self-report and evidence in headache diary of lessened or absent pain.
2. The student will comply with referral recommended by school nurse.

3. The student will comply with the treatment approach outlined by the healthcare provider.

4. The student will demonstrate knowledge of his/her own headache process and understanding of the treatment approach as shown by report of same to school nurse.

5. The student will attend follow-up meetings with the school nurse to monitor progress and success of treatment as well as to determine student's emotional status.

REFERENCES

1. Neinstein LS. Headaches. In: *Adolescent Healthcare: A Practical Guide.* Baltimore: Urban and Schwarzenberg, 1984: 263–271.

2. McGrath PJ, Humphreys P. Recurrent headaches in children and adolescents: diagnosis and treatment. *Pediatrician* 1989; 16 (1–2); 71–77.

3. Linet MS, et al. An epidemiologic study of headache among adolescents and young adults. JAMA 1989; 261 (15): 2211–16.

4. Larsson B, Melin L. Follow-up on behavioral treatment of recurrent headache in adolescents. *Headache* 1989; 29 (4): 250–54.

5. Larsson B, Melin L. The psychological treatment of recurrent headache in adolescents—short-term outcome and its prediction. *Headache* 1988; 28 (3): 187–95.

6. Solbach P, et al. Tension headache: a comparison of menstrual and non-menstrual occurrences. *Headache* 1988; 28 (2): 108–10.

7. Chow MP, et al. Headache. In: *Handbook of Pediatric Primary Care.* 2nd ed. New York: J Wiley, 1984: 918–921.

8. Duckro PN, Cantwell-Simmons E. A review of studies evaluating biofeedback and relaxation training in the management of pediatric headache. *Headache* 1989; 29 (7): 428–33.

9. Grazzi L, et al. A therapeutic alternative for tension headache in children: treatment and 1-year follow-up results. *Biofeedback Self Regul* 1990; 15 (1): 1–6.

10. Labbé EE. Childhood muscle contraction headache: current issues in assessment and treatment. *Headache* 1988; 28 (6): 430–34.

30 IHP: Hearing Deficit

Cynthia K. Silkworth

INTRODUCTION

Hearing loss is a sensory deficit that directly affects a child's ability to learn. Estimates indicate that the prevalence of hearing loss in children is between 3 and 6 percent,[1] and that each year in the United States, 1 in 750 infants is born with a significant hearing problem.[2] A hearing deficit may affect both ears or just one, may be mild or severe, and may be permanent or fluctuate over time. It can create enormous problems for the young child learning speech, as well as for the school-aged child or adolescent who may miss parts of instructions, classroom discussions, and other learning opportunities because of the inability to hear. Early detection and intervention of a hearing deficit can help prevent related problems in speech, social development and educational progress.

Pathophysiology

Hearing loss can be classified into three main types.

Conductive: The loss is due to problems in the outer or middle ear. In the outer ear, accumulation of wax in the canal, foreign objects in the canal, and infection of the ear canal (external otitis) can cause hearing loss. In the middle ear, infection of the middle ear (acute otitis media, chronic otitis media), fluid buildup in the middle ear (serous otitis media), tumors, and trauma to the tympanic membrane can cause hearing loss.

Sensorineural: The loss is due to dysfunction of the inner ear, auditory nerve damage, or damage to the auditory centers in the temporal lobes of the brain. Causes for this type of hearing loss include those that are noise-induced (gunfire, loud music, machinery), and those that result from head trauma, ototoxic drugs (gentamycin, streptomycin, neomycin), tumors, meningitis, viral diseases (measles, mumps), congenital perinatal infections (TORCH infections), anoxia at birth, or Meniere's disease.

Mixed: The loss is a combination of both conductive and sensorineural hearing loss.

Hearing loss is also classified by severity of loss.

Mild: 20–40 dB, quiet speech is inaudible.
Moderate: 40–60 dB, average conversational speech is inaudible.
Severe: 60–80 dB, loud speech is inaudible.
Profound: greater than 80 dB, all speech is inaudible.

Behaviors indicating a student may have a hearing deficit include[2-5]:

1. inattention or daydreaming
2. failure to respond to questions
3. saying "what" frequently
4. requests for directions to be repeated
5. continually misunderstanding directions
6. waiting to visually check with other student(s) before starting a task or assignment
7. watches speaker's face, especially the lips
8. misarticulation of common words
9. confusing words that sound alike
10. using immature speech or language
11. speaks abnormally loud or soft
12. body language that may indicate straining to hear
13. withdrawn, low self-esteem

Hearing Deficit Management

Medical interventions:

- medications—to treat infections
- surgery—remove tumors, repair tympanic membrane, insert p.e. tubes, repair or replace bones in the middle ear, other

Amplification:

- hearing aids
- personal FM systems (phonic ear)

Educational interventions:

- preferential seating in the classroom
- special teaching strategies—visual cues and reinforcement, repetition of instructions, facing the student when speaking, and so on
- special educational services—speech and language, hearing impaired program
- alternative language system—sign language

Adapted from Feinstein,[2] Bleck and Nagel,[3] Wold,[5] and Silkworth et.al.[6]

INDIVIDUALIZED HEALTHCARE PLAN

History

- When was the hearing deficit identified?
- What is the probable cause for the deficit?
- Health conditions associated with the hearing deficit
- History of ear infections—when, treatment, outcome
- Healthcare providers involved in assessment and treatment of the student's hearing deficit
- Past audiological findings
- Past tympanometry findings
- Past otoscopic assessment findings
- Current medical management
- Past and current use of amplification and its effectiveness
- Student's speech and language development

- Ability to communicate with family and friends—usual patterns of communication, methods used and their effectiveness
- Past and current educational interventions—preferential seating, special education services, other, and their effectiveness
- Past and current school experiences—academic, social
- Student's academic progress

Assessment

- Student and parents'/guardian's knowledge of the hearing deficit
- Teacher(s)' knowledge about the student's hearing deficit and teaching strategies for hearing impaired students
- Student's perception of his/her hearing deficit
- Parents'/guardian's perception of their child's hearing deficit
- Current audiological status—audiometric (with and without amplification), tympanometric, and otoscopic assessments
- Ability to communicate with others—receptive and expressive
- Ability to hear and function in the mainstream classroom setting—classroom observation
- Proper use and care of hearing aids, if applicable
- Self-care skills—testing hearing aid functioning and batteries
- Decision-making skills
- Social skills
- Classroom environment(s)—noise (from other classrooms, hallway, fans from the heating system, and so on), seating arrangement that allows the student to see the teacher's and other student's faces when they are talking, and so on

Nursing Diagnoses (N.D.)

N.D. 1 Sensory–perceptual alteration—auditory, (NANDA 7.2)* related to (specific cause of the hearing deficit).

N.D. 2 (Potential for) impaired communication, (NANDA 2.1.1.1) related to hearing deficit.

N.D. 3 (Potential for) alteration in learning related to hearing deficit.

N.D. 4 Knowledge deficit about use and care of amplification devices for hearing deficit (hearing aids, personal FM system), (NANDA 8.1.1) related to:
  - lack of information.
  - lack of interest or motivation to learn.
  - developmentally not ready for receiving the information or performing the tasks.

N.D. 5 (Potential for) impaired social interactions, (NANDA 3.1.1) related to hearing deficit.

* (See chapter 2, page 38 for explanation of the NANDA approved numerical system.)

Goals

Achieve and maintain maximum potential for hearing. (N.D. 1)

Decrease or eliminate causative or contributing factors to the hearing deficit. (N.D. 1)

Reduce or eliminate barriers to communication in the classroom setting. (N.D. 2)

Improve communication ability and skills. (N.D. 2)

Maximize and maintain the student's ability to learn. (N.D. 3)

Remove or decrease hearing-related barriers to learning. (N.D. 3)

Increase knowledge and skills in use and care of amplification devices (hearing aids, personal FM system). (N.D. 4)

Effective social interaction in the school, home, and community environments. (N.D. 5)

Nursing Interventions

Determine current hearing status and maximum potential for hearing (with and without amplification). (N.D. 1)

Discuss with the student, parents/guardians, healthcare provider, teachers, speech clinician, and teacher of the hearing impaired: (N.D. 1–3)

- Type, cause, and severity of the hearing deficit.

- Ways to maximize the student's hearing (hearing aids, other).

- How the hearing deficit does or may impact the student's ability to communicate and learn.

Utilize measures to reduce or eliminate causative or contributing factors to the hearing deficit. (N.D. 1–3)

- Monitor hearing in students with recurrent ear infections and serous otitis media—refer to healthcare provider if hearing deficit is present.

- If the student needs to take medication during the school day to treat or prevent ear infections, assist the student to take the medication.

- If amplification devices are used (hearing aids, personal FM device), make sure they are functioning properly.

- Reduce or eliminate as much background noise as possible (for example, by closing the door to the hallway during class time, turning off machines in the classroom when they are not being used for the learning task at hand, giving directions and *then* passing out the worksheets so paper shuffle noise doesn't interfere with the verbal message, and so on).

In-service teachers and other school staff who work with the student. Discuss ways to enhance the student's ability to learn and communicate. (N.D. 2, 3)

- Preferential seating in the classroom—front two rows with the best hearing ear toward the teacher and other students.

- Talk distinctly and clearly, facing the student.

- New vocabulary words should be written on the blackboard and pronounced clearly.

- Use visual as well as verbal cues to assist the student to understand the message.

- Reinforce important instructions or information by also writing it down (on an overhead, blackboard, top of the worksheet, etc.).

- If television programs, films, or filmstrips are going to be used as part of the curriculum, assist in arranging for closed captioning services for those materials.
- Encourage the student to ask for clarification if he/she does not understand what a person said.
- Encourage the development of active listening skills for all students in the class.
- If the student uses amplification devices, include: what the devices are, how they work, how they assist the student to communicate and learn, how the devices need to be used in the classroom and other activities, and how the devices will be monitored and stored.
- If the student uses lip reading, make sure the student can see the speaker's face and that his/her eyes are on the speaker before the speaker starts.
- If the student only understands sign language, have an interpreter with the student in all his/her classes, and assist the teacher(s) and other students to learn and use sign language.

Provide positive reinforcement to the student, teachers, and other school personnel for demonstration of skills and strategies that increase the student's ability to communicate and learn. (N.D. 2, 3)

If the student currently receives special educational services, review the student's individual educational plan (IEP) to determine if the student's needs are being addressed and/or met. (N.D. 2, 3)

Refer to the Child Study Team if the student's hearing deficit seems to negatively affect his/her ability to learn—further academic assessment, speech and language assessment, hearing impaired assessment, and so on. (N.D. 2, 3)

Refer to the Child Study Team for speech and language assessment if the student exhibits the following behaviors: (N.D. 2, 3)

- unable to respond to verbal questions in the classroom
- difficulty following directions
- asks for directions to be repeated
- difficulty learning new words
- misarticulation of words
- confusing words that sound alike
- using immature speech or language
- speaks abnormally loud or soft
- difficulty expressing thoughts and ideas

Refer to the Child Study Team if the student is demonstrating learning needs that are not being met by his/her current educational program. (N.D. 2, 3)

Discuss with the student the reason he/she needs to use amplification devices to hear and learn (at a developmentally appropriate level). (N.D. 4)

Provide health education opportunities to the student (at developmentally appropriate level). (N.D. 4)

- what a hearing aid or personal FM system is and how it works
- how to determine if batteries are charged
- how to change the batteries if they are dead

- how to clean the ear molds
- how to adjust the volume so people who are speaking can be heard well, without also having a lot of background noise

Keep extra batteries at school, stored in a cool, dry place. (N.D. 1, 4)

If the personal FM system batteries are rechargeable, assist the student by designating a permanent place to recharge the batteries at the end of each day and teach them how to plug them in so they will recharge. (N.D. 4)

Encourage the student to tell his/her teacher and parents if the hearing aid or personal FM system is not working properly. (N.D. 2–4)

Monitor the proper functioning of the student's hearing aids and personal FM system daily. (N.D. 1–4)

Monitor proper use of amplification devices by the student. (N.D. 2–4)

- observation
- teacher report
- student report

Provide positive reinforcement to the student for demonstrating new knowledge and skills in the use and care of his/her hearing aids or personal FM system. (N.D. 4)

Discuss with the student, parents/guardians, and teacher(s): (N.D. 5)

- past and current social interactions the student has in school, in his/her neighborhood with other children, and participation in community organizations and activities (scouts, sports teams, church groups, other).
- importance of the development and maintenance of good social skills for all children.
- the student's social skills and ability to use them.
- the student's weaknesses in social skills (such as, won't talk unless the other person does first, etc.).

Provide support for the development and maintenance of social skills and communicating with others: (N.D. 5)

- individual (instruction with demonstration and practice)
- social skills group (demonstration and practice with a peer group)
- classroom social skills development activities (such as, cooperative group learning, buddy system for some classroom assignments, and so on)

Encourage the student to become involved in social activities at school (clubs, sports) and in the community (scouts, 4H, church groups, other). (N.D. 5)

Expected Student Outcomes

The student will:

- State the type, cause, and severity of his/her hearing deficit (dependent on developmental ability). (N.D. 1, 4)
- Describe how his/her hearing deficit can affect his/her ability to communicate and learn. (N.D. 1–3)

- Take prescribed medication for the treatment or prevention of ear infections, as prescribed (if applicable). (N.D. 1)
- Name the teacher(s) and other school personnel (speech clinician, special learning disabilities teacher, teacher of the hearing impaired, school nurse) who can help him/her to communicate and learn. (N.D. 2–4)
- List ways he/she can increase his/her ability to communicate with others. (N.D. 2)
- List ways to reduce or eliminate unnecessary noise. (N.D. 1–3)
- Demonstrate ways that increase his/her ability to communicate with others. (N.D. 2)
- Tell his/her parents/teachers/other students if he/she is having trouble hearing or does not understand what was said. (N.D. 2–5)
- Communicate effectively with his/her teacher. (N.D. 2)
- Communicate effectively with his/her classmates. (N.D. 2)
- Demonstrate ability to learn in the classroom. (N.D. 3)
- List ways to decrease hearing-related barriers in (N.D. 3) the classroom.
- Name the amplification devices he/she uses to (N.D. 1,4) improve his/her ability to hear.
- Describe how a hearing aid and/or a personal FM system works to help him/her hear better (at a developmentally appropriate level). (N.D. 4)
- Describe why hearing aids and/or a personal FM system are necessary for him/her to hear and learn (at a developmentally appropriate level). (N.D. 4)
- Demonstrate how to use his/her hearing aids and personal FM system. (N.D. 1–4)
- Wear hearing aids at home and at school everyday. (N.D. 1-4)
- Demonstrate correct care of hearing aids: how to tell if batteries are charged, how to replace dead batteries, how to check and clean ear molds, how to set the volume control. (N.D. 4)
- Tell parents/teachers if his/her amplification devices are not working properly. (N.D. 4)
- Place the volume of the hearing aids at a level where he/she can hear the best. (N.D. 4)
- Place the volume of the personal FM system at a level where he/she can hear the best. (N.D. 4)
- Recharge the batteries for his/her personal FM system at the end of the school day. (N.D. 4)
- Name his/her friends at home and at school. (N.D. 5)
- List activities he/she likes to do with friends: at school, in his/her neighborhood, in community groups. (N.D. 5)
- Demonstrate use of good social skills in the classroom and during social time at school (such as at lunch, during noon recess, before and after school). (N.D. 5)
- Be involved in at least one activity that requires social interactions outside of the school day (such as a club, sport, or organization). (N.D. 5)

REFERENCES

1. American Academy of Pediatrics. *School Health: A Guide for Health Professionals.* Evanston, IL: American Academy of Pediatrics, 1977.
2. Feinstein SC. Hearing loss in infants and children. *Topics in Pediatrics* 1990; 8 (1): 6–9.
3. Bleck EE, Nagel DA. *Physically Handicapped Children: A Medical Atlas for Teachers.* 2nd ed. New York: Grune and Stratton, 1982.
4. E.A.R.S. (Educational/Audiological and Related Services) Program publications, 1989. Available from: Intermediate School District 916, 70 W. Co. Rd. B2, Little Canada, MN 55117.
5. Wold SJ. *School Nursing: A Framework for Practice.* North Branch, MN: Sunrise River Press, 1981.
6. Silkworth C, Gray C, Phillips J. Hearing impairment: assessment and management. In: Larson G, ed. *Managing the School Aged Child with a Chronic Health Condition: A Practical Guide for Schools, Families and Organizations.* Wayzata, MN: DCI Publishing, 1988 (available from Sunrise River Press, 11481 Kost Dam Rd, North Branch, MN 55056, 612-583-3239).
7. Bess FH. The minimally hearing-impaired child. *Ear Hearing* 1985; 6 (1): 43–47.
8. Levine MD, Brooks R, Shonkoff J. *A Pediatric Approach to Learning Disorders.* New York: Wiley, 1980.
9. Oberklaid F, Harris C, Keir E. Auditory dysfunction: in children with school problems. *Clin Pediatrics* 1989; 28 (9): 397–403.

31 | IHP: Hemophilia

Cynthia K. Silkworth

INTRODUCTION

Hemophilia is an inherited, chronic blood clotting disorder. It occurs in approximately 1:10,000 male births in the United States and affects all races and socioeconomic groups equally.[1] Persons with hemophilia do not bleed harder or faster than normal. However, they bleed longer because their body cannot make a firm blood clot. The severity of bleeding differs from person to person, and the seriousness of a bleeding episode depends on the site of the bleed and the type and extent of injury that caused the bleed to start. Prolonged bleeding into joints and muscle tissues or repeated bleeding into specific sites may eventually cause deformity and loss of function. Prompt treatment following an injury can prevent this long-term complication of hemophilia.[1]

Pathophysiology

Hemophilia is caused by an abnormality of blood clotting proteins that are present in blood plasma, one of the plasma proteins needed to form a clot is missing or reduced.[1] Persons with hemophilia bleed longer than persons who do not have the disorder.

The most common forms of hemophilia[2] are:

Hemophilia A (classic hemophilia)—factor VIII deficiency, 80 percent of all persons with hemophilia

Hemophilia B (Christmas disease)—factor IX deficiency, 10 percent of all persons with hemophilia

Von Willebrand's disease—abnormality of platelet function and mild to severe factor VIII deficiency, 5 percent of all persons with hemophilia

Hemophilia A and B are sex-linked hereditary bleeding disorders transmitted on a gene of the X chromosome. For this reason, hemophilia usually affects only males; however, very rarely a female is born with hemophilia if her mother is a carrier and her father has hemophilia. It may be the result of a spontaneous genetic mutation or inherited from one generation to another. Von Willebrand's disease is an autosomal dominant trait, and occurs equally in males and females.

Severity of hemophilia is described as severe, moderate, or mild. These categories are based on the amount of active clotting factor in the blood.

Mild:
- clotting factor activity level between 5 to 50 percent of normal
- usually only have a problem after major injuries or surgery

Moderate:
- clotting factor activity level greater than 1 percent, but below 5 percent of normal
- occasional bleeding episodes after injuries

Severe:
- clotting factor activity level is less than 1 percent of normal
- may have bleeding without apparent cause or with only slight injury

The severity of bleeding remains constant throughout the person's life.[2]

The most common bleeding problem is bleeding into the joints (most often the ankles, knees, and elbows) and muscles. About 80 percent of people with hemophilia have some musculoskeletal complications.[2] Less common, but potentially serious, are bleeding in the head, eye, throat, neck, abdomen, hip, and groin.

Hemophilia Management

Minor injuries, small cuts, abrasions, and nosebleeds are usually not serious, but should be observed to make sure the bleeding has stopped. Internal bleeding into joints, muscles, abdomen, head, neck, eye, lower back, and groin requires replacement of the deficient clotting factor and medical attention.

Acute management

- Factor replacement—raising the factor activity level high enough to stop bleeding.
- Joint support—use of sling, splint, crutches, other, to prevent or decrease deformity.
- Rest the affected area—initially, however, begin moving the area to exercise the muscles as soon after the bleeding episode as pain allows.

Pain management

- Ice—relieves pain, decreases size of leaking blood vessels, and limits the amount of bleeding (will not stop the bleeding and should not take the place of factor replacement therapy).
- Acetaminophen—never aspirin because it can hinder platelet plug formation.
- Narcotic pain medication—codeine, demerol, other.
- Antiinflammatory nonsteroidal medications—naprosyn, motrin, other.

Subacute management

- Exercise—will strengthen muscles that can protect joints and reduce joint bleeding.
- Physical therapy—restoration of muscles and joints to prehemorrhage functional status.
- Medical therapy—joint aspiration, debridement and/or synovectomy, osteotomy, etc.
- Child and family education—hemophilia education program
- Counseling—assistance with coping, individual and/or family

INDIVIDUALIZED HEALTHCARE PLAN

History

- Type of hemophilia
- Severity of hemophilia
- Usual bleeding pattern—including last bleeding episode
- Usual results of bleeding episodes
- Healthcare providers involved in the management of the student's hemophilia and regular health management
- Hemophilia management plan: measures used to control bleeding, pain management, exercise, physical therapy, medical therapy, child and family education, and counseling
- Student's participation in developing and implementing hemophilia management plan
- Assistance needed to implement the management plan
- Effectiveness of the management plan—student's, parents'/guardian's and healthcare provider's perspectives
- Procedure for factor replacement therapy
- Prevention and safety measures used and their effectiveness
- Involvement of support persons/systems
- Experience with self-care at home: recognizing signs and symptoms of a bleeding episode, factor replacement, pain management, exercise, and physical therapy
- Past experiences with bleeding episodes: at home and school
- Past school attendance patterns—specifically the number of days missed due to hemophilia
- Participation in regular school activities
- Participation in physical education activities—regular or modified
- Participation in regular exercise program—sports or leisure, school-related or non-school-related

Assessment

- Knowledge about hemophilia—student, parents/guardians, and teachers
- Student's perception of his/her health and hemophilia
- Parents'/guardian's perception of the student's health and hemophilia
- Student's locus of control—health, school, family, and activities of daily living
- Student's ability to do self-care: basic first aid for small external wounds, recognizing signs and symptoms of a bleeding episode, factor replacement, pain management, exercise, and physical therapy
- Motivation for self-care

- Barriers to self-care
- Decision-making skills
- General health status
- Joint swelling, deformity, limitation of movement
- Muscle atrophy
- Discoloration of skin—bruising
- Current height and weight
- Exercise tolerance and endurance
- Posture
- Gait
- Coordination and balance
- Environmental assessment: school building and grounds, potential sources of injury, safety rules and equipment already in place, safety rules and equipment that need to be added, protective equipment or padding that would reduce the chance of injury

Nursing Diagnoses (N.D.)

N.D. 1 (Potential for) tissue injury (NANDA 1.6.1)* related to deficiency in clotting factor.

N.D. 2 (Potential for) alteration in comfort (pain), (NANDA 9.1.1) related to:
- bleeding episode
- swelling
- joint deformity (arthropathy)

N.D. 3 (Potential for) alteration in mobility (NANDA 6.1.1.1) due to bleeding episode(s).

N.D. 4 Knowledge deficit (NANDA 8.1.1) about: (hemophilia, bleeding episodes, hemophilia management plan, safety/risk reduction measures) related to:
- lack of information
- lack of interest/motivation
- no experience with using the information

N.D. 5 (Potential for) noncompliance (NANDA 5.2.1.1) with hemophilia management plan, related to:
- knowledge deficit
- denial of illness
- perceived nonsusceptibility
- perceived ineffectiveness of management plan or treatments

N.D. 6 (Potential for) alteration in student role, (NANDA 3.2.1) related to:
- absences from school due to bleeding episodes.
- recurrent restriction of participation in school and classroom activities due to potential for injury, recuperation period needed for recent bleeding episode, and so on).

---

* (See chapter 2, page 38 for explanation of the NANDA approved numerical system.)

Goals

Prevent injuries and bleeding episodes. (N.D. 1, 3)

Institute safety measures that will decrease risk of injuries. (N.D. 1)

Develop and implement an emergency management plan addressing what to do if a bleeding episode occurs in school. (N.D. 1, 2)

Treat bleeding episodes promptly and adequately. (N.D. 1, 2, 5)

Good pain management. (N.D. 2)

Develop regular exercise pattern to develop strong muscles that can reduce bleeding episodes. (N.D. 3)

Increase knowledge about: (hemophilia, bleeding episodes, treatment measures, safety/risk reduction measures). (N.D. 1–6)

Use knowledge to make good decisions about his/her hemophilia. (N.D. 1, 4, 5)

Comply with prevention measures. (N.D. 1, 3, 5)

Comply with treatment measures. (N.D. 1–3, 5)

Good school attendance pattern. (N.D. 6)

Maximum participation in classroom activities in accordance with health status. (N.D. 4, 6)

Nursing Interventions

Discuss potential sources of injury (based on the environmental assessment), with the student, parents/guardians, and teachers: (N.D. 1)
- where they are located: classroom, hallway, gymnasium, playground, other.
- type of activity: physical education class, recess,passing time between classes, other.

Develop safety measures to be implemented at school (based on potential sources of injury). (N.D. 1)
- environment-specific: playground equipment, classroom, hallways, etc.
- safety rules: general and those that are specific to a particular activity or sport
- use of protective equipment or padding

Develop an emergency care plan for bleeding episodes that occur at school and on school-related activities. (N.D. 1)
- include the student, parents/guardians, teachers and healthcare providers
- coordinate and incorporate with hemophilia management plan at home and with healthcare providers
- list and describe treatment measures to follow
- set guidelines for seeking assistance if a bleeding episode occurs (any bleeding or specific types of injuries, notifying parents/guardians, notifying healthcare providers)
- special considerations for field trips
- make modifications in the plan as needed

Treat all bleeding episodes as promptly and adequately as possible. (N.D. 1)

Discuss pain management measures with the student, parents/guardians, and healthcare providers: (N.D. 2)
- pain-relieving medications
- ice

- exercise after bleeding episodes
- pain of an acute bleeding episode
- pain of chronic arthropathy

Assist the student to describe any pain he/she is experiencing: (N.D. 2)

- type
- intensity
- pain of acute bleeding episode versus chronic pain from arthropathy

Assist the student to make decisions regarding utilization of pain-relieving management measures. (N.D. 2)

- Acetaminophen or other prescribed pain-relieving medications (aspirin and any derivatives *should not* be used by persons with hemophilia because it inhibits platelet functions)
- use of ice to relieve pain
- importance of beginning to move the affected limb to exercise the muscles after treatment as soon as possible as the pain lets up (strong muscles help protect joints)

Obtain medication and specialized healthcare procedure orders and authorization for any management measures that need to be done at school from healthcare providers and parents/guardians. (N.D. 1–3)

Obtain any equipment, supplies, and/or medications that are needed to carry out prescribed and authorized management measures. (N.D. 1–3)

Keep accurate bleeding episode and management records. (N.D. 1, 2)

- time of onset of symptoms or injury
- type of injury (cause, body area affected)
- nature of pain
- management measures done at school and when they were done
- effectiveness of management measures
- who was notified and when they were notified
- sequelae from the bleeding episode (swelling, need for supportive devices, effect on range of motion in a joint)

Discuss with student, parents/guardians, and teachers the ways that bleeding episodes into joints and muscles can be prevented: (N.D. 3)

- develop strong muscles to assist in protecting joints through participation in regular exercise.
- regular exercise also can assist in developing agility, coordination, and endurance that can reduce the risk of injury during physical activities.
- use of protective equipment or padding in activities, when appropriate, to decrease the risk of injury.
- follow safety rules.
- avoid activities that will put excessive stress on joints and muscles (such as wrestling, heavy weightlifting, racquetball, etc.).
- achieve and/or maintain appropriate weight for height (extra weight puts extra load and stress on joints).

If a bleeding episode occurs in a lower limb joint or muscle, the student may need to use crutches for mobility around school for one to several days following an episode. (N.D. 3)

- inform the student's teachers
- allow extra passing time between classes
- student should wear a sturdy, non-slip soled shoe on the unaffected foot, observe crutch walking and stair climbing ability on crutches, and reinforce proper technique as needed

In-service for teachers and other appropriate school staff (such as the principal, health aide, playground supervisor, lunchroom supervisor, secretary, and others). (N.D. 1–4, 6)
- what hemophilia is
- the type and severity of the student's hemophilia
- signs and symptoms of a bleeding episode—spontaneous or injury-induced: (tingling or bubbling sensation, pain/tenderness, swelling, stiffness/limited movement of a joint, feeling of warmth in an area, blueness or discoloration of the skin, fresh or old blood passing from body openings, double or blurred vision [eyebleeds], trouble swallowing/trouble breathing [neck or throat bleeding], signs or symptoms of a head injury or history of a recent injury)
- what to do if an injury occurs
- what to do if they suspect a bleeding episode is occurring
- importance of prompt and adequate management of bleeding episodes
- need to resume activities gradually after a bleeding episode
- importance of exercise to build strong muscles that can help protect the student's joints
- any need for restriction or modification in activities (specific, such as contact sports, certain playground equipment, skateboarding)
- need for flexible educational programming (such as past and advance assignments, hospital or home tutoring, temporary classroom or physical education adjustment)

Provide health education opportunities: individual, dependent on knowledge level and developmental level. It may be new information or reinforcement for a previous learning experience. (N.D. 1–5)
- what hemophilia is
- the type and severity of his/her asthma
- signs and symptoms of a bleeding episode (spontaneous or injury-induced)
- what happens when a bleeding episode occurs in a joint (hemarthrosis) or muscle
- signs and symptoms of a bleeding episode into a joint: (bubbling or tingling feeling in the joint, feeling of warmth in the joint, swelling, decreased range of motion, pain or tenderness in the joint)
- possible joint changes that can occur if the joint bleeds are not adequately treated: (muscle wasting, cartilage destruction, morning stiffness, chronic pain, limited movement)
- signs and symptoms of bleeding into muscles: (gradually intensifying pain, limitation of movement in surrounding joints, numbness or loss of sensation in the limb, muscle feels tight and swollen)
- possible muscle changes that can occur if muscle bleeds are not adequately treated: (destruction or wasting of muscle tissue, nerve damage due to pressure on nerves)
- what to do if a bleeding episode occurs
- need for prompt and adequate treatment of bleeding episodes
- need for gradual resumption of activities after a bleeding episode

- how to get help for bleeding episodes (at home, at school, at a friend's house, other)
- what to do when a bleeding episode occurs (per hemophilia emergency care plan)
- identification of potential sources of injury
- safety and injury risk reduction measures that will assist in preventing bleeding episodes (dependent on specific activity and/or environment)
- need to follow safety rules and use safety equipment or padding (depending on specific activity)

Discuss the school-related prevention and management measures with the student. (N.D. 1–5)
- prevention measures
- prescribed bleeding episode management measures
- need for the measures
- importance of his/her participation in implementing the measures
- his/her role in implementing the measures: (follows established prevention measures, early identification of bleeding episode symptoms, reports signs/symptoms of a bleeding episode promptly to his/her teacher and school nurse, participates in providing bleeding episode care, and so on)
- other people who will be included: parents/guardians, healthcare providers, school personnel
- importance of his/her participation
- how the school prevention and management measures fit in with measures at home and with their healthcare providers
- benefits of compliance
- consequences of noncompliance
- motivators and barriers to compliance

Assist the student to participate in managing a bleeding episode (depending on his/her knowledge and skills). (N.D. 1, 5)

Choose and implement motivators to compliance. (N.D. 5)

Remove as many barriers to compliance as possible. (N.D. 5)

Discuss the need to wear a bracelet or necklace that indicates he/she has hemophilia. (N.D. 1, 5)

Monitor the student's ability to: (N.D. 1, 3, 5)
- follow safety rules
- utilize protective equipment and padding
- recognize the signs and symptoms of bleeding episodes
- seek and implement prompt and adequate management of bleeding episodes
- participate in providing bleeding episode management measures

Monitor attendance pattern and reasons for absences. (N.D. 6)

Encourage regular school attendance with environmental and educational modifications made as needed. (N.D. 6)

Monitor academic performance—referral to child study team as needed. (N.D. 6)

Expected Student Outcomes

The student will:

- Describe what hemophilia is. (N.D. 1, 4)
- State the type and severity of hemophilia he/she has. (N.D. 1, 4)
- List the signs and symptoms of a bleeding episode. (N.D. 1–4)
- Describe what to do if he/she is injured. (N.D. 1, 4)
- Describe what to do if he/she thinks a bleeding episode is occurring. (N.D. 1, 4)
- Describe how to get help for bleeding episodes: at home, at school, at a friend's house, other. (N.D. 1, 4)
- Describe his/her management measures for a bleeding episode. (N.D. 1–5)
- Report signs and symptoms of a bleeding episode to his/her teacher, school nurse, and parents/guardians promptly. (N.D. 1)
- Seek care for a bleeding episode promptly. (N.D. 1, 3, 5)
- Demonstrate what to do if a bleeding episode occurs. (N.D. 1, 4)
- Participate in implementing his/her bleeding episode management measures. (N.D. 1, 5)
- Describe the pain he/she is feeling by type, intensity, and whether it feels like a bleeding episode versus chronic arthropathy. (N.D. 1, 2)
- List ways to manage pain resulting from hemophilia (acute bleeding episode and chronic arthropathy). (N.D. 2)
- List physical exercise/activities that would develop strong muscles. (N.D. 3)
- List physical exercise/activities he/she participates in. (N.D. 3)
- State the safety rules for sports and other physical activities he/she participates in. (N.D. 3–5)
- List the activities that would put excessive stress on joints and muscles. (N.D. 3)
- Participate in regular physical exercise/activities. (N.D. 3, 5, 6)
- Achieve and maintain appropriate weight for height and age. (N.D. 3, 5)
- State what happens when a bleeding episode occurs in a joint or muscle. (N.D. 3, 4)
- List signs and symptoms of a bleeding episode in a joint and muscle. (N.D. 3, 4)
- Describe what to do if a bleeding episode occurs in a joint or muscle. (N.D. 3, 4)
- List places and activities at school that may cause an increased risk of injury. (N.D. 1, 4)
- List safety measures he/she can do to decrease the risk of being injured. (N.D. 1, 3–5)
- State safety rules for activities he/she participates in. (N.D. 1, 3–5)
- Follow safety rules for the activity he/she is participating in. (N.D. 1, 3–5)
- Wear and/or correctly utilize the protective equipment or padding for the activity he/she is participating in. (N.D. 1, 5)

- Wear a necklace or bracelet indicating he/she has hemophilia. (N.D. 1, 5)
- List the benefits of complying with prevention and management measures. (N.D. 5)
- List the consequences of not complying with prevention and management measures. (N.D. 5)
- List the motivators and barriers to complying with prevention and treatment measures. (N.D. 5)
- Maintain a good school attendance record. (N.D. 6)
- Participate in regular classroom activities as fully as possible (depending on health status). (N.D. 6)
- Participate in physical education activities (regular or modified). (N.D. 4, 6)

REFERENCES

1. Eckert E. *Your Child and Hemophilia.* New York: National Hemophilia Foundation, 1990.
2. Cotta S, Jutras M, McQuarrie A. *Physical Therapy in Hemophilia.* New York: National Hemophilia Foundation and Canadian Hemophilia Society, 1987.

BIBLIOGRAPHY

American Red Cross and the National Hemophilia Foundation. *Hemophilia and Sports.* New York: National Hemophilia Foundation, Dec 1984.

Brown R. *The Hemophilia Handbook.* Atlanta, GA: Hemophilia Association of Georgia, 1988.

Inman M, Corrigan JJ Jr. Hemophilia: information for school personnel. *J School Health* 1980; 50 (4): 137–40.

32 | IHP: Hepatitis—Viral

Wanda R. Miller

INTRODUCTION

Hepatitis is a diffuse inflammatory response of the liver resulting from tissue damage. This occurs in viral hepatitis, as well as in other infectious diseases or as the result of chemical toxins in the liver. At least five viral types are classified in the viral hepatitis group: hepatitis A, hepatitis B, hepatitis C, hepatitis D (delta virus), and hepatitis E. Clinically these viral diseases are similar, but epidemiologically they are significantly different.

Hepatitis A

Formerly known as infectious hepatitis, hepatitis A is caused by the hepatitis A virus (HAV). Estimates indicate the incidence of HAV in the United States to be in the hundreds of thousands, but asymtomatic cases make the actual numbers impossible to determine. Following a decade of decreased incidence in hepatitis A in the United States, from 1970 to 1980, a sharp increase of 26 percent occurred from 1983 to 1988. During 1988, 28,500 cases of hepatitis A were reported in the United States.[1] Hepatitis A is commonly reported in older children and young adults and makes up 50 percent of the reported cases of all hepatitis.[1] Of the reported cases of hepatitis A, the case fatality rate is 0.6 percent.

Hepatitis B

Formerly called serum hepatitis, this infection is caused by the hepatitis B virus (HBV). The incidence of acute cases of hepatitis B has increased over the past decade to a peak in 1985. In 1988, 23,200 cases of hepatitis B were reported in the United States; however, it is estimated that nearly 300,000 persons, predominantly young adults, contract hepatitis B annually. There may be as many as one million hepatitis B carriers in the United States, a quarter of whom will eventually develop chronic active hepatitis. Hepatitis B carriers are at high risk for developing cirrhosis and primary liver cancer.[1]

Hepatitis C (non-A, non-B hepatitis)

Hepatitis C is a parenterally transmitted hepatitis virus. More than one agent may cause non-A, non-B hepatitis, but one of the organism's antibodies has been identified as hepatitis C. A recently demonstrated hepatitis C viral antigen has established that hepatitis C accounts for most of the non-A, non-B posttransfusion hepatitis. One or more additional agents causes approximately 10 percent of the non-A, non-B posttransfusion hepatitis. A total of 2,470 parenterally transmitted non-A, non-

B type acute viral hepatitis cases were reported in the United States in 1988. Parenteral non-A, non-B hepatitis is transmitted as a sporadic acute hepatitis or as the result of transfusion. Approximately 50 percent of the patients with acute non-A, non-B hepatitis infection will develop chronic hepatitis.

Hepatitis D (delta virus)

Hepatitis D occurs in conjunction with acute hepatitis B infection or as a carrier state of hepatitis B. Delta hepatitis is believed to be a defective virus that is dependent on hepatitis B to become a whole virus and when whole becomes exceptionally virulent. The virus almost exclusively affects parenteral drug abusers and persons with hemophilia.

Hepatitis E

Hepatitis E is an enterically transmitted virus formerly included in the non-A, non-B hepatitis group. Hepatitis E is spread by the fecal-oral route and is found in countries with poor standards of hygiene and sanitation. Hepatitis E has not been identified in the United States.

Pathophysiology

The clinical course of viral hepatitis disease varies widely from the absence of any signs to severe fulminating symptoms. Infected children, especially those under three years of age, are frequently asymptomatic but the severity of the disease increases with the age of the individual infected. In older children and adults onset is usually abrupt, including fever (38 to 39 degrees C/ 100 to 102 degrees F), malaise, anorexia, nausea, and abdominal discomfort. Commonly, but not exclusively, in acute hepatitis B, flu-like symptoms such as, headache, myalgia, and coryza may also occur early in the course

of the infection, followed by symptoms of serum sickness, such as rash, petechias, pruritus, arthralgias, or symmetrical migratory arthritis. As the disease continues, liver involvement becomes evident in both hepatitis A and B, first with dark urine and clay-colored stools which precede jaundice by one to five days, enlargement of the liver, and splenomegaly. Convalescence with fatigue and weakness for weeks or months may follow.

Hepatitis A is primarily transmitted by person-to-person contact, through oral ingestion of fecal contaminants. Transmission is frequent where poor personal hygiene and poor sanitation exist, in the intimate grouping of a family, and where intimate sexual contact occurs. Water contaminated with infected feces and food contaminated by infected food handlers have also contributed to outbreaks of HAV.

The incubation period for hepatitis A is commonly twenty-eight days but can range from fifteen to fifty days. The feces of infected individuals contain high concentrations of HAV during the last two weeks of the incubation period and during the days just prior to the onset of jaundice. Viremia probably occurs during this same period and the disease has rarely been transmitted by blood transfusion. HAV has not been found in urine, nor has a chronic carrier state been demonstrated.[2]

Hepatitis B infection is a major nosocomial problem with serious sequelae. Exposure to hepatitis B occurs by inoculation of contaminated serum or plasma into the skin through needlestick injuries or illicit intravenous drug use, to mucous membranes through accidental splashes, sexual contact, and perinatally from mother to child during the delivery process or possibly in utero. Transmission of hepatitis B has also been associated with contaminated platforms of spring-loaded finger-stick devices. The incubation period of hepatitis B is commonly 120 days, but may occur from 45 to 160 days after exposure. The chronic carrier state of HBV is inversely related to the age at which infection occurs. Up to 90 percent of the newborns who are infected at birth from hepatitis-positive mothers will be carriers of HBV. Twenty-five to fifty percent of children infected before five years of age will become carriers, whereas only 6 to 10 percent of individuals infected as adults will become carriers.[3]

The hepatitis B virus is a double-shelled DNA virus. It has several antigen-antibody systems that can be detected by serologic tests. These systems are important in making a diagnosis and in determining infection control decisions:

Hepatitis B surface antigen (HBsAg) is produced in large amounts usually beginning 30 to 60 days after exposure. The antigen begins to decline toward the end of the acute phase of the disease. HBsAg establishes the diagnosis and as long as it is detectable in the blood the person is considered infectious. The persistence of HBsAg for longer than six months signifies a carrier or chronic hepatitis.

Antibodies to hepatitis B surface antigen (anti-HBs) become detectable one to six months after HBsAg and indicate immunity to HBV. Individuals who are positive for anti-HBs do not need prophylaxis against the disease.

Hepatitis B core antigen (HBcAg) is detectable shortly after HBsAg and before anti-HBs appear. The advantage to this antigen is that a period of time exists between the decline of HBsAg levels in an acute case and the appearance of

anti-HBs. This period of time, labeled a "window" by some,[4,5] can last for up to three months. The presence of HBcAg signifies recovery and usually immunity.

Anti-HBc is the most sensitive index of the presence of hepatitis B and is useful in diagnosis of HBV in the "window."

Hepatitis B "e" antigen (HBeAg) is an indicator of high infectivity and individuals who are positive for this antigen have very high titers of HBV circulating in their body. HBeAg's persistence after the acute disease is associated with chronic hepatitis and indicative during the chronic stage of the severity of the chronicity.

Antibody HBe (anti-HBe) conversely indicates less severity.

Prophylactic strategies against hepatitis B include two genetically engineered yeast vaccines, Recom bivax HB and Engerix-B, developed for HBV that produce antibodies to HBsAg in 95 percent of those vaccinated.[6] The vaccine has no effect on carriers to reduce or eliminate the carrier state. Postexposure immune globulin (IG) or hepatitis B immune globulin (HBIG) may also be effectively administered to unvaccinated persons exposed to hepatitis B. HBIG is the prophylaxis of choice when a person is exposed to blood that is known to be HBsAg positive. When the status of the blood is unknown immune globulin (IG) is administered immediately and the blood of the source tested for HBsAg. Immune globulin is an alternative when HBIG is unavailable, or when an exposure to hepatitis may not have occurred.

The Advisory Committee for Immunization Practices (ACIP) of the United States Public Health Service has recommended prevention of perinatal hepatitis B virus infection by universal screening of all pregnant women for HBsAg and administration of hepatitis B vaccine and HBIG to infants of HBsAg positive mothers within twelve hours of birth; universal vaccination of infants born to HBsAg-negative mothers; vaccination of selected high-risk adolescents; and vaccination of selected high-risk groups.[7] The American Academy of Pediatrics (AAP) has recommended universal immunization of all infants against hepatitis B disease. [8] Over the next few years, school nurses will undoubtedly need to stay abreast of the ACIP and AAP's recommendations to determine if changes have occurred in state laws requiring a hepatitis B immunization series for adolescents and/or young children. The preliminary hepatitis B serum draft recommendations for infants are one dose at birth, at one month of age, and at six months of age. In the near future combination vaccines for hepatitis B and haemophilus influenza b should be available.

Hepatitis C has epidemiological characteristics similar to those of HBV. It is transmitted primarily through blood and is known to be transmitted to transfusion recipients, parenteral drug users, and dialysis patients.[1] The importance of sexual transmission is unclear.[1] Half of the people with acute hepatitis C will develop chronic hepatitis.

Hepatitis D (delta virus) is epidemiologically similar to HBV. The infection most commonly affects parenteral drug abusers and persons with hemophilia.

Hepatitis E is transmitted enterically and has an incubation period of six to eight weeks.[8] Hepatitis E is primarily reported in tropical and subtropical countries. The course of the disease is rapidly progressive in the acute stage with a high fatality rate.

INDIVIDUALIZED HEALTHCARE PLAN

IHP: Hepatitis A

History for Hepatitis A

Assessment of hepatitis A is based on a history of exposure to disease in the family, in early childhood educational settings for children with special educational needs, in daycare settings located in a high school, or through sexual contacts. The diagnosis is confirmed by demonstration of hepatitis A IgM antibody. Obtain a history of exposure to disease and history of current illness.

- Have you or anyone in your family traveled recently in a rural area or in backcountry, or eaten in a foreign country where poor sanitation exists?

- Do any of the children in your family attend daycare?

- Does anyone in your family live in a custodial care setting and periodically visit the family?

- Has anyone else in the family been ill?

- Have you eaten food or drunk any water that is unique to you?

- How many students in the school setting are ill?

- Do the students who are ill eat in the school cafeteria?

- Do any of the food service personnel have now or in the recent past had symptoms of fever, malaise, anorexia, nausea, and vomiting?

Assessment for Hepatitis A

- Observe for fever of 38-39 degrees C/ 100-102 degrees F, malaise, anorexia, nausea, and vomiting.
- Observe for jaundice one to five days following the onset of flu-like symptoms. In cases where more than one student is involved obtain the history of the food service personnel in the school.
- The medical diagnosis of acute hepatitis A is made by identifying IgM anti-HAV in serum collected during the acute phase or early convalescence. IgG anti-HAV appears in the convalescent period of the disease, when the person is no longer infectious, and remains in the serum conferring protection against the disease.

Nursing Diagnoses (N.D.)

N.D. 1 Potential for infection related to susceptible group at high risk for infection such as early education, day care, special student populations, or hepatitis A in an individual. (NANDA 1.2.1.1)*

N.D. 2 Alteration in socialization due to isolation during the infectious stage of hepatitis A. (NANDA 3.1.2)

N.D. 3 Altered family processes related to a child with hepatitis A. (NANDA 3.2.2)

Goals

Prevent hepatitis A disease. (N.D. 1)
Prevent the spread of hepatitis A. (N.D. 1)
Maintain social contacts with the teacher and classmates. (N.D. 2)
Provide emotional support. (N.D. 3)

Nursing Interventions

- Provide accurate, complete information to teachers and staff who work with non-toilet-trained or fecally incontinent children about the spread of hepatitis A by the fecal-oral route. (N.D. 1)
- Provide information to the food service personnel about their need to remain at home if they are ill and for consultation in the event they become ill at school. (N.D. 1)
- Identify children for whom the risk of exposure to hepatitis A is realistically higher than for other children, such as diapered children, young children, and children with developmental delays. (N.D. 1)
- Provide information to the parents of these children about the spread of the disease, the potential for fecal-oral transmission to occur, and the availability of immune globulin (IG) as a prophylaxis. (N.D. 1)
- Provide developmentally appropriate hand-washing curriculum to the teaching staff for implementation at various grade levels. (N.D. 1)
- In-service staff about the importance of hand washing and the care of fecal excretion. (N.D. 1)
- Reinforce the teacher's plan for prevention of horizontal infection. (N.D. 1)

---

* (See chapter 2, page 38 for explanation of the NANDA approved numerical system.)

- In-service staff about the importance of disinfecting instructional materials or toys that may be mouthed by young children. (N.D. 1)
- Make referral to public health nurse or make a home visit to ensure appropriate procedures in the home. (N.D. 1)
- Report hepatitis to the local, county, or state health department. (N.D. 1)
- Provide information to high-school daycare centers about the need to administer IG to staff and children in the event of a diagnosis of hepatitis A in one or more children or staff from the center. (N.D. 1)
- Provide information to classroom students about hepatitis A and assure them of protective behaviors. (N.D. 2)
- Encourage classroom drawings/get well cards or telephone conversations. (N.D. 2)
- Reinforce family's plan to protect other family members from contracting hepatitis A. (N.D. 3)
- Stress rapidity of recovery in most cases of hepatitis A. (N.D. 3)
- Explain the usual disease course, include usual recovery process. (N.D. 3)

Expected Student Outcomes

- Susceptible students do not contract hepatitis A. (N.D. 1)
- Staff wash hands before and after eating, toileting, or assisting a child with toileting. (N.D. 1)
- Students wash hands before and after eating or toileting. (N.D. 1)
- Students and staff exposed to hepatitis A receive immune globulin. (N.D. 1)
- Student returns to school knowledgeable of events that have occurred at school and feels welcome. (N.D. 2)
- Family continues to support the psychosocial needs of the student and meets expectations of health promotion and prevention. (N.D. 3)

IHP: Hepatitis B

History for Hepatitis B

Assessment of hepatitis B is based on a history of exposure to the blood, semen, or saliva of an HBsAg positive person. An HBsAg positive person is frequently an immigrant or refugee from countries where HBV is prevalent, the child of an HBsAg positive biological mother, institutionalized for a developmental disability, a user of illicit parenteral drugs, a homosexually active male, a sexual contact of a carrier, or a patient in hemodialysis units.

- Where were you born? If born in a foreign country, when did you come to this country? Is your mother HBsAg positive?
- Are you sexually active? How many different sexual partners have you had?
- Do you use a condom every time you have sexual intercourse?
- Has your sexual partner been ill within the last five and a half months?

- Have you ever used intravenous drugs or used drugs to "shoot up"? If so, do you use clean needles every time you use drugs?

- Are you currently receiving intravenous therapy for a health condition?

Assessment for Hepatitis B

- Observe for fever of 38-39 degrees C/ 100-102 degrees F, malaise, anorexia, nausea, and vomiting.

- Observe for jaundice one to five days following the onset of flu-like symptoms.

- Three antigens indicate acute hepatitis B: HBsAg, HBcAg, and HBeAg. A prolonged HBsAg for longer than six months indicates a carrier state.

- Do you have any rashes on your skin?

- Have you had any aches or pain in your joints?

Nursing Diagnoses (N.D.)

N.D. 1 Potential for infection related to susceptible hosts and infectious hepatitis B agent as related to exposure to blood or bodily fluids. (NANDA 1.2.1.1)*

N.D. 2 Alteration in socialization due to isolation during the infectious stage of hepatitis B. (NANDA 3.1.2)

N.D. 3 Altered family processes related to a child with hepatitis B. (NANDA 3.2.2)

N.D. 4 Alteration in self-concept due to contracting a sexually transmitted or drug related disease resulting in situational low self-esteem. (NANDA 7.1.2.2)

Goals

Prevent hepatitis B disease. (N.D. 1)
Prevent the spread of hepatitis B. (N.D. 1)
Maintain social contact with the teacher and classmates. (N.D. 2)
Provide emotional support to the family. (N.D. 3)
Provide emotional support to the student. (N.D. 4)

Nursing Interventions

- Provide accurate, complete information to teachers and staff who are exposed to blood or to bodily fluids that may contain blood contaminated with hepatitis B. (N.D. 1)

- Provide information to adolescent mothers about the risk of transmitting hepatitis B to an unborn child, the need to determine their HBsAg status, and the availability of immune globulin or HB immune globulin as a prophylaxis and hepatitis B vaccine as a preventive. (N.D. 1)

- In-service staff about the importance of caring for potentially infectious waste and for disinfecting counters, floors, or objects contaminated with blood with hydrochloride, bacteriocides, or 70 percent alcohol. (N.D. 1)

- Provide information to healthcare workers, hemodialysis patients, sexually active homosexual males, intravenous drug users, and household and sexual contacts of HBV carriers on the need to obtain HBIG and hepatitis B vaccine. (N.D. 1)

* (See chapter 2, page 38 for explanation of NANDA approved numerical system.)

- Make referral to public health nurse or make a home visit to ensure appropriate procedures in the home. (N.D. 1)

- Report hepatitis B to the local, county, or state health department. (N.D. 1)

- Provide information to classroom students, without divulging private information, about hepatitis B and encourage them to use protective behaviors. (N.D. 2)

- Encourage classroom drawings/get well cards or telephone conversations to staff and students infected with hepatitis B. (N.D. 2)

- Reinforce family's plan to protect other family members from contracting hepatitis B. (N.D. 3)

- Stress rapidity of recovery in most cases of hepatitis B. (N.D. 3)

- Explain the usual disease course, include usual recovery process. (N.D. 3)

- Provide health counseling for the student which allows him/her to gain a perception of self and restore confidence. (N.D. 4)

Expected Student Outcomes

- Susceptible staff and students do not contract hepatitis B. (N.D. 1)

- Staff will treat all blood spills as if the blood is contaminated with hepatitis B. (N.D. 1)

- Staff and students will wash hands thoroughly following any exposure to blood. (N.D. 1)

- Students and staff exposed to potential hepatitis B will receive immune globulin immediately and HBIG if the potential blood source is determined to be HBsAg positive. (N.D. 1)

- Student returns to school knowledgeable of events that have occurred at school and feels welcome. (N.D. 2)

- Family continues to comply with expectations. (N.D. 3)

- The student is responsible for his/her own behavior and makes choices in his/her best interest. (N.D. 4)

REFERENCES

1. Centers for Disease Control. Recommendations and reports. *MMWR* 1990; 39: 1–26.
2. Minnesota Department of Health. Protection against viral hepatitis type A, delta hepatitis, and non-A non-B hepatitis: recommendations of the Immunization Practices Advisory Committee (ACIP). *Disease Control Newsletter—CDC* 1990; 18 (8): 73–80.
3. Minnesota Department of Health. Protection against viral hepatitis, type B; recommendations of the Immunization Practices Advisory Committee (ACIP). *Disease Control Newsletter—CDC* 1990; 18 (7): 61–72.
4. Dong B, Barton EC, Mancini BA. Viral hepatitis. *Nurse Practitioner: Primary Health Care Am J* 1984; 9 (Mar): 27–8, 30, 32.
5. Gurevich I. Viral hepatitis. *Am J Nursing* 1983; (Apr): 571–86.
6. Szmuness W, Stevens CE, Harley EJ. Hepatitis B vaccine: demonstration of efficacy in a controlled clinical trial in a high-risk population in the United States. *N Engl J Med* 1980; 303: 833–41.
7. Committee (Advisory Committee for Immigration Practices—ACIP) outlines universal strategy to counter hepatitis B. *American Academy of Pediatrics News* 1991; 7 (7): 1, 11.
8. Gitnick G. Hepatitis 1990. *Scand J. Gastroenterol* 1990; 175: 113–17.

33 | IHP: Immunodeficiency Diseases

Cynthia K. Silkworth

INTRODUCTION

Immunodeficiency diseases result when part of the immune system is absent or does not function properly.[1,2] Because the immune system is composed of many parts (different types of cells and serum proteins), there are many different immunodeficiency diseases. An immunodeficiency disease can be specific to one cell type or generalized to several components of the immune system. Some diseases may be mild, whereas others can be severe. Some are permanent and others can be temporary. In some immunodeficiency diseases, the cause is genetic, in others the cause is unknown. Some immunodeficiency diseases are common and others are relatively rare. Complications associated with some immunodeficiency diseases may be life-threatening, whereas other immunodeficiency diseases may be cured with new treatments such as bone marrow transplants. Most cases of immunodeficiency disease are viewed as chronic and not terminal.[3]

The exact frequency of each immune deficiency disease is not known; however, it is estimated to be 1:10,000 persons in the United States.[4] One disease, Selective Immunoglobulin A Deficiency, may be found as frequently as 1:400 individuals. Severe Combined Immunodeficiency Disease, on the other hand, is found in only 30 to 50 persons each year in the United States.[1,4]

Pathophysiology

Primary Immunodeficiency Diseases

X-linked Agammaglobulinemia—lack of ability to produce immunoglobulins, failure of the pre-B lymphocytes to mature into B-cells, all the immunoglobulins are markedly reduced or absent.

- Infections frequently occur at or near mucous membranes (such as inner ear, sinuses, eyes, and respiratory tract), and can also involve the bloodstream and internal organs.
- Most common bacterial infections: pneumococcus, *Streptococcus, Staphylococcus,* and *Haemophilus influenzae.*
- Particular susceptibility to common viruses that cause diarrhea and respiratory infections (colds and flu).
- Genetic disease—can be inherited.

Selective IgA Deficiency—total absence or severe deficiency of IgA class of immunoglobulins; B-lymphocytes are unable to change into IgA-producing plasma cells.

- Common presentations are chronic or recurrent infections (especially ear infections, sinusitis and pneumonia), allergies, asthma, autoimmune disease (rheumatoid arthritis, systemic lupus erythematosis), or chronic diarrhea.

- Most common immune deficiency disease.
- Cause or causes are unknown.

Common Variable Immunodeficiency— characterized by unusual infections and low levels of serum immunoglobulins (hypogammaglobulinemia), degree and type of deficiency of serum immunoglobulins varies from person to person, not caused by a single defect: some have few or nonfunctional B-lymphocytes, others lack helper T-lymphocytes, and others have excessive numbers of suppressor T-lymphocytes (acquired agammaglobulinemia).

- Most common presentation is recurrent bacterial infections, especially involving ears, sinuses, nose, bronchi and lungs, caused by *Haemophilus influenzae,* pneumococci, and staphlococci.
- Common form of immune deficiency disease.
- Cause or causes are unknown.

Severe Combined Immunodeficiency (SCID)—severe defect in both the T-lymphocyte and B-lymphocyte systems causing a marked susceptibility to infections, caused by absence or poor functioning of T-helper cells; the thymus gland is absent or functions poorly, and/or the bone marrow cells (stem cells) are defective or absent; in most cases all immunoglobulin levels are usually very low.

- Most serious of the immune deficiency disorders.
- Onset of infections in the first few months of life,
- Severe infections and complications, such as pneumonia, meningitis, and bloodstream infections.
- Most cases are inherited, autosomal recessive or x-linked recessive.

DiGeorge syndrome—T-cells are decreased with B-cells normal to elevated, usually with normal immunoglobulins; poor development of the thymus gland results in T-cell deficiency, also poor development of the parathryoid gland results in hypocalcemia.

- Associated congenital malformations are common.
- Extreme susceptibility to infection with viruses and opportunistic organisms.
- Cause or causes are unknown.

Wiskott-Aldrich syndrome—serum IgM level is low; deteriorating T-cell function and thrombocytopenia, inability to produce antibodies to polysaccharide antigens.

- Recurrent episodes of otitis media, sinusitis, pneumonia, and sepsis.
- X-linked recessive disorder.

Chronic Granulomatous Disease (CGD)—group of rare disorders causing inability of the person's phagocytic cells (polymorphonuclear leucocytes and monocytes) to kill certain microorganisms, most infections result in granulomas (localized swollen collections of infected tissue).

- Syndrome is usually recognized during childhood.
- Common presentation consists of frequent and unusually severe infections by staphylococci or by unusual bacterial species.
- Most granulomas occur in skin, lungs, lymph nodes, liver, and bone.
- Genetic disease—can be inherited.

Secondary Immunodeficiency Diseases

Secondary immunodeficiency diseases are a diverse group of immunologic disorders that result from another illness, such as an

(Adapted from Geha, [5], Pachman et al., [3] Rader, [1] Selekman, [2] and Wood.[4])

infectious disease, malignancy, or metabolic disease, or its therapy, such as immunosuppressive agents or splenectomy. They may be temporary and resolve when the primary illness resolves or they may be permanent.

Management of Immunodeficiency Diseases

General health measures that maximize the body's natural defences against infections are important as well as specific medical therapies.[1, 3]

General health measures include:

- Nutrition—adequate diet that provides essential nutrients for normal growth and development, body repair and maintenance.

- Hygiene—good hand-washing practices, good dental hygiene practices, good skin care, and proper care of minor injuries.

Specific medical therapies include:

- Antibiotics—directed at the specific organism causing the infection and/or broad spectrum, long- and short-term.

- Gammaglobulin—intramuscular or intravenous, dose and frequency individualized to the requirements of each person.

- Bone marrow transplant—administration of bone marrow cells from a donor, most often used to treat SCID.

- Antiinflammatory medications—treatment in autoimmune diseases.

- Replacement of missing biochemical—in ADA Deficiency/SCID.

- Human gene therapy (experimental)—in ADA Deficiency/SCID.

- Special diets and dietary procedures—in times of infection, illness, or food intolerance the normal diet may need to be modified or special methods of providing nutrition used, such as parenteral or enteral nutrition.

- Counseling—assistance with coping, individual and/or family.

INDIVIDUALIZED HEALTHCARE PLAN

History

- Student's specific immunodeficiency disease

- When the diagnosis was made

- Severity of the immunodeficiency disease

- Healthcare providers involved in management of the student's immunodeficiency disorder and regular health maintenance

- Immunodeficiency management plan (past and current)—general health measures, antibiotic therapy, special diet and/or dietary procedures, gammaglobulin therapy, bone marrow transplant, counseling, and others

- Student's participation in the development and implementation of the management plan

- Assistance needed to implement the management plan—student and/or family

- Involvement of support persons/systems

- Compliance with the immunodeficiency management plan

- Effectiveness of the immunodeficiency management plan—student's, parents'/guardian's and healthcare provider's perspectives
- Immunization status—immunizations that have been given, titer levels, plans for future immunizations
- Past experiences with infections—including communicable diseases
- Past experiences with hospitalizations
- Experience with self-care at home—medications, physical activity, dietary management, special procedures
- Past school attendance patterns—specifically the number of days missed due to infections or need for treatment of the immunodeficiency disease
- Participation in regular school activities
- Participation in regular physical education activities
- Special education services the student has received in the past or is currently receiving

Assessment

- Knowledge about the specific immunodeficiency disease—student, parents/guardians, and teachers
- Student's perception of his/her health and immunodeficiency disease
- Parents'/guardian's perception of the student's health and immunodeficiency disease
- Student's locus of control—health, school, family, and activities of daily living
- Daily activity schedule—morning to night, school and home
- Current nutritional intake, special nutritional or dietary needs
- Hand-washing technique
- Ability to do self-care—medications, physical activity, dietary management, special procedures
- Motivation for self-care
- Barriers to self-care
- Decision-making skills

Nursing Diagnoses (N.D.)

N.D. 1 (Potential for) infections (NANDA 1.2.1.1)* due to an alteration in the immune system (or) specific immunodeficiency disease.

N.D. 2 Alteration in health maintenance (immunizations) (NANDA 6.4.2) related to (specific) immunodeficiency disease.

N.D. 3 (Potential for) alteration in nutrition, less than body requirements, (NANDA 1.1.2.2) related to:
- infection
- illness
- food intolerance

---

* (See chapter 2, page 38 for explanation of the NANDA approved numerical system.)

N.D. 4 (Potential for) alteration in activity tolerance (NANDA 6.1.1.2) related to recurrent infections.

N.D. 5 (Potential for) noncompliance with prescribed medication(s) (NANDA 5.2.1.1) related to:
- knowledge deficit
- denial of need for medication(s)
- perceived ineffectiveness of the medication(s)
- unpleasantness of medication administration

N.D. 6 (Potential for) alteration in student role (NANDA 3.2.1) related to:
- absences from school due to frequent infections
- absences from school due to need for therapy with healthcare provider
- absences from school due to need for exclusion because of high potential risk of infection from other students (or) occurrence of a particular communicable disease in the school population

Goals

Prevent infections. (N.D. 1)

Maintain good hygiene practices. (N.D. 1)

Reduce unnecessary exposure to communicable diseases. (N.D. 1)

Maintain appropriate immunization status. (N.D. 2)

Maintain adequate nutritional intake. (N.D. 3)

Maintain adequate growth and weight gain pattern. (N.D. 3)

Base daily school schedule and activities on his/her activity tolerance. (N.D. 4)

Participate in regular school/classroom activities, with modifications made as necessary. (N.D. 4, 6)

Increase knowledge about his/her prescribed medication(s). (N.D. 5)

Compliance with prescribed medication(s). (N.D. 5)

Good school attendance pattern (relative to health status). (N.D. 6)

Conduct management measures during school hours with the least amount of educational disruption possible. (N.D. 6)

Nursing Interventions

Observe for signs and symptoms of infection in the student. (N.D. 1)

- fever/chills
- swollen glands
- fatigue
- pain
- nasal congestion or drainage
- headache
- cough
- muscle aches
- nausea/vomiting/diarrhea
- rash
- other symptoms specific to the student

Set guidelines for notifying parents/guardian and healthcare providers: (N.D. 1)

- Occurrence of specific diseases in the classroom, such as chicken pox or strep throat (In some cases, gammaglobulin-containing antibodies to those diseases may need to be given to prevent the student from acquiring the disease.)

- Increase in incidence of specific diseases in the school or community, such as influenza or pneumonia.

- Signs and symptoms of infection in the student.

Monitor communicable disease within the school and community. (N.D. 1)

Obtain medication orders and authorization for any medications that need to be taken at school (parent/guardian, and healthcare provider). (N.D. 1)

In-service teachers and other appropriate school staff. (N.D. 1, 3, 4, 6)

- specific immunodeficiency disease the student has

- severity of the disease

- signs and symptoms of an infection

- what to do if they suspect the student has signs or symptoms of an infection

- how an immunodeficiency disease can cause problems with eating and digesting food

- importance of maintaining a well-balanced diet

- need for snacks during the school day (if needed)

- allowing snacks to be eaten in the classroom and/or hallway between classes

- need for special diet or special dietary procedure and how it will be implemented at school

- how infections affect a person's activity tolerance

- signs and symptoms the student may be reaching his/her maximum activity tolerance (feeling weak and tired, headache, stomachache, crying for no apparent reason, and so on)

- medications the student will need to take during the school day and why these medications are necessary

- the necessity of absences from school due to: frequent infections, need for visits and therapy with his/her healthcare provider, exclusion from school because the incidence of specific illnesses in school places the student at risk for severe or fatal infection (such as chicken pox)

- need for flexible educational programming (such as classroom and physical education adjustments, past and future assignments, hospital and home tutoring, other)

- encourage teachers to ask questions and/or raise concerns if they have them

Assist parents/guardians to talk with their child's teachers about their child's immunodeficiency disease. (N.D. 1, 3, 4, 6)

Discuss the student's immunization status with the student's parents/guardians and healthcare providers. (N.D. 2)

- immunizations that have been given

- immunizations that are contraindicated (NO LIVE VACCINES should be given to students with certain types of immunodeficiency disorders.)

- immunizations that are planned for the future

- immunization status of siblings (In some cases, live vaccines should not be given to siblings either.)

Obtain a written statement from the physician explaining why the student cannot be in compliance with mandated state immunization laws. (N.D. 2)

Document that the medical exemption from mandated immunization requirements exists and the reason for the exemption on the student's school health record. (N.D. 2)

Inform the student's teacher(s) of the student's immunization status and explain why certain immunizations cannot be given. (N.D. 2)

Assist the student and his/her parents/guardians to assure an adequate diet is maintained. (N.D. 3)

- discuss what makes a diet well-balanced
- encourage the student to eat well-balanced meals
- discuss the importance of not skipping meals
- assist the student to supplement his/her diet with snacks during the school day, as needed

Assist the student and his/her parents/guardians to implement a special diet (full liquid, bland, or soft diet), if it is indicated. (Some infections or conditions may cause difficulty chewing, swallowing, or digesting foods.) (N.D. 3)

- discuss the reason(s) for needing a special diet
- specific kinds of foods that need to be included and excluded from the diet
- foods that need to be eaten at school
- short- or long-term (if long-term, have the healthcare provider provide a written order for the special diet)

Monitor the student's: (N.D. 3)

- tolerance of the special diet
- compliance with the special diet
- attitude about needing to eat the special diet

If special dietary procedures are necessary (enteral or parenteral nutrition): (N.D. 3)

- obtain orders and authorization for the specialized healthcare procedure to be done, from healthcare provider and parents/guardians
- obtain necessary equipment and liquid feedings or parenteral solutions

  (These procedures are used when the person is unable to eat sufficient foods to meet his/her energy needs or whose gastrointestinal function is inadequate.)

Monitor growth, height and weight, at specified intervals of time (such as every three months). (N.D. 3)

Assist parents/guardians, teachers, and healthcare providers in understanding the need of the student to participate in regular classroom activities and discuss classroom modifications that may need to be made (such as half-day school program to start with when a child is returning to school after an absence because of an infection, need for rest periods in the health office during the school day, potential need for intermittent homebound or hospital instruction if a serious infection develops, other) (N.D. 4, 6)

Assist physical education teachers to modify physical education activities and requirements, as necessary. (N.D. 4)

Monitor classroom and physical education activity tolerance. (N.D. 4)

Provide health education opportunities (appropriate to the student's developmental level): (N.D. 1–4)

- what an immunodeficiency disease is

- his/her specific immunodeficiency disease

- why persons with immunodeficiency diseases are at greater risk for infections than persons who do not have an immunodeficiency disease

- general measures to reduce risk of infection—good hand-washing technique and practice, skin and hair care, dental hygiene, and nutritional intake pattern

- measures to reduce or avoid exposure to persons with known communicable diseases

- what immunizations are

- why persons with immunodeficiency diseases cannot receive some immunizations

- immunizations he/she cannot receive

- importance of participating in classroom and physical education activities

- signs and symptoms he/she may be reaching his/her maximum tolerance—feeling weak or tired, headache, stomachache, crying for no apparent reason, other

- what to do if he/she has signs and symptoms mentioned

- identification of his/her medication(s) and how they work

- correct administration of the medication(s)

Discuss with the student: (N.D. 5)

- why he/she needs to take the medication

- need to take the medications as prescribed (on time, at designated intervals, specific dose, using the correct technique)

- importance of his/her participation in medication administration

- benefits of compliance

- consequences of noncompliance

- motivators and barriers to compliance

Choose and implement motivators to compliance. (N.D. 5)

Remove as many barriers to compliance as possible.(N.D. 5)

Assist the student to administer prescribed medications. (N.D. 1, 5)

- medications are available at the specified times
- self-medication program
- least amount of classroom disruption, as necessary

Monitor medication administration, reinforce proper technique as needed. (N.D. 1,5)

Monitor compliance with prescribed medication(s). (N.D. 5)

Assist the student and parent(s)/guardian(s) to obtain prescribed management measures with their healthcare provider (such as informing teachers and administrators of the student's absence and why the absence and management measures are necessary). (N.D. 1, 6)

Monitor attendance pattern and reasons for absences. (N.D. 6)

Monitor academic performance—referral to child study team as needed. (N.D. 6)

Expected Student Outcomes

The student will:

- Describe why he/she is at greater risk for getting infections than other persons who don't have an immunodeficiency disease. (N.D. 1)
- List measures he/she can do to prevent or reduce risk of infection. (N.D. 1)
- List signs and symptoms of infection. (N.D. 1)
- Demonstrate good personal hygiene practices—handwashing, skin and hair care, and dental hygiene. (N.D. 1)
- State why he/she cannot receive immunizations. (N.D. 2)
- Demonstrate adequate nutritional intake. (N.D. 3)
- State the reason why a well-balanced diet is important. (N.D. 3)
- Describe what makes a diet well-balanced. (N.D. 3)
- Eat a well-balanced diet. (N.D. 3)
- State why his/her special diet is necessary (if a special diet is needed). (N.D. 3)
- Demonstrate compliance with the special diet. (N.D. 3)
- Demonstrate adequate height and weight gain. (N.D. 3)
- Participate in regular classroom activities, with modifications made as necessary. (N.D. 4, 6)
- Participate in regular physical education activities, with modifications made as necessary. (N.D. 4)
- Identify signs and symptoms that indicate he/she is reaching his/her maximum activity tolerance. (N.D. 4)
- List the medication(s) he/she is taking. (N.D. 1, 5)
- Describe how the medication(s) work. (N.D. 1, 5)
- Demonstrate proper administration of his/her medication as prescribed (dose, interval, time, and technique). (N.D. 1, 5)
- State why he/she needs to take the medication(s). (N.D. 5)
- Describe how he/she participates in administration of his/her medication(s). (N.D. 5)
- Describe the benefits of taking the medication(s) as prescribed. (N.D. 5)
- Describe the consequences of not taking the medication(s) as prescribed. (N.D. 5)
- List motivators and barriers to compliance with taking medication(s) as prescribed. (N.D. 5)
- Demonstrate compliance with prescribed medication(s). (N.D. 5)
- Maintain a good school attendance pattern. (N.D. 6)

REFERENCES

1. Rader M, ed. *Patient and Family Handbook.* Columbia, MD: Immune Deficiency Foundation, 1987.
2. Selekman J. The multiple faces of immune deficiency in children. *Pediatr Nursing* 1990; 16 (4): 351–55.
3. Pachman L, Lynch P, Silver R, Ozog D, Poznanski A. Primary immunodeficiency disease in children: an update. *Curr Probl Pediatr* 1989; 19 (1): 8–55.
4. Wood R, Sampson H. The child with frequent infections. *Curr Probl Pediatrics* 1989; 19 (May): 234–81.
5. Geha R. Antibody deficiency syndromes and novel immunodeficiencies. *Pediatr Infect Dis J* 1988; 7 (May): S57–S60.

BIBLIOGRAPHY

Albano E, Pizzo P. The evolving population of immunocompromised children. *Pediatr Infect Dis J* 1988; 7 (May): S79–S86.

Buckley R. Advances in the diagnosis and treatment of primary immunodeficiency diseases. *Arch Intern Med* 1986; 146 (Feb): 377–84.

Stiehm ER. Clinical and laboratory evaluation of the child with suspected immunodeficiency. *Pediatrics in Review* 1985; 7 (2): 53–61.

34 | IHP: Lice

Wanda R. Miller

INTRODUCTION

Lice, or pediculosis, have tormented human beings since ancient times. Evidence of the louse has been found on the scalps of prehistoric American Indian mummies and appeared in ancient Egyptian and Greek writings.[1] Probably the most famous accounting in the literature occurred in England in the twelfth century when Thomas Becket was killed. As his cooling body lay in the cathedral for reviewal "vermin boiled over like water simmering in a cauldron." Historically, lice have been associated with periods of upheaval and poor hygienic conditions; however, in recent years, there has been a resurgence in the incidence of lice infestation that is unrelated to social upheaval or poor hygiene. Some believe the increase has paralleled the banning in 1973 of DDT and may be related.[1, 2]

Surveys conducted from 1973 to 1976 indicate that three to six million cases of head lice occurred in the United States in those years,[1, 3, 4] and many public health practitioners believe the prevalence of head lice is increasing. Estimates in 1980, based on the purchase of medicated shampoo, indicate that the incidence had jumped to ten to twelve million cases per year of head lice.[1] Despite the efforts of school nurses to maintain high standards of public health, studies indicate between one to three percent of school children are infested with lice.[5–7] In fact, one reference reports that as high as seven to ten percent of children in kindergarten through sixth grade may be infested.[1] There is evidence that head lice are more commonly found on girls rather than boys, on children in kindergarten through second grade rather than older children, on whites rather than blacks, and on children from low-income families where crowded housing accommodations exist; however, lice are not limited to any one sex, age, social, ethnic or economic group of children.[5]

Body lice are not as prevalent in the United States as the other two types of the species. They have caused more serious public health problems in Europe, however, where the body louse has played a significant role as a carrier of disease in epidemics of louse-borne typhus, trench fever, and relapsing fever.

Pubic lice are a common sexually transmitted disease. Incidence is estimated at one to two million cases annually in the United States.[8] The steady increase in pubic lice is more likely the result of increased sexual freedom than the banning of DDT.

Pathophysiology

Lice are human parasites that suck blood, crawl on human beings, and require warmth and humidity to survive. Three types of lice infest humans—head lice (*Pediculus humanus capitis*), body lice (*Pediculus humanus corporis*), and pubic or crab lice (*Pthirus pubis*). Identification of the specific type of louse is essential for the nurse in determining appropriate treatment.

Head lice and body lice are closely related in characteristics. They are translucent grey-white in color. The mature adult has an elongated body with three parts: a head, a thorax, and a segmented abdomen that makes up three-fifths of the body length. The male is smaller than the female, which is 2.0-4.0 mm in length. Immature lice may be as short as 1.0 mm in length. They have hooked claws at the end of each of their six legs. Head lice can be distinguished from body lice by their preferred habitat. Adult and immature head lice are found on the hairy surface of the scalp of humans, and the eggs (nits) are usually found fastened to the hair shafts at the nape of the neck and the area behind the ears. They may be found anywhere on the scalp but are not characteristically found on the eyebrows or eyelashes of the host. In contrast, body lice prefer to live in the inside seams of clothing, lay their eggs on material fibers, and move to the skin of the body to feed.[9] They are more numerous where clothing is in continuous contact with the body.

Pubic lice have a shorter abdomen than head or body lice. Their second and third set of legs are larger and appear crab-like. They are commonly found on hairs in the pubic area, but may live in the hairy areas of the armpits and chest, or on the eyebrows and eyelashes. In young children, infestations almost always occur in the eyebrows and eyelashes.

When ready to feed, the louse attaches its mouth to the skin, incises an opening, pours saliva into the wound to prevent clotting, and pumps blood from the injury into its digestive system. The most common symptom caused by the feeding of lice is itching. It is caused by the saliva of the louse on the skin.[2, 10] Some people who are highly sensitized to the louse's saliva develop intense itching and inflammation at the site of the louse bite. If only a few lice are present, itching symptoms may be absent.

The eggs (nits) are yellowish-brown to white-colored ovals, slightly less than 1 mm long with a cap at one end. They are cemented onto the hair shaft close to the skin where they incubate for about one week. Since human hair grows about 1/4 inch per week, eggs greater than 1/4 inch from the scalp have either hatched or are infertile and will never hatch. Temperatures above 100 degrees F. and below 75 degrees F. greatly reduce or prevent entirely the hatching process. Once hatched, the louse nymph molts three times within a period of eight to nine days before becoming a mature adult. (See Table 1).

The primary transmission of head lice from one person to another is by direct contact. They may in some cases be transmitted indirectly or by fomites, such as combs, hairbrushes, clothing, hats and bedding. Body lice are frequently transmitted in clothing. Pubic lice are transmitted chiefly by sexual contact, although they may be acquired from bedding and close personal contact. Animal lice normally do not infest people.

Treatment

Treatment consists of topical shampoos or lotions derived primarily from three chemical ingredients: 1% Lindane, 1% Permethrin (Pyrethrin) and 0.5% Malathion. See Table 2 for specifics on the various treatments.

Table 1. Clinically Useful Biologic Data on Lice

Biologic Characteristics	Body Louse	Head Louse	Pubic Louse
Most common habitat	Clothing	Head hair	Groin, eyelashes
Average number on host	10–15	10–15	10–15
Incubation period for eggs	7–10 days	7–10 days	7–10 days
Maturation period *	10 days	10 days	10 days
Life span of adults on host	35 days	30 days	30 days
Life span of adults away from host at 22 deg. C	4–7 days	2 days	1 day
Life span of eggs away from host	30 days	10 days +	No data
Temperatures lethal to adults and eggs	5 min. at 51.5 deg. C	5 min. at 51.5 deg. C	? assume same as other lice
Vector of disease	Yes ≠	No	No

* Period of time required for a newly hatched nymph to become an egg-laying adult.
+ Louse eggs will not hatch at or below room temperature (20–24 deg. C).
≠ Typhus (*Rickettsia rickettsii*), trench fever (*Rickettsia quintana*), relapsing fever (*Treponema recurrentis*)

Reprinted from Juranek.[9]

Table 2. Common Pediculicide Treatments

Generic/Trade Name	Kill Time *	Ovicidal Effect +	Residual ≠
Lindane/Kwell	186.2	45–70%	None
Permethrin/Nix	10–15	70–80%	Up to 10 days
Pyrethrin/Rid	10.5	74%	None
Pyrethrin/R&C	18.6	75%	None
Malathion/Ovide	4.4	95%	Up to 4 weeks

* Kill Time—The time required to kill every louse measured in minutes.
+ Ovicidal Effect—The percent of eggs (nits) killed in the prescribed treatment time.
≠ Residual—The length of any residual effect in killing lice.

Most of the medicated shampoos are readily accessible over the counter with the exception of Kwell and Ovide, which are prescription medications. The application time for medication to be on the hair is 10 minutes for all products except Ovide, which is applied and left on the hair for 8 to 12 hours. Compliance with the manufacturer's instructions for application time is important for effective treatment. Although Malathion has the greatest efficacy as an ovicidal agent, all of the pediculicides demonstrated hatch rate kill times. The recommended medication schedule is for a single application of shampoo followed seven to ten days later by a second application. Of concern, however, is the frequent reapplication of the medication, one of the most common abuses that occurs with pediculicide shampoos. Students may attend school in between treatment regimes. As described in the chart, 0.5 percent malathion lotion is a highly effective, rapid-acting pediculicide with a 95 percent ovicide killing rate.[11]

Kwell's longevity on the market and name recognition continue to make it a favorite among physicians; however, lindane is more toxic to mammals than either permethrin (pyrethrin) or malathion[12] and fails to equal the effectiveness of products made from the other two chemicals.[11] Kwell is contraindicated for preterm infants and is not approved for children under 2 years of age. Nix and Ovide have not been approved for children under 2 years of age either. None of these three shampoos is recommended by the Centers for Disease Control for use by pregnant women or by nursing women. There are no recommendations for RID or for R & C.

Eurax (10% Crotamiton) has been shown to be effective in the treatment of head lice but is not commonly used in the United States.

Reports of resistance to the three commonly used pediculicides have been noted in the literature. Given the past history of adaptability of insects to insecticides and the increasing widespread use in the United States of these three pediculicides, it seems feasible that resistance to the current medicated shampoos will occur. Maunder[10] believes that the development of resistance is inevitable following ten to twenty years of widespread use.

INDIVIDUALIZED HEALTHCARE PLAN

History

Review the student's health record to determine previous episodes of lice infestation and update the history information. Pertinent information may be obtained through the following questions:

- How long has the student been infested with lice and how many times has the student already been treated?
- Does anyone else in the family have lice?
- Who are the child's siblings and closest friends?
- Do any of the child's closest friends or siblings have lice?
- Are the siblings or friends under three years of age?
- Does the child attend a daycare, an after-school group program, or babysitting facility?

- Has anyone in your family ever had lice before?
- If so, how did you treat it?
- Is the person who will be applying the shampoo pregnant or nursing?

Assessment

Current Status

Determine if the student has any itching. If so, where on the body does the itching occur and how long has it been occurring? Discuss the student's current lice infestation and determine all possible sources of transmission.

Assess the knowledge, attitudes, and beliefs of the student's parent (s) to determine the extent of health education and counseling needed. Determine whether the parent (s) are reliable sources of information and whether they are able to comply with the treatment procedure accurately. If the parent (s) already know about the infestation, determine what they have already done to stop the infestation.

Determine the student's emotional response to the infestation.

Physical Assessment

- Inspect all areas of the scalp covered by hair using wood applicator sticks, forceps, or a fine-tooth comb (discard or sterilize the instrument in between each student).
- Inspect areas of the body where itching has occurred.
- Document observation of lice or nits.
- Describe nits observed in terms of location on the body or clothing, color, approximate numbers, and the location of the nits on the hair shaft. Carefully differentiate dandruff, hair spray globules, and hair casts. Inspect the head for excoriations produced from itching and/or secondary infections that may have occurred at the primary site.

Nursing Diagnoses (N.D.)

N.D. 1 Alteration in knowledge: deficit in information. (NANDA 8.1.1)*

N.D. 2 Alterations in self-concept: disturbance in self-esteem due to the perceived shame for having lice. (NANDA 7.1.2.2)

N.D. 3 Alteration in physical integrity through impairment of the skin integrity that may be actual or potential due to insect bites or secondary infection from scratching. (NANDA 1.6.2.1.2.1, 1.6.2.1.2.2)

N.D. 4 Alterations in coping of the family in ineffective and compromised behavior due to noncompliance with the procedures. (NANDA 5.1.2.1.2)

Goals

The family and student are knowledgeable in identifying, preventing, and treating pediculosis. (N.D. 1)

The student understands the pediculosis condition and assumes an appropriate level of responsibility for its prevention. (N.D. 2)

---

* (See chapter 2, page 38 for explanation of the NANDA approved numuerical system.)

The type of louse involved is known, treatment of pediculosis is effective, and lice and nits are eradicated. (N.D. 3)

The family establishes effective coping skills. (N.D. 4)

Nursing Interventions

Update the above history to provide foundation for nursing assessment and intervention. (N.D. 1)

Provide information to parent (s) about methods for disinfection of fomites, clothing, and bed clothing, including machine washing, machine drying, dry cleaning, ironing, and storage in plastic bags for a period of time that exceeds the life span of crawling lice and eggs off the host. For example: (N.D. 1)

- temperatures exceeding 52 degrees C (125 degrees F) for 5 to 10 minutes will kill lice and their eggs

- industrial hot water heaters maintain water temperatures at 60 degrees C; however, some cannot sustain water at that temperature when consecutive loads of wash are run

- run articles through the hottest setting on the dryer for at least twenty minutes

- personal articles of clothing may be dry cleaned

- nonwashables may be sealed in a plastic bag for fourteen days

- combs and brushes may be heated to 150 degrees F in water for 5 to 10 minutes or soaked in a pediculicide for one hour

- vacuum rugs and upholstered furniture

Inform the parents of treatment myths, such as: (N.D. 1)

- fumigating rooms and using insecticidal sprays on furniture and carpets to kill lice and eggs are not effective

- cutting hair does not reduce the risk of infestation

Discuss head lice with the teacher so that prevention principles are known. (N.D. 1)

- Assign coat hooks to individual students

- Assign permanent resting mats, soft toys, towels, pillows or blankets to each student

- Review classroom activities involving dress-up hats or other head gear

- Keep students' hats in coat sleeves or pockets away from other students' hats

Discuss head lice with the student so he/she knows about the prevalence of the condition. (N.D. 2)

Determine the need for and efficacy of screening the entire classroom for lice. (N.D. 2)

Explain common types of medication available to the parent (s), their effectiveness in killing lice, the application time required in order for the medicated shampoo to be effective, and the precautions necessary for children under 2 years of age and for pregnant and nursing women. (N.D. 3)

Apply, or teach the family to apply, pediculicide shampoo by reading directions several times and following directions described on the label. (N.D. 3)

Make child as comfortable as possible during procedure by using plastic drape to protect clothing, instructing child to shut eyes tightly during application, and using a fine-tooth comb on dry or slightly damp hair to remove the empty nit case. (N.D. 3)

Instruct the parents to restrict use of the medication to the two applications indicated in treatment of the condition. (N.D. 3)

Discuss the effect of removal of all the nits to insure that any eggs that are still living after the medicated shampoo will not hatch. (N.D. 4)

Follow up with the student upon return to school after the first treatment and seven to ten days later after the second treatment to determine that all the lice have been killed.

Expected Student Outcomes

The parent (s) identify lice infestations in their children and apply a medicated shampoo that is safe for both the student and those administering the medication. (N.D. 1)

The student complies with a follow-up schedule as evidenced by keeping appointments with the nurse. (N.D. 2)

The student accepts intervention with no evidence of self-consciousness. (N.D. 2)

The parent (s) report future infestations to the nurse in order to enhance surveillance of students in the school. (N.D. 3)

The student complies with prescribed treatment as shown by the absence of lice and nits. (N.D. 4)

REFERENCES

1. Robinson RR, Lawson DW. Head Lice: A Community-Based Epidemiological Control Manual. Pfipharmecs-Division of Pfizer, Inc. 1981.
2. Pratt HD, Littig KS. *Lice—Public Health Importance and Their Control.* Atlanta: Centers for Disease Control, 1976 (DHEW publication no. [CDC] 76–8265).
3. Gratz NG. The current status of louse infestations throughout the world. Proceedings of the International Symposium of the Control of Lice and Louseborne Diseases. Washington, DC: US Gov Print Off, 1973: 23–31.
4. Orkin M. Pediculosis today. *Minn Med* 1974; 57: 848–52.
5. Billstein S, Laone P. Demographic study of head lice infestations in Sacramento County school children. *Int J Dermatol* 1979; 18: 301–04.
6. Donaldson RJ. The Head Louse in England: Prevalence Amongst School Children. London: Health Education Council United Kingdom, 1975.
7. Slonka GF, McKinley TW, McCroan JE, et al. Epidemiology of an outbreak of head lice in Georgia. *Am J Trop Med Hyg* 1976; 25: 739–43.
8. Newsom JH, Foire JL, Hackett E. Treatment of infestation with *Phthirus Pubis:* comparative efficacies of synergized pyrethrins and benzene hexachloride. *Sex Transm Dis* 1979; 6 (3): 203–205.
9. Juranek DD. Pediculicides and scabicides. In: *Handbook of Drug Therapy.* DHEW publication, 1979.
10. Maunder JW. Resistance to organochlorine insecticides in head lice and trials using alternative compounds. *Medical Officer* 1971; 125: 27–29.
11. Meinking TL, Taplin D, Chester Kalter DC, Eberle MW. Comparative efficacy of treatments for pediculosis capitis infestations. *Arch Dermatol* 1986; 122: 267–71.
12. Taplin D, Castillero PM, Spiegel J, et al. Malathion for treatment of *Pediculus humanus var capitis* infestation. *JAMA* 1982; 247: 3103–05.
13. Whaley LF, Wong DL. *Nursing Care of Infants and Children.* St. Louis: CV Mosby, 1983: 650.

IHP: Nutrition—Growth Deficiencies and Children with Chronic Conditions

Mary J. Villars Gerber

INTRODUCTION

Nutrition concerns in children with developmental disabilities are prevalent. Concerns about nutrient requirements, intake and utilization are frequently present.

Poor growth is generally a multifaceted problem with contributing factors that are physiologic, biologic, behavioral, and environmental. Many syndromes have associated growth abnormalities. It is important to identify factors that are treatable. Some conditions/developmental disabilities with related growth lags include athetoid cerebral palsy, other encephalopathies, Down syndrome, nonspecific developmental delays and mental retardation, autism, craniofacial anomalies, metabolic disorders, renal failure, nerve and muscular disorders, failure to thrive, and child abuse and neglect. Mechanical problems include difficulty chewing and swallowing. Behavioral concerns include food refusal and food preferences that do not provide balanced nutri-

tion. Environmental concerns include feeding/eating routines, responses of caregivers, and feeding environments.

Nutritional intervention is focused on increasing intake of energy and nutrients. Caloric content of regular food can be increased by the addition of fat, protein and/or carbohydrate. It is very often a challenge to increase calorie content while maintaining a volume of food that the child can manage, from both a physiologic and mechanical perspective.

Planning for feeding of these children must be individualized and include realistic recommendations for intake as well as development of feeding skills. Small frequent meals and dietary supplements are common. The school will be involved in providing this type of accommodation in the child's educational program because of the length of time spent in school and the energy demands of school activities.

INDIVIDUALIZED HEALTHCARE PLAN

History

History of nutrition concerns and feeding problems:
- Have there been any digestive difficulties?
- Has there been difficulty with chewing/swallowing?
- Has the student had a poor appetite? Describe.
- Is there a history of food refusal? Describe.

- Has the student demonstrated food preferences? Describe.
- Have you ever consulted with a nutritionist? Date and results.
- What nutrition interventions have been utilized?
- Historical growth curves (height, weight, height for weight)

Assessment

- Current growth measurements. Obtain height, weight, and height for weight measurements. Plot on appropriate growth charts. For students with down syndrome, use a Down syndrome growth chart.[1] Growth charts for males and females with Down syndrome appear as a supplement to this chapter. If the child falls within the 5th to 95th percentile, there is not a height/weight discrepancy of more than 25 percent, and the historical growth curve shows a growth spurt in infancy and adolescence, the child's growth is considered within normal limits. Measurements outside those parameters should be referred for further investigation.

- Observe student's eating behavior. Environmental, situational, physical, and developmental problems should be assessed for contributing factors.

- Interview caregiver for routine dietary intake and concerns. What have caregivers been told about the child's nutrition status? What are the usual feeding/eating routines at home? Obtain three-day diet diary or 24-hour recall.

- Observe condition of hair, teeth, gums, skin, and muscle tone. Hair loss and dull, dry, thin hair can be a sign of protein and calorie deficiency. Skin should be smooth, elastic, firm, free from lesions, and appropriately pigmented. Muscle tone should be firm and well developed. Dental disorders may create difficulty with chewing.

- Dental condition. Dental cavities, infected gums, oral infections, misaligned teeth, or missing teeth can contribute to pain and subsequent reduced oral intake.

- Obtain medical diagnosis and medical history. Some conditions and syndromes have associated growth delays.

- Review of medication effects and side effects. Stimulants and anticonvulsant medications may cause appetite depression.

- Determine level of physical activity.

Nursing Diagnoses (N.D.)

N.D. 1   Altered nutrition: less than body requirements (NANDA 1.1.2.2)* related to: (specify)

> Neuromuscular impairment
> Loss of appetite
> Refusal to eat
> Impaired swallowing or chewing
> Physical disability
> Other

---

* (See chapter 2, page 38 for explanation of the NANDA approved numerical system.)

Goals

Provide balanced nourishment. (N.D. 1)
Promote nutritional intake. (N.D. 1)
Promote self-feeding. (N.D. 1)

Nursing Interventions

- For students below the 5th percentile or above the 95th percentile, or with a height/weight discrepancy of more than 25 percent, refer for complete nutritional assessment to pediatrician, pediatric nurse practitioner, or registered dietitian. This will include health and feeding history, dietary assessment, physical exam, lab tests, feeding assessment, and anthropometric measurements. (N.D. 1)

- Facilitate referral to school or consulting occupational therapist or speech and language clinician for feeding and oral motor assessment. (N.D. 1)

- Assist in establishing feeding program, recommended by occupational therapist, in school setting. (N.D. 1)

- Provide supplements and or high calorie/nutritious snacks as appropriate. Because the student is in school for a significant part of his/her day, these supplements and snacks will need to be provided during school as well as at home. Establish a home/school communication system. (N.D. 1)

- Monitor growth with regular weight and height measurements. This should be conducted at least monthly, and plotted on a standard growth grid. (N.D. 1)

- Refer for dental care as needed. (N.D. 1)

- Case management: Refer and follow up for healthcare if needed. Coordinate services. (N.D. 1)

Expected Student Outcomes

- Student consumes adequate amount of appropriate food with minimum effort. (N.D. 1)
- Student assists with feeding to the extent possible within limitations. (N.D. 1)
- Student gains weight. (N.D. 1)

REFERENCES

1. Cronk C, Crocker AC, Pueschel SM, Shea AM, Zackai E, Pickens G, Reed RB. Growth charts for children with Down syndrome one month to 18 years of age. *Pediatrics* 1988; 81: 102–10.

RESOURCES

Brizee LS, Sophos CM, McLaughlin JF. Nutrition issues in developmental disabilities. *Infants Young Children* 1990; 2 (Jan): 10–21.
Carpenito LJ. *Handbook of Nursing Diagnosis*. Philadelphia: JB Lippincott, 1989.
Carpenito LJ. *Nursing Diagnosis, Application To Clinical Practice*. Philadelphia: JB Lippincott, 1989.
Fee MA, Charney EB, Robertson WW. Nutritional assessment of the young child with cerebral palsy. *Infants Young Children* 1988; 1 (Jul): 33–40.
Springer N. *Nutrition Casebook on Developmental Disabilities*. Syracuse Un. Press, Syracuse, NY, 1982.
U.S. Department of Health and Human Services, Public Health Service. *Nutritional Screening of Children, A Manual for Screening and Follow-up*. Available from: Public Health Service, Health Service Administration, Bureau of Community Health Services, 5600 Fishers Lane, Rockville, MD, 20857.

United Cerebral Palsy of Minnesota. *Nutrition for Children With Special Needs* 1985. Available from UCP of
     Minnesota, S-233 Griggs-Midway Building, 1821 University Ave., St. Paul, MN 55104.
Whaley LF, Wong DL. *Nursing Care of Infants And Children.* St. Louis: CV Mosby, 1987.
Wong DL, Whaley LF. *Clinical Manual of Pediatric Nursing.* St. Louis: CV Mosby, 1990.

SUPPLEMENT 1A. Percentiles for stature and weight of boys with Downsyndrome, 1 to 36 months of age.

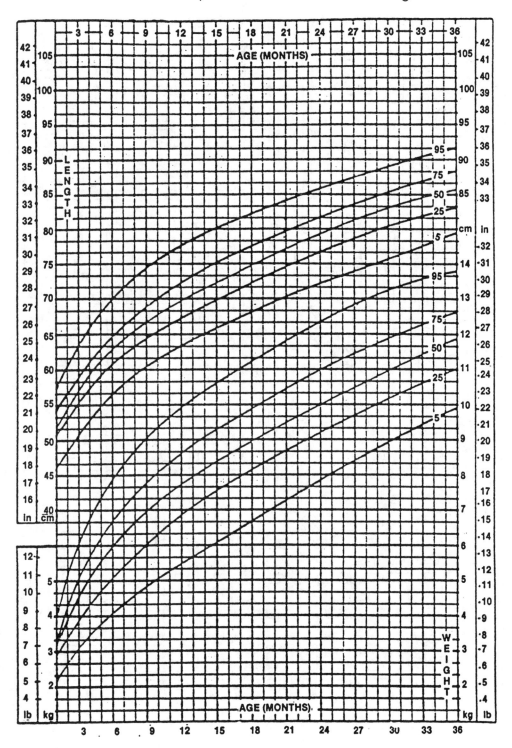

Reproduced by permission from Cronk C, Crocker A, Pueschel S, Shea A, Zackai E, Pickens G, Reed R. Growth charts for children with Down Syndrome: 1 month to 18 years of age. *Pediatric* 1988; 81(1): 107-108.

SUPPLEMENT 1B. Percentiles for stature an dweight of boys with Down syndrome, 2 to 18 years of age.

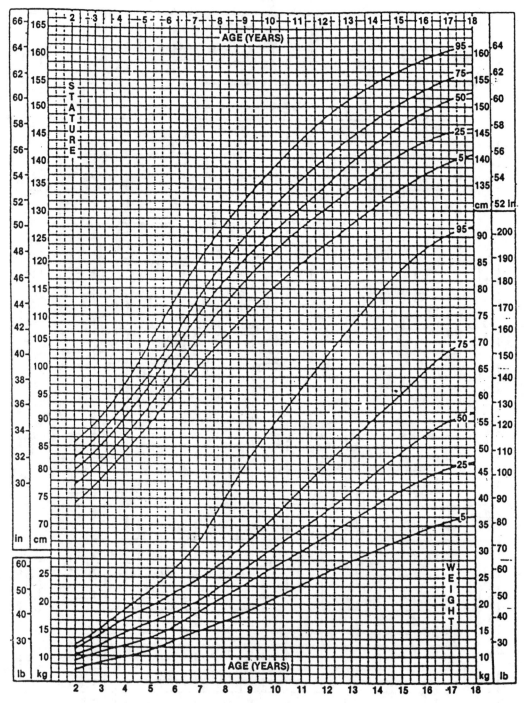

Reproduced by permission from Cronk C, Crocker A, Pueschel S, Shea A, Zackai E, Pickens G, Reed R. Growth charts for children with Down Syndrome: 1 month to 18 years of age. *Pediatric* 1988; 81(1): 107-108.

SUPPLEMENT 2A. Percentiles for stature and weight of girls with Downsyndrome, 1 to 36 months of age.

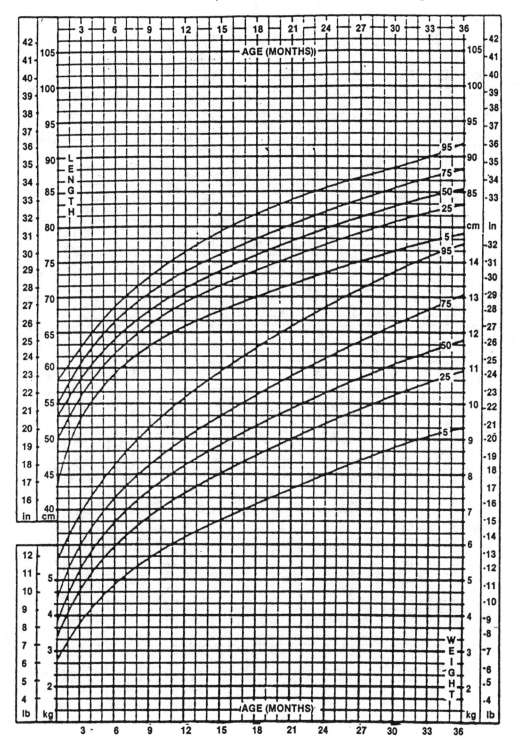

Reproduced by permission from Cronk C, Crocker A, Pueschel S, Shea A, Zackai E, Pickens G, Reed R. Growth charts for children with Down Syndrome: 1 month to 18 years of age. *Pediatric* 1988; 81(1): 107-108.

SUPPLEMENT 2B. Percentiles for stature and weight of girls with Downsyndrome, 2 to 18 years of age.

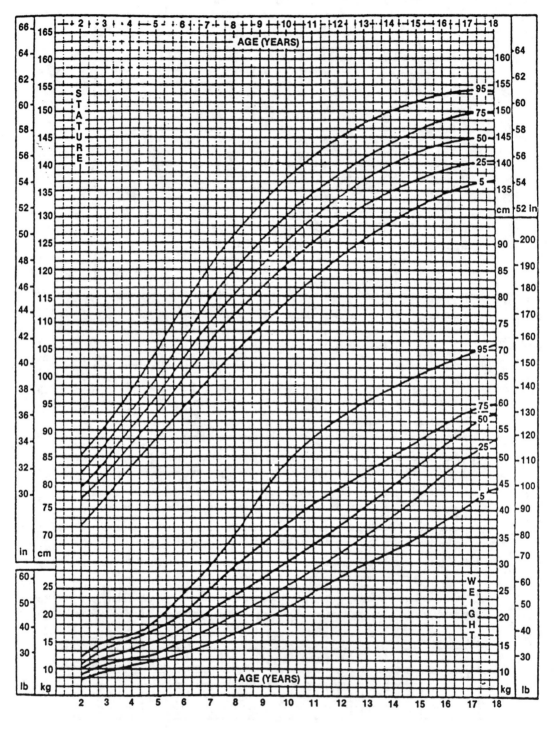

Reproduced by permission from Cronk C, Crocker A, Pueschel S, Shea A, Zackai E, Pickens G, Reed R. Growth charts for children with Down Syndrome: 1 month to 18 years of age. *Pediatric* 1988; 81(1): 107-108.

36 | IHP: Otitis Media

Wanda R. Miller

INTRODUCTION

Otitis media is the generic term for one of the most frequent disease conditions of early childhood. It can, and often does, overlap and represent a continuum of one disease process beginning with the initial onset of acute otitis media (AOM), frequently progressing through subacute or serous otitis media (SOM), and continuing on in a small number of children to develop destructive and long-standing chronic otitis media (COM). Considerable controversy exists surrounding the cause, incidence, and management of this complex disease condition. School nurses will continue to find their practice interventions in the midst of the controversies between physicians, specialists in ENT, pediatricians, and audiologists, until the research defines more specifically the cause(s), sequelae, and effective management of otitis media.

Both the incidence and prevalence of otitis media are related strongly to the age of the child. Fiellau-Nikolajsen[1] reported that, "Serous otitis media does not occur in newborns and is relatively uncommon during the first 4 to 6 months of life. In the 6 to 12 month age group there is such an explosive increase in the number of new cases that 13 percent to 15 percent of all children have SOM around 12 months of age. The frequency of SOM, all factors being equal, peaks at ages 2 to 4 years, during which 20 percent of all 'normal' children have SOM." Two-thirds of three-year-old children will have experienced at least one episode of acute otitis media and a third have had three or more infections by age three.[2]

Pathophysiology

The most commonly identified symptom of otitis media is middle ear effusion, or fluid in the middle ear. It is always present in AOM and SOM and is often present in COM also. Acute otitis media frequently begins with symptoms of ear pain and fever and the signs of a red and bulging tympanic membrane, which are evident only on otological examination as pressure from effusion increases. Acute otitis media can, however, be elusive and totally asymptomatic, with the middle ear effusion of AOM resolving itself. Serous otitis media is asymptomatic except for mild-to-moderate conductive hearing loss. The middle ear effusions of SOM have high viscosity, are cloudy, and persist for four weeks or longer. Long-standing middle ear inflammations are purulent with low viscosity. The slow, recurring, insidious inflammation that lasts for three months or longer is called chronic otitis media.

Three etiological factors interact with one another and contribute to the initiation, maintenance, and aggravation of otitis media: dysfunction of the eustachian tube, the pathogenesis of otitis media in the upper respiratory tract from viral and bacterial infections, and the role of allergies in middle ear disease.[3]

The single most important factor in the development of otitis media is dysfunction of the eustachian tube. The eustachian tube has three major functions: protection from nasopharyngeal sound, pressure, and secretions; drainage of secretions into the nasopharynx; and ventilation of the middle ear to replenish gases that have been absorbed. Either a functional or mechanical obstruction of the tube will result in dysfunction and otitis media with effusion. Functional obstructions occur when the eustachian tube is too compliant and remains persistently collapsed, inadequately opens, or both. Negative pressure develops in the middle ear resulting in serum hypersecretion and accumulation of fluid. Finally, reflux of bacterial or viral infected nasopharyngeal secretions occurs when the tube does open due to the highly negative pressure in the middle ear. Functional obstruction of the eustachian tube is common in infants and young children because their tubal cartilage is more compliant. Mechanical obstruction of the eustachian tube results from inflammation of the tube during upper respiratory tract infections and from enlarged adenoids or nasopharyngeal tumors.

The second most important factor in the pathogenesis of otitis media is upper respiratory tract viral and bacterial infections. There is initial indication that respiratory viral infections and pharyngeal bacterial infections increase the frequency of otitis media. Epithelial cell injury during influenza illnesses may enhance attachment of pneumococci to mucosal cells.[4]

Finally, the role of allergies in middle ear disease has not been determined, however, several deficiencies in immunoglobulin appear to have a relationship to the disease process.

There is extreme variability in the course of untreated otitis media, making it difficult to characterize. The approximate characteristics of five typical responses to untreated courses of otitis media have been described by Fiellau-Nikolajsen[1] as:

- 15 percent of children experience a single occurrence of the disease lasting one to three months;
- 25 percent of children experience multiple occurrences of the disease lasting for one to three months;
- 15 percent of children experience a single occurrence of the disease lasting for three to nine months;
- 15 percent of children experience multiple occurrences of the disease lasting for three to nine months; and finally,
- 10 percent of children experience multiple occurrences of the disease lasting one or more years.

Serous otitis media occurs primarily in the winter, in premature infants, in children with cleft palates, in children enrolled in daycare, in children with allergies, in boys, in certain families, and in certain populations, such as American Indians, Alaskan Eskimos, and some Southeast Asian groups.

School nurse intervention is crucial to young children if continuity of care and successful treatment are to occur. Compliance with medication regimes and adherence to scheduled medical appointments greatly affect the prognosis of otitis media. Susan L. Jones has published a study of nursing intervention utilizing the Health Belief Model to obtain compliance in the treatment of otitis media.[5] Jones evaluates two forms of nursing intervention designed to increase compliance for scheduling a follow-up referral appointment and for keeping the appointment. The nursing intervention consists of a standardized assessment of the subject's perceived susceptibility, seriousness, and benefits versus costs. Compliance of the parent in the medication regime and follow-up of medical and audiological care are related to the parents' perception that the child is at risk for having AOM again, the otitis is serious for the child's health and educational status, and the time and money expended versus the benefit of freedom from middle ear disease.

Medication/Treatment

The treatment of choice for acute otitis media is systemic antimicrobial drugs. Surgical procedures should be reserved for situations in which the disease does not respond to medical treatment or when the disease process persists or frequently reoccurs.

The two causative bacterial agents found most frequently in AOM are *Streptococcus pneumoniae* (29%) and *Haemophilus influenzae* (23%). *Branhamella catarrhalis,* in the past, has represented about 5 percent of the incidence, but recently has been found in 12 to 22 percent of the cases. Group A beta-hemolytic streptococcus and *Staphylococcus aureus* each represent less than 5 percent of the cases.[6,7] In COM 25 percent of the cases are sterile and *Haemophilus influenzae* is cultured in 13 percent of the cases. All other bacterial organisms cultured in COM are represented in less than 10 percent of the cases.

Amoxicillin (or ampicillin) is the preferred drug for initial therapy of acute otitis media because it is active against *S. pneumoniae* and most strains of *H. influenzae*. Amoxicillin is administered for ten days on a t.i.d. or q.i.d. regime based on weight. Erythromycin and sulfisoxazole are combined for children who are allergic to penicillins. Ampicillin is not effective against beta-lactamase-producing organisms. Cefaclor or the combination amoxicillin-clavulanate are administered if beta-lactamase-producing *H. influenzae* or *B. catarrhalis* are isolated from middle ear fluid. Two new cephalosporins, cefuroxime axetil and cefixime, are also available if resistant organisms are present. Children should show significant improvement within 48 to 72 hours if therapy has been maintained. If signs and symptoms persist, children should be reevaluated by day five.[6] Few adverse effects have been noted; however, skin rashes and gastrointestinal tract upset are occasionally observed in all of the drugs cited. Abdominal cramping and vomiting have been noted in as many as 40 percent of the children taking erythomycin. These drugs should be discontinued at the first appearance of a skin rash or sign of adverse reaction.

Coexisting respiratory virus infection frequently precedes AOM. Rhinovirus and respiratory syncytial virus were the two most frequently detected organisms.[8] Fever, restlessness, poor appetite, rhinitis and cough preceded AOM by an average of six days. Cough and rhinitis persisted for seven days after the onset of antimicrobial treatment. The persistence of respiratory symptoms may not indicate the failure of treatment but the persistence of the viral infection. This prolonged viral infection in the middle ear of some patients may lead to the development of SOM.

The need for surgery should be individually assessed if the antimicrobial prophylaxis fails and otitis recurs. Recent studies have indicated that myringotomy alone has minimal efficacy. If a generalized anesthesia is necessary to perform myringotomy, the addition of tympanostomy tubes provides a longer effusion-free period, fewer medical treatments, fewer required surgical retreatments, and a shorter period of time with abnormal hearing in the better ear.[9] Offsetting the benefits of tube placement is the high rate of sclerotic or atrophic scarring of the eardrum. Although tonsillectomy has proven to be ineffective in reducing otitis media, adenoidectomy offers long lasting benefits with no known long-term sequelae.

INDIVIDUALIZED HEALTHCARE PLAN

History

Assessment of otitis media is based on history information, observation with a pneumatic otoscope, tympanometry, and audiometry. Review the student's health record to determine a previous history of ear pain, or serosanguineous drainage from the ear.

- Has your child had a fever, cough, or runny nose or been irritable within the last two weeks?
- Has your child ever had episodes of pain in the ear, tugged at the ears, or had fever?
- Have you ever suspected a hearing loss in your child?
- Has your child had three documented episodes of otitis media in six months or four episodes in twelve months?
- How long did the fluid remain in the child's ear? Has the fluid persisted for two to three months (see characteristics of untreated cases described earlier)?
- What kinds of medical intervention were previously used?
- When was the child's most resent episode of otitis media? How long did it last?
- Is your child's speech intelligible? Is your child receiving speech therapy?

Assessment

The part of the ear that protrudes from the head is called the auricle or pinna. The rigidity of the auricle is due to its cartilaginous structure. In contrast, the ear lobe, consisting of fatty tissue, is flexible. The external ear collects and funnels sound waves through the tympanic membrane to the middle ear. The opening from the outside of the ear to the tympanic membrane is called the auditory canal or external meatus. The external auditory canal is about one inch long with a slight curve. It has a skeleton of cartilage in the outer one third to one half of the canal which becomes a skeleton of bone as it nears the tympanic membrane. The skin of the inner part of the canal is exceedingly thin and sensitive. The external ear ends at the tympanic membrane. This membrane is considered part of the middle ear, and is made up of layers of skin, fibrous tissue, and mucous membrane. On otoscopic examination a healthy tympanic membrane is shiny, translucent, and pearly gray in color. The tympanic membrane is positioned at a slant with the lower anterior quadrant farthest away from the examiner. Most of the membrane is slightly concave and taunt, pulled inward near the center by one of the ossicle bones of the middle ear, the malleus. The short process of the malleus protrudes against the membrane at the center near the top of the membrane. The handle of the malleus extends downward from the short process to the umbo. A small part of the membrane is located over the short process and is flaccid, hence the name pars flaccida. A light reflex or cone of light is present on the membrane. The apex of the cone, beginning at the umbo, fans out onto the anterioinferior quadrant of the healthy tympanic membrane.

In the early stages of acute otitis media vascularization of the blood vessels along the periphery of the membrane, across the pars flaccida, and down the malleus handle is evident. (Crying or sneezing will also cause hypervascularization.) Retraction of the membrane occurs with negative pressure drawing the umbo at the center of the membrane into the middle ear and causing the short process to become more prominent, or may as the disease progresses, bulge, become fiery red in color, and spontaneously rupture. Pneumatic otoscopy is a useful tool in the young child in determining middle ear effusion. The procedure is performed with an otoscope, enclosed otoscope head, and insufflator attachment. The otoscope is placed in the ear canal and an airtight seal is obtained. Then the insufflator bulb is pressed while the tympanic membrane is observed. The healthy membrane will fluctuate in response to the air pressure. In serous otitis media the membrane is retracted and shows decreased mobility with pneumatic otoscopy. (A soft-tipped specula will provide a more reliable seal in performing a pneumatic otoscopic examination. As children advance in age the reliability of the seal decreases. Air leaks may also occur in the equipment, producing false negatives, and can be checked by compressing the insufflator bulb and then placing a finger over the end of the speculum.[10] The handle of the malleus is usually shortened and chalky in color, and the lateral process is prominent. The presence of a thin, serous effusion within the middle ear gives the tympanic membrane a dull yellowish or bluish color and opaque appearance. In cases of incomplete eustachian tube obstruction, air bubbles or an air level may be seen. The light reflex is distorted or missing.

Immediate medical care is needed for acute otitis particularly when accompanied by pain. Differentiation for external otitis and otitis media would be helpful and can be made by observation or palpation of the tragus. Children with external otitis may have so much pain that otoscopic examination is not possible.

Tympanometry can identify from 75 to 98 percent of children with middle ear effusion.[11] However, in 1987 the American Academy of Pediatrics issued a statement that impedance audiometry (one aspect of which is tympanometry) should not be used in mass screening programs for the detection of hearing loss or middle ear effusion; not be used as a replacement for audiometric screening, because it will not detect sensorineural hearing loss and may lead to overreferral of children with asymptomatic middle ear effusion.[11] Although tympanometry does not identify sensorineural hearing losses and should not be used in place of the pure-tone audiometric hearing testing that should occur in schools, it is a useful testing procedure to gain additional information in children who are too young or incapable of responding to the audiometric tones and in the management of children known to have otitis media. The equipment is expensive and requires some inservice training to provide accurate testing results, but should be considered for the management of children with otitis media.

Nursing Diagnoses (N.D.)

N.D. 1 Altered physiologic processes in the middle ear due to effusion resulting in impaired sensory or conductive hearing function. (NANDA 7.2.2)*

N.D. 2 Altered human response patterns in perception processes: auditory. (NANDA 7.2)

---

* (See chapter 2, page 38 for explanation of the NANDA approved numerical system.)

N.D. 3   Altered comfort due to pain related to pressure on the tympanic membrane caused by inflammatory process. (NANDA 9.1.1)

N.D. 4   Alterations in participation family noncompliance with prescribed medication regime resulting in continued disease process. (NANDA 5.2.1.1)

N.D. 5   Alterations in participation family noncompliance with follow-up of medical examinations resulting in loss of hearing acuity and potential for infective organism. (NANDA 5.2.1.1)

Goals

The student's middle ears are free from fluid. (N.D. 1)

The student hears within the normal conversational range. (N.D. 2)

The student is free from pain. (N.D. 3)

The student maintains the prescribed protocols for medication. (N.D. 4)

The student follows up health appointments with the school nurse, physician, or audiologist. (N.D. 4)

Reinfection is prevented. (N.D. 5)

Nursing Interventions

- Obtain a complete health history of upper respiratory infections, ear infections, and previous medical interventions. (N.D. 1)

- Examine the child by observation of the throat, palpation of the cervical nodes, otoscopic and pneumatic observation of the tympanic membrane, pure-tone threshold audiometric testing and acoustic immittance by tympanometry. (N.D. 1)

- Refer children with AOM to their primary healthcare provider immediately for medical intervention with a microbial medication. (N.D. 1)

- Obtain a reciprocal release of information from the parent. (s) and maintain a cooperative working relationship with the primary healthcare provider, sharing the progress notes from the ongoing assessment observations. (N.D. 2)

- Position the student toward the front of the classroom and directly in front of the teacher as often as possible. (N.D. 2)

- Assess the status of the middle ear every two weeks following an episode of AOM or SOM with pneumatic otoscopy, audiometer and typanometer, until the effusion is resolved and then monthly during the months from November through April until the child has been clear of SOM for one full year. (N.D. 2)

- Position for comfort according to needs of individual child. (N.D. 3)

- Position with affected ear in dependent position lying on the affected side for relief of pain. (N.D. 3)

- Administer oral liquids or soft foods. (N.D. 3)

- Obtain current medication orders for acute otitis. (N.D. 4)

- Provide the parent(s) of the child, at least once during the ten-day medication regime, health education about the susceptibility of their child to otitis media, its severity, and the effects of noncompliance with the medication regime, and diligent observations of the child for conductive hearing loss versus the benefits to good health management. (N.D. 4)

- Explain the limited nature of treatment by medication only and the need for ongoing supervision by a healthcare professional. (N.D. 4)

- Explain the role of the healthcare profession in curing or controlling symptoms, reducing risk of factors in recurrence, preventing complications, and preventing irreversible or chronic conditions.[5] (N.D. 5)

- Stress importance of follow-up in two or three weeks with the school nurse for monitoring of the infection and referral back to the healthcare provider if the infection is not resolved. (N.D. 5)

- If SOM persists for more than three months urge the parent to request a consultation with the primary healthcare provider and possible referral to an ENT specialist for treatment to resolve the persisting conductive hearing loss. (N.D. 5)

- Refer the child to an educational audiologist if the hearing loss persists past three months. (N.D. 5)

- Assist in obtaining financial assistance if needed. (N.D. 5)

- Promote aeration of middle ear by having child sit upright to eat, gently blow nose, use blowing games, chew gum, and employ the Valsalva procedure of pinching the nose and closing the lips while air is forced up the eustachian tube. (N.D. 5)

- Eliminate tobacco smoke and known allergens from child's environment. (N.D. 5)

Expected Student Outcomes

- The student does not have a conductive hearing loss that persists for more than three months without aggressive medical and audiological intervention. (N.D. 1)

- When the child has a middle ear effusion the student sits close to the teacher in order to hear the educational program during the school day. (N.D. 2)

- A student who has tympanometry tubes is knowledgeable about the potential for infection from exposure to swimming. (N.D. 2)

- Parents are aware of the services provided by the school nurse and seek consultation for issues related to SOM and conductive hearing loss. (N.D. 2)

- Teachers are alerted to the potential for this child to develop SOM at any time and watch for disinterest or lack of attention and refer the child to the school nurse for periodic assessments following upper respiratory infections. (N.D. 2)

- The length of time that a conductive hearing loss continues is reduced. (N.D. 2)

- The student rests quietly during episodes of pain and demonstrates no signs of discomfort. (N.D. 3)

- The student completes the full medication regime prescribed for AOM. (N.D. 4)

- Documentation of nursing care is complete: medication administration is recorded daily, hearing audiometry and tympanometry are recorded, referrals are recorded, and a system of follow-up is maintained. (N.D. 4)

- The student maintains a schedule of nursing, medical, and audiological health maintenance appointments. (N.D. 5)

- Child remains free of infection. (N.D. 5)

REFERENCES

1. Fiellau-Nikolajsen M. Danish approach to the treatment of secretory otitis media. *Ann Otol Rhinol Laryngol* 1990; 146: 1–28.
2. Teele GW, Klein JO, Rosner BA. Epidemiology of otitis media in children. *Ann Otol Rhinol Laryngol* 1980; 89 (Suppl 68): 5-6.
3. Tos M. Danish approach to the treatment of secretory otitis media. *Ann Otol Rhinol Laryngol* 1990; 146: 6.
4. Henderson FW. A longitudinal study of respiratory viruses and bacteria in the etiology of acute otitis media with effusion. *N Engl J Med* 1982; 306: 1377–83.
5. Jones S. A nursing intervention to increase compliance in otitis media patients. *Appl Nursing Res* 1989; 2 (2): 68–73.
6. Bluestone C. Modern management of otitis media. *Pediatr Clin North Am* 1989; 36 (6): 12.
7. Giebink GS, Canafax DM. Controversies in the management of acute otitis media. *Adv Pediatr Infect Dis* 1988; 3: 47–64.
8. Arola M, Ruuskanen O, Ziegler T, Mertsola J, Nanto-Salonen K, Putto-Laurila A, Viljanen MK, Halonen P. Clinical role of respiratory virus infection in acute otitis media. *Pediatrics* 1990; 86 (6): 848–55.
9. Gates G, Wachterdorf C, Hearne E, Holt G. Treatment of chronic otitis media with effusion: results of tympanostomy tubes. *Am J Otolaryngol* 1985; 6: 249–53.
10. Cavanaugh RM. Obtaining a seal with otic specula: must we rely on an air of uncertainty? *Pediatrics* 1991; 87 (1): 114–16.
11. Zanga JR, Butts FM. Sights and sounds: tympanometry in the schools—is it worth the effort? *School Nurse* 1991; 7 (2): 36–38.

37 | IHP: Pregnancy— Adolescent

Wanda R. Miller

INTRODUCTION

Whether it is Arthur Cambell's frequently quoted 1968 statement, "The girl who has an illegitimate child at the age of 16 suddenly has 90% of her life's script written for her,"[1] or Frank Furstenberg Jr's more recent one, "The costs of premature parenthood are evident,"[2] it is clear the consequences of adolescent pregnancy and parenting are multifaceted and extensive. They impact on the physical, educational, economic, social, and emotional status of the adolescent mother, and to a lesser degree, on the father. Ultimately, they impact on the child's physical, cognitive, behavioral, and emotional status, as well. The young women who choose to parent their babies are disadvantaged in a variety of areas—age, socioeconomic class, academic performance, vocational aspirations, and psychological health—even prior to the baby's arrival. Pregnancy further jeopardizes the mother's status and ultimately that of the child's.[3]

Despite the risks of becoming a parent, there has been an increase in adolescent sexual behavior over the past decade. Describing the trends for age at first premarital sexual intercourse of adolescent women (15 to 19 years of age) in the United States, the Centers for Disease Control's National Survey of Family Growth (NSFG) reported three, five-year

periods, from 1970 to 1985, in which the sexual activity increase had been steadily declining (i.e.,during 1970-75 the increase was 7.8 percentage points; during 1976-80, 5.6; and during 1981-85, 2.1). In the 1988 NSFG study, however, sexual activity increased by 7.4 percent, bringing the overall percentage to 51.5 percent of adolescent women who reported having had premarital sexual intercourse. The greatest increase, however, occurred in women aged 15 years old who increased more than five times their percentage of sexual intercourse from 4.6 to 25.6 points.[4]

A portion of the increase in percentage is also attributable to the increase in white adolescent's sexual intercourse. In 1975, slightly more than half of white females and three-fourths of black females in the 18 to 19 year age group had had intercourse.[2] Although the proportion of black adolescents who report having had sexual intercourse is consistently higher than the proportion of white adolescents who report having had sexual intercourse, the difference narrowed substantially over time because of a greater relative increase in sexual intercourse among white adolescents. By 1988 the NSFG found 72.6 percent of white women and 75.6 percent of black women aged 18 to 19 who reported having had premarital sexual intercourse.[4]

More likely than not, the difference will continue to decrease, because the situation of young whites is becoming more like that of young blacks. More white teens have been engaging in early intercourse, using contraception only casually, and showing great reluctance to marry in the event of a premarital conception.[5]

In comparing sexual behaviors of adolescent women in six developed countries, Elise Jones found that the median age at first intercourse was similar in France, Great Britain, the Netherlands, and the United States. In Sweden and Canada the median age at first intercourse was one year younger and one year older, respectively.[6] In spite of proportionate data for adolescent women who reported having first intercourse in all six of the countries, Jones found that the abortion, pregnancy, and birth rates for teenagers in the United States were higher than the rates found in any of the other five developed countries.[6] Although the United States birth rates declined over the ten-year period from 1970 to 1980, they continued to be much higher than the birth rates for each of the five other countries. The birth rate of 32.6 per 1,000 for adolescents 15 to 17 years of age in the United States was more than twice that of Canada, the country with the next highest rate, and six times higher than Sweden, the country with the lowest rate. The birth rate of 82.6 per 1,000 for women 18 to 19 years of age was 25 points higher than that of England, the country with the next highest rate for that age group.[7]

The abortion rates paralleled the birth rates for adolescent women 15 to 17 years of age in the United States and exceed the rate of the other five countries by 31 points in adolescent women 18 to 19 years of age.[7] Abortions occur more commonly in younger age groups than in older age groups and among white adolescent women more commonly than among blacks. Approximately 40 percent of all pregnancies to adolescents end in abortion.[2] Adolescents who choose to abort are more educationally ambitious and more likely to be from higher socioeconomic backgrounds. Their families are less religious, the attitude of their mothers and peers toward abortion is more positive, and they are less likely to have friends or relatives who are teenage single parents.[2] Both abortion and contraceptive services for adolescents are more accessible to adolescents in the other countries through national healthcare programs. The United States' system of clinics results in the lowest level of utilization of services and the poorest contraceptive practice among adolescents of all six countries.[6]

In spite of the lack of accessible clinics for adolescents in the United States, there is some indication of change occurring in the utilization of contraceptives. Mosher and McNally [8] reported that the percent of women who used a contraceptive method at first intercourse rose from 47 percent in 1975–79 to 65 percent in 1983-88. This change resulted almost entirely from the increased use of condoms by partners. The portion of women using a contraceptive method at first intercourse varied according to the individual characteristics of the woman. An important predictor of contraceptive use by adolescents was the adolescent mother's level of education. Whether education is the predictor of socioeconomic level for the family or a model of the process to adulthood is not clear. However, if the adolescent perceives the goal of delayed childbearing, completing an education, and obtaining a good job as the only way to attain a respected adult status, early parenthood is unacceptable and use of contraception more likely.[8]

The rate of marriages in adolescent parents has changed significantly also. Single-parent families doubled between 1959 and 1983, and by 1986, more than half of all black children in the United States lived in single-parent households.

Early sexual activity has been found by several researchers to be a primary cause of early, unplanned pregnancy.[6, 9] The adolescent at risk for pregnancy is one involved in early sexual and other adult activities, who also has poor performance in school. Franklin reports that race (being black), going steady, and cigarette smoking were the strongest predictors for early initiation into sexual activity.[9]

To recap three important behavior changes have occurred in the adolescent population within the past decade: a greater percentage of adolescent women are sexually active, a significant increase in the number of younger women and white women who report having had sexual intercourse has occurred, and fewer adolescent women who are parenting are marrying.

Completion of School

Prior to conception, adolescents who become pregnant are below average in school performance and achievement test scores.[3] Their poor academic record is preceded by a history of absenteeism, class failures, credit losses, and difficulties and disinterest in school. Given this profile, the added stress of early childbearing adversely affects the life chances of young mothers to complete school and attain economic self-sufficiency.[5] Adolescent pregnancy is the major cause for female students to drop out of school. Eight out of every ten adolescent mothers, 17 years of age and under, do not complete high school.[3] Although high school completion rates were 95 percent in 1983 for all women, rates were from 53 percent among women who gave birth within seven months after leaving school, to 79 percent among those who became pregnant after leaving school.[10]

Within the black community, there is a strong commitment to provide assistance to pregnant teens to discourage them from leaving school.[5] It is less clear whether white teens derive this same support. When whites do not marry, their schooling is somewhat more likely to be curtailed than blacks, resulting in a higher probability of white mothers not completing high school. [5] Adolescent mothers, white and black, who live at home with their parents until the child is three years old, are more likely to return to school.[3]

Economics

Female-headed families are at considerable economic disadvantage in comparison with two-parent families and father-headed families. For instance, in 1987 the median income for two-parent families was $34,800, for father-headed families $21,500, and for mother-headed families $15,800.[11] This economic disadvantage is consistent with information from 1984 which showed that 54 percent of families headed by a single woman were below the poverty level, compared to 12.5 percent of two-parent families.[12] There is further evidence that a greater disadvantage exists when the first birth occurred before the women was age 20, a finding that is consistent in both whites and blacks.[5]

The cost to the public of teenage childbearing for 1985 was $16.65 billion in Aid to Families and Dependent Children, food stamps, and Medicaid. The calculations in 1985 indicate the public will pay an average of $13,902 per year over the next 20 years for a family begun by each first birth to a teenager.[13]

Marriage

The number of single-parent families doubled between 1959 and 1983, and by 1986, more than half of all black children lived in single-parent households. The rate of adolescent fathers living apart from at least one of their children tripled between 1979 and 1983.[12] The most distinctive racial differences occur in the area of marriage patterns. Although these patterns are changing, whites are more likely to enter marriage and remain wed than blacks. Both blacks and whites who become teen mothers and marry are more likely to divorce eventually. These differences in marriage patterns have important implications for the economic situation of black and white mothers.[5]

Fathers

Although it would seem that family commitments early in life could decrease educational attainment and economic achievement in later life for males, there is little supporting evidence for this position, and living with their children (for whites) and marrying the mother (for blacks) increase the odds that adolescent males will finish school.[5, 12] Since very few adolescents are choosing to marry, this affects only a small decreasing number of males. Rising rates of unemployment among young black males and poor economic prospects for poorly educated men have affected the pool of marriage-eligible men for black females. In addition, young men in low socioeconomic communities, particularly young men of color, are afflicted with a variety of social ills—drug use, alcoholism, delinquency and crime, and mental disabilities.[5]

Family Size

The single area in which the consequences for black and white women appear to be identical is family size. Early childbearers averaged between 0.5 and 1.0 more children than later childbearers.[5] Nationwide, one third of women under the age of eighteen who have been pregnant become pregnant again within twenty-four months,[14] and one-half of all adolescent mothers will experience a second pregnancy within thirty-two months of delivery.[15] The fact that 50 percent of teenage mothers have a second child within thirty-six months of the first further limits their work or educational opportunities.[3]

Medical Issues

Adolescent pregnant women suffered a higher incidence of anemia ,[16] but had no higher incidence of hypertensive disorders or hospital admissions and were as likely as older mothers to have had a normal delivery. However, mothers 15 years and under are at increased risk for cephalopelvic disproportion, anemia, toxemia, hypertension, and vaginal infections.[10] The incidence of eclampsia was twice as high among these women as among older teenagers.

Whether or not they were firstborn children, the infants of teenage mothers were more likely than those of older women to be born preterm (9 percent versus 5 percent) and to be underweight. Prematurity is ascribed to socioeconomic causes, while low weight for gestational age is not.[16] Perinatal death rates were highest among babies whose mothers were younger than 15 years of age and diminished progressively by age of mother among those infants whose mothers were aged 15–19, but after control for socioeconomic status, the outcomes were not significantly different.[16] Young maternal age is strongly associated with both sudden infant death and other postneonatal deaths, while social class is much less strongly associated with sudden infant death. Sudden infant death appears to be related to extremes in the mother's circumstance—very low socioeconomic status, young motherhood, and high parity. Although there is an increased risk of accidents in the home and outdoors due to the mother's lack of experience and maturity,[16] willful neglect and child abuse are not more common among the children of teenagers.

The postpartum linear growth of women less than 16 years of age, delivering their first child, was found to be minimal or absent one to seven years after delivery. Nutrition, as well as estrogen effect on epiphyseal closure, may be affecting final diminished heights in adolescent mothers.[3]

Children

The mother's age has a small, but significant, effect on her child's cognitive development when background characteristics are controlled; however, the social and emotional development are less clear. [16] The educational and economic consequences that early childbearing imposes on young mothers creates a family environment for their offspring that impedes their chances of success.[5] Cognitive delays in the children of adolescents have been documented on IQ, vocabulary, and block tests. The main variable being the mother's level of academic proficiency at the time of her pregnancy. Later on, these children have more dramatic problems, requiring remedial help, repeating grades, and dropping out of school at a higher rate than other children.[12] Hechtman found that children of adolescent mothers, at seven and 12 years of age, performed less well in school and had a reading age 0.4 years below children of older mothers.[3]

Children of adolescent mothers were found to be overly conforming and somewhat noncommunicative at age four, and at age seven were more hostile, resentful of authority, subject to some speech problems in relating to peers, and had low frustration tolerance.[3] At age eight and ten they were more dependent on their mothers and more distractible.[3] Mild emotional problems, including aggressiveness, impulsiveness, rebelliousness, and poor control of anger, also have been documented.[12] Children from families of four or more children were at significantly greater risk of becoming delinquent or developing conduct disorders. In contrast, the resilient children of Kauai, an island of Hawaii, who performed well above the norm despite a history of family poverty and instability typically were born more than two years apart from their siblings.[14]

It has been suggested that some of the adverse cognitive, behavioral, social and emotional effects of the child of the adolescent mother stem from inadequate and suboptimal mothering. Young mothers exhibit significantly less verbal interaction than older mothers and tend to be slower in responding to the infant's needs. They look at and talk to their babies less frequently than did older mothers. Most of the responses young mothers made to their infants were authoritative, rigid, and highly punitive, reflecting little sensitivity or parenting knowledge.[3]

Cognitive and Psychosocial Development

Adolescent reasoning about sexuality, sexual decision-making, and sexual behavior are often oversimplified. The reasoning is examined as a function of age rather than cognitive development; although, we know that cognitive growth lags behind physical growth. Younger adolescents, 15 to 17 years of age, may be functioning at the concrete level of cognitive development. In fact, neither sex education nor knowledge are related to postponement of sexual intercourse or use of contraceptives in this age group.[17]

Reasoning concepts, including: generating or envisioning alternatives, evaluating alternatives, engaging in perspective-taking, and reasoning about chance and probability help the formal operational thinker to explore all the possible options. This process requires the thinker to explore the boundaries of reality and to creatively envision the unknown.

The formal operational thinker can systematically conceptualize all the changes or combinations possible when presented with the facts of a situation. The ability to consider options and combinations is crucial to the process of decision making. The adolescent will not or cannot make use of available contraceptives unless they can envision sexual encounters, curb impulsive responses, seek out needed information, and apply the information to their own behavior. Interventions to develop decision-making skills should encourage consideration of all the options available.

The evaluation of alternatives requires the thinker to formulate events or situations into hypothetical questions. "If such-in-such happens, then I will do thus-and-so." This process increases the capability of the thinker for planfulness.[18] Cobliner[19] explains that without the ability to evaluate the consequences of behavior or the capacity for planfulness in reasoning, the adolescent will fail to use contraceptives. Likewise, the ability to anticipate the future is of prime importance in sexual decision-making.[8, 20]

The ability to perceive another person's viewpoint depends on the ability of the thinker to continually refocus their perspective on the other person's needs. The capacity to consider and understand the need of another person is tied to perspective-taking or understanding. The need of a female partner to contracept, from the male's point of view, and a disregard for the needs of the child, from the adolescent mother's point of view,[18] describes this reasoning. Newberger describes a more egocentric level of parental interpretation of the child's behavior as, "my child should stop crying because it is unpleasant for me to hear."[18]

Formal cognitive thinkers, when given the appropriate information, can better estimate the odds of an event occurring. Understanding the idea of chance and probability may be an important factor in sexual risk-taking. Adolescents believe that the chance of pregnancy is cumulative rather than independent for each act of sexual intercourse. The adolescent may construct what Elkind[21] has called a "personal fable" of themselves as special, unique, and ultimately an invincible person untouchable by the reality of probability.

Stress frequently results in disorganization and regression of the thinker to an earlier stage of cognitive development. Learner outcomes that target fourth and fifth graders to learn the decision-making model are limited by the cognitive developmental stage of the individual child and cannot be expected to be implemented effectively in a stressful situation such as initial dating or dating of older males.

INDIVIDUALIZED HEALTHCARE PLAN

History

The initial history to determine the potential of a pregnancy should focus on the occurrence of sexual intercourse, the menstrual history, and signs of pregnancy. If the woman is sexually active and may be pregnant, additional history information in the area of school history, family life, father of the baby, substance abuse, emotional, physical and sexual abuse, rape, medical history, and activities will be helpful.[22] Pertinent information should be collected through the following questions:

- How long have you been menstruating?

- When was your last menstrual period? What is the usual length of time in between your periods?

- Have you had sexual intercourse? How often do you have intercourse and when was the last time you had intercourse?

- Have you ever taken birth control pills? If so, do you take birth control pills regularly now?

- Do you use a condom when you have intercourse? Do you use a condom every time you have intercourse? When does your partner put the condom on?

- Do you use any other birth control method?

- Have you ever had a sexually transmitted disease?

- What signs do you have that make you think you might be pregnant? Are you nauseated, more lethargic or active, or has your weight changed?

- Are your breasts tender or engorged?

- What are your thoughts and feelings about pregnancy?

- Is the pregnancy planned?

- Do you feel positively or negatively about the pregnancy or are you ambivalent?

- Are you thinking about carrying the child to term and parenting the child or placing the child for adoption? Or are you thinking about obtaining an abortion?

- What grade are you in? How many grades have you repeated? Are you in special education or do you have an IEP?

- How many days of school have you missed? Have you ever run away? Been in court?

- Who do you live with? Do you live alone, with your parents, with a friend, or with a spouse or partner?

- How old was your mother at her first pregnancy?

- How old is the father of the baby? What is his education? How long have you known him? What type of work does he do?

- What is your relationship to the father of the baby? Is the relationship with you positive, are you having problems in the relationship, or is the relationship ended?

- How does the father of the baby feel about the pregnancy? Is he supportive or nonsupportive?

- Who else is available to you as a support system? Family? Friends?

- Has anyone ever emotionally, physically, or sexually abused you? Who? When? (This question should be preceded by a candid explanation of the child abuse reporting requirements in your state in order to maintain the integrity of the interview confidentiality.) Have you ever been raped?

- What kind of chemicals do you use? Cigarettes? Alcohol? Marijuana? Other?

If a pregnancy exists the following health history questions will assist the school nurse to manage the health status of the student at school and to appropriately refer the student for prenatal care.

- What do you eat during a typical 24-hour period? Are you able to eat as you did previously or are you nauseated?
- Have you ever been anemic?
- Do you have dizzy periods now or feel faint?
- Are your ankles swelling?
- Do you have varicose veins developing?
- Are you experiencing any shortness of breath?
- Do you have any numbness or tingling in your hands?
- Are you currently or have you been nauseated or vomited?
- Are you constipated? Have hemorrhoids?
- Do you crave certain foods?
- Do you have dental caries?
- Are you having striae gravidarum? Do you have pruritus?
- Are you experiencing any joint or back pain? Leg cramps?
- Have you ever had genital herpes, gonorrhea, syphilis, chlamydia, or vaginitis?
- Are you having urinary frequency? Do you have cystitis or nephritis?
- Have you ever had hepatitis or have the whites of your eyes turned yellow?
- Are you experiencing any pain? If so, where, when did it begin, how long does it last, what precipitates the pain and what alleviates it?
- Do you have any spotting? If so, how much, when, and is it accompanied by pain?

Assessment

Initial assessment of pregnancy may be obtained through a pregnancy test, however, confirmation of the test should be made by a physician or nurse midwife who will follow the woman through the pregnancy.

Early referral to a healthcare facility for prenatal and delivery care is essential.

Determine relationship between weight for height. Document information on a growth grid.

Determine the dietary intake for the past week, preferably. If unable to remember the week's intake obtain as much information as possible.

Determine tenderness if there is abdominal pain.

Nursing Diagnoses (N.D.)

N.D. 1 Alteration in coping due to the stress of a new pregnancy, decision process, and the conflict of the parenting role. (NANDA 5.1.1.1)*

N.D. 2 Alteration in knowledge deficit due to teenage pregnancy. (NANDA 8.1.1)

---

* (See chapter 2, page 38 for explanation of the NANDA approved numerical system.)

N.D. 3   Alteration in socialization due to isolation from parents, friends, and community agencies that provide support services. (NANDA 3.1.2)

N.D. 4   Alteration in nutrition due to "morning sickness" and to the increasing nutritional needs of a pregnant woman. (NANDA 1.1.2.2)

N.D. 5   Knowledge deficit related to parenting and infant care. (NANDA 8.1.1)

N.D. 6   Anticipatory grieving related to plans to obtain an abortion or to place the infant up for adoption. (NANDA 9.2.1.2)

N.D. 7   Knowledge deficit related to birth control. (NANDA 8.1.1)

Goals

The student will review the options available to her and make a decision about her role as a parent. (N.D. 1)

The student will know the positive and negative aspects of each alternative. (N.D. 1)

The student will choose the option that is the best alternative for her and will be able to work out the issues that arise because of the decision with confidence in the choice that she has made. (N.D. 1)

The student will be knowledgeable about the changes in her body due to the pregnancy, the signs of potential problems, and the labor and delivery process. (N.D. 2)

The student will develop a broad-based support system of social and professional people. (N.D. 3)

The pregnant woman will know the foods needed to provide adequate nutrition during pregnancy. (N.D. 4)

The pregnant woman will eat a balanced nutritional diet throughout the pregnancy and lactation period. (N.D. 4)

The student will demonstrate knowledge of the concept of parenting and infant care. (N.D. 5)

The student will obtain support during the grieving process. (N.D. 6)

The student will be knowledgeable of family planning methods. (N.D. 7)

Nursing Interventions

Assist the student in informing her parents of the pregnancy. (N.D. 1)

Review the options of abortion, giving birth and placing the child for adoption, and giving birth and keeping the child. (N.D. 1)

Encourage the student to visualize the positive and negative aspects of each of the options, including the responsibilities and the effects of the decision. (N.D. 1)

Provide developmentally appropriate cooperative learning situations where student can assess the opportunities and problems and make decisions based on scientific information. (N.D. 1)

Assist the student to develop a plan of action that is realistic and that is attainable for the student. (N.D. 1)

Provide health, social service, and educational resource agencies and support system referrals to assist the student to attain her goal. (N.D. 1)

Provide peer-group sessions for social support, mutual problem solving, and affirmation of program goals. (N.D. 1)

Provide groups that focus on issues related to achieving independence. (N.D. 1)

Assess the student's reaction to her pregnancy by establishing a therapeutic relationship. (N.D. 2)

Assist the student to minimize barriers to healthcare, such as financial hardship or accessibility, which prevent the teenager from obtaining primary healthcare. (N.D. 2)

Assess the student for physiological and psychological effects of pregnancy, such as pregnancy-induced hypertension, intrauterine growth retardation, denial, and a delay in prenatal attachment behaviors. (N.D. 2)

Provide education on prenatal healthcare and fetal development. (N.D. 2)

Teach the student the importance of nutrition to the fetus during pregnancy. Assist the student to develop a meal plan and food budget and encourage her to practice proper nutrition. (N.D. 2)

Teach the student the effects of smoking, alcohol, and drugs on the unborn fetus. (N.D. 2)

Provide primary nursing care in a nonjudgmental manner. Direct the student to classes, demonstrations, and literature that increase the students knowledge and choices for care. (N.D. 2)

Assess the educational needs of the patient and develop an individual educational plan for the student that meets her needs to complete her high school education. Consider alternative educational plans as the need arises in order to assist the student to become self-sufficient. (N.D. 2)

Teach the family and father (if present) about the physical and psychological changes that occur during pregnancy. (N.D. 3)

Refer the student to appropriate community services, such as a Women, Infants and Children (WIC) program, daycare center, women's center, counseling service, and religious group. (N.D. 3)

If the student has "morning sickness," assist the student to determine when and for how long in the morning she is nauseated, if necessary, arrange for the student to enter school at a later class hour for a limited period of time or provide a resting place in the health room for the student in the morning, and provide the student with bland food as tolerated to reduce the nausea. (N.D. 4)

For the pregnant adolescent: instruct the student in the nutrients and the calories needed in the daily diet to maintain a healthy mother and fetus, determine the food likes and intake of the student. (N.D. 4)

Determine student's knowledge deficiencies before delivery. (N.D. 5)

Teach the student concepts of personal hygiene, exercise, rest, nutrition, and breast care. (N.D. 5)

Assess the student's understanding of medical information received from the primary healthcare provider and the need to comply with the prescribed care. (N.D. 5)

Assess the student for mood changes and level of self-esteem. (N.D. 5)

Encourage the student to express her concerns and needs. (N.D. 5)

Determine if plans have been made for the infant's care during the school day. (N.D. 5)

Assist the student to obtain child care prior to delivery. More and more frequently secondary schools are providing infant and toddler child care facilities on the high school site. (N.D. 5)

Teach the unique characteristics of the infant's behavior. Assist the student to anticipate the developmental needs of the child on a monthly periodicity for the first six months and then every three months thereafter. (N.D. 5)

Determine the student's decision. The student may change her mind or have serious misgivings about her decision. Encourage her to talk with her parents, a counselor, the father of the infant, and/or a religious advisor. (N.D. 6)

Approach the decision-making process in a nonjudgmental manner. If the nurse's personal beliefs do not allow a nonjudgmental approach, inform the student of the need to withdraw from the client-nurse relationship and provide the student with a readily accessible support professional to continue services for the student. (N.D. 6)

Assist her in locating an agency and in establishing a relationship with the agency's nurse or social worker. (N.D. 6)

Observe the patient for signs of loss and grief, such as anxiety, depression, or crying. Determine if more in-depth crisis intervention is needed. (N.D. 6)

Determine the student's interest in family planning and knowledge of birth control methods. (N.D. 7)

Encourage the student to delay sexual intercourse. If the student chooses to be sexually active, teach the student contraceptive devices and methods of birth control. (N.D. 7)

Focus attention on long-term outcomes to project the adolescent into the future. (N.D. 7)

Role-play tasks that stress perspective-taking activities, such as caring for infants and toddlers, engaging in simulation exercises involving birth and motherhood, or carrying around an uncooked egg to simulate the fragility of an infant. (N.D. 7)

Stress the importance of using birth control while breastfeeding. (N.D. 7)

Expected Student Outcome

The student made an independent decision with the support of her family and loved ones and is carrying out the plan successfully. (N.D. 1)

The adolescent parent is a knowledgeable consumer of the healthcare system and obtained early prenatal care, maintained a nutritious diet and is continuing her education. (N.D. 2)

Family members are better prepared and provide support to meet the physical and emotional needs of the student. (N.D. 3)

Community resources constitute an integral part of the patient's support network. (N.D. 3)

The student eats a well-balanced and nutritious diet for an adolescent woman who is pregnant. (N.D. 4)

The student understands the needs of her child and adapts to the role of parent. (N.D. 5)

The parent recognizes age-appropriate infant behaviors and identifies those behaviors. (N.D. 5)

The mother and infant bond. (N.D. 5)

The student is able to verbalize her loss to the nurse, assure herself that the decision she made was the best decision for her at this time, and gradually resumes her functions. (N.D. 6)

The student prevents unwanted pregnancies in the future. (N.D. 7)

REFERENCES

1. Cambell AA. The role of family planning in the reduction of poverty. *J Marriage Family* 1968; 30 (2): 236–45.
2. Furstenberg FF Jr, Brooks-Gull J, Chase-Lansdale L. Teenaged pregnancy and childbearing. *Am Psychologist* 1989; 44 (2): 313–20.
3. Hechtman L. Teenage mothers and their children: risks and problems: a review. *Can J Psychiatry* 1989; 34 (6): 569–75.
4. Centers for Disease Control. Premarital sexual experience among adolescent women—United States, 1970–1988. *MMWR* 1991; 39 (51 and 52): 929–32.
5. Furstenberg FF Jr, Herceg-Baron R, Mann D, Shea J. Parental involvement: selling family planning clinics short. *Fam Plan Perspect* 1987; 14 (3): 140–44.
6. Jones EF, Forrest JD, Goldman N, Henshaw SK, Lincoln R, Rosoff JI, Westoff CF, Wulf D. Teenage pregnancy in developed countries: determinants and policy implications. *Fam Plan Perspect* 1985; 17 (2): 53–63.
7. Lee KS, Corpuz M. Teenage pregnancy: trend and impact on rates of low birth weight and fetal, maternal, and neonatal mortality in the United States. *Clin Perinatol* 1988; 15 (4): 929–42.
8. Mosher WD, McNally JW. Contraceptive use at first premarital intercourse: United States 1965–1988. *Fam Plan Perspect* 1991; 23 (3): 108–16.
9. Franklin D. Race, class, and adolescent pregnancy: an ecological analysis. *Am J Orthopsychiatry* 1988; 58 (3): 339–54.
10. Mott FL, Marsiglio W. Early childbearing and completion of high school. *Fam Plan Perspect* 1985; 17 (5): 234–237.
11. *Current Populations Report.* Money, Income, and Poverty Status in the U.S.; 1987. Bureau of the Census, Dept. of Commerce. 1987; Series P60: 161.
12. Davis S. Pregnancy in adolescents. *Pediatr Clin North Am* 1989; 36 (3): 665–80.
13. Burt MR. Estimating the public costs of teenage childbearing. *Fam Plan Perspect* 1986; 18 (5): 221–26.
14. Schorr LB. Within Our Reach: Breaking the Cycle of Disadvantage. New York: Anchor Press, 1988.
15. Nelson PB. Repeat pregnancy among adolescent mothers: a review of the literature. *J Natl Black Nurses Assoc* 1990; Fall/Winter 9 (1): 28–34.
16. Makinson C. The health consequences of teenage fertility. *Fam Plan Perspect* 1985; 17: 132.
17. Howard M, McCabe J. Helping teenagers postpone sexual involvement. *Fam Plan Perspect* 1990; 22 (1): 21–26.
18. Gordon DE. Formal operational thinking: the role of cognitive-developmental processes in adolescent decision-making about pregnancy and contraception. *Am J Orthopsychiatry* 1990; 60 (3): 346–56.
19. Cobliner WG. Pregnancy in the single adolescent girl: the role of cognitive functions. *J Youth Adolescence* 1974; 3: 17–29.
20. Baizerman M. Can the first pregnancy of a young adolescent be prevented? A question which must be answered. *J Youth Adolescence* 1977; 6: 343–51.
21. Elkind D. Egocentrism in adolescence. *Child Development* 1967; 38: 1025–34.
22. Palmore S, Millar K, Millar M. An interview for pregnant teens: identifying special needs in a school setting. *School Nurse* 1990; 6 (4): 18–21.

38 | IHP: Respiratory Dysfunction

Mary J. Villars Gerber

INTRODUCTION

Respiratory dysfunction has a variety of causes that can result in ventilatory failure in children and that are a significant cause of childhood illness.

Three types of functional disorders[1] are:

1. Obstructive lung disease. There is an increase in resistance to upper or lower respiratory tract.
2. Restrictive lung disease. There is impaired lung expansion resulting from loss of lung volume, decreased distensibility, or chest wall disturbance.
3. Primary inefficient gas transfer. There is insufficient ventilation for carbon dioxide removal or impaired oxygenation of pulmonary capillary blood as a dysfunction of the respiratory control mechanism or a diffusion defect.

Students with respiratory dysfunction in a school setting are generally stable, but may require certain procedures that will necessitate healthcare planning. These procedures may include bronchial drainage, suctioning, or monitoring of a tracheostomy.

Bronchial drainage is indicated whenever there is excess fluid or mucus in the bronchi that is not being removed by normal ciliary activity and cough.

Suctioning of the nose and mouth is simply done to clear mucus from the airway. It may be conducted with a suction machine or nasal aspirator.

Tracheostomies are performed for a variety of reasons, including mechanical obstruction, disease of the central nervous system, neuromuscular disease, secretional obstruction, or disturbances of gas diffusion.

All school staff working with a student with significant respiratory dysfunction need training in cardiopulmonary resuscitation.

INDIVIDUALIZED HEALTHCARE PLAN

History

What is the history of symptoms related to respiratory dysfunction?
Were there contributing or causative factors?
What medications have been utilized and to what extent were they effective?
What is the medical/surgical history?

Assessment

Physical examination is needed to determine baseline:
- Respiratory
    Respiratory rate, rhythm, depth
    Cough
    Sputum
    Breath sounds

- Circulatory
    Pulse
    Blood pressure
    Skin color

- Current medication therapy, side effects, and action on symptoms

- Current procedures utilized to maintain optimal respiratory function. Determine student's tolerance to the procedure and extent to which it is effective.

Nursing Diagnoses (N.D.)

N.D. 1 Potential for infection (NANDA 1.2.1.1)* related to excessive pooling of secretions.

N.D. 2 Potential ineffective airway clearance (NANDA 1.5.1.2) related to increased secretions.

N.D. 3 Ineffective airway clearance (NANDA 1.5.1.2) related to perceptual and cognitive impairment.

N.D. 4 Ineffective breathing pattern (NANDA 1.5.1.3) related to neurologic or musculoskeletal impairment.

N.D. 5 Potential ineffective airway clearance (NANDA 1.5.1.2) related to increased secretions secondary to tracheostomy, obstruction of inner cannula, or displacement of tracheostomy tube.

N.D. 6 Impaired verbal communication (NANDA 2.1.1.1) related to inability to produce speech secondary to tracheostomy.

Goals

Prevent pooling of secretions and possible development of infection. (N.D. 1)

Maintain patent airway. (N.D. 2–5)

Increase oxygen supply to lungs. (N.D. 1–5)

Ease respiratory efforts. (N.D. 3, 4)

Promote expectoration of mucous secretions. (N.D. 1, 2, 5)

Facilitate communication. (N. D. 6)

---

* (See chapter 2, page 38 for explanation of the NANDA approved numerical system.)

Nursing Interventions

Suction secretions from airway as needed to clear airway and stimulate cough reflex. (N.D. 1–5)

Position to prevent aspiration of secretions, provide for comfort, and maximize lung expansion. (N.D. 2–5)

Assist student to expectorate sputum. (N.D. 1–5)

Provide nebulization with appropriate solution and equipment as prescribed. (N.D. 2–4)

Perform percussion, vibrations, and postural drainage if prescribed. (N.D. 1, 2, 5)

Maintain adequate hydration to thin secretions. (N.D. 1–5)

Maintain adequate humidity of air to promote thinning of secretions. (N.D. 1–5)

Instruct on proper method of controlled coughing. (N. D. 1–5)

Administer medications as ordered. (N.D. 1, 2, 5)

Case management: Refer and follow up for medical care if needed, coordinate service providers. (N.D. 1–5)

Obtain current medical orders for medications or procedures that are needed in school. (See Supplement to this chapter for sample forms.) (N.D. 1–5)

Maintain records to document medications or procedures administered at school. (See Supplement to this chapter for special forms.) (N.D. 1–5)

Utilize a method of communication by which the student can make his/her needs known. (N.D. 6)

Identify and utilize factors that promote communication. (N.D. 6)

Refer to speech/language/communication specialist to assess and facilitate methods of communication. (N.D. 6)

Expected Student Outcomes

Will remain free of infection. (N.D. 1)

Airway remains clear. (N.D. 1–5)

Student breathes easily. (N.D. 2–5)

Respirations are within normal limits and are not labored. (N.D. 2–5)

Will not experience aspiration. (N.D. 2–5)

Student will communicate needs. (N.D. 6)

REFERENCES

1. Whaley LF, Wong DL. *Nursing Care of Infants and Children.* St. Louis: CV Mosby, 1987.

RESOURCES

Carpenito LJ. *Nursing Diagnosis, Application to Clinical Practice.* Philadelphia: JB Lippincott, 1989.
Colorado Department of Health, Colorado Department of Education. *Procedure Guidelines for Healthcare of Special Needs Students in the School Setting.* Denver, 1988.

Larson G, ed. *Managing the School Age Child With a Chronic Health Condition: A Practical Guide For Schools, Families and Organizations*. DCI Publishing, 1988 (available from Sunrise River Press, Wayzata, MN: 11481 Kost Dam Rd, North Branch, MN 55056, 612-583-3239).

Wong DL, Whaley LF. *Clinical Manual of Pediatric Nursing*. St. Louis: CV Mosby, 1990.

Supplement – Chapter 38

Health Care Action Plan
Physician Information

Dear Physician:

Your patient _____, D.O.B. _____,
is attending _____. The parents are
requesting that specific health care procedures be provided while the student is at
school. We are requesting your assistance in identifying the health information and
services which need to be provided in the school setting. Any cost incurred for your
participation is at the expense of the family. Members of the school team include the
parent, school administrator, school nurse and other school personnel with direct
responsibility for the educational care of the student. We look forward to working with
you to provide an optimal educational experience in a safe environment for your
patient.

Diagnosis(es): _____
_____

Physical condition for which the procedure is to be performed: _____

Medical orders for procedures and medication which are to be done at school: _____
_____
_____

Precautions, possible untoward reactions, and interventions: _____
_____
_____

Time schedule and/or indication for the procedure: _____
_____

The procedure is to be continued as above until (date): _____
_____

Other _____
_____
_____
_____
_____

Physician's Signature _____ Date _____ 19_____
Address _____ Phone _____

copies: School

Reprinted, with permission, from Colorado Department of Health, Colorado Department of Education. *Procedure
Guidelines for Health Care of Special Needs Students in the School Setting.* Denver, 1988.

Sample Form

School Health Flow Sheet
For Planning Treatments in the School Setting*

Student's Name: _____ Birthdate: _____

Physician: _____ Phone: _____

	Treatment to be Given	Quantity/ Duration	Provider
Day: Time:			
Day: Time:			
Day: Time:			
Day: Time:			
Day: Time:			
Day: Time:			
Day: Time:			
Day: Time:			
Day: Time:			
Day: Time:			
Day: Time:			
Day: Time:			

* To plan the schedule of the student's healthcare, list the different types of treatment with frequency, e.g.: medication, feeding, postural drainage, catheterization, suctioning.

Reprinted, with permission, from Colorado Department of Health, Colorado Department of Education. *Procedure Guidelines for Health Care of Special Needs Students in the School Setting.* Denver, 1988.

Sample Form

Daily Log of Treatment Given by School Personnel

Student's Name: _____ Birthdate:_____

Procedure: _____From _____ 19 _____ To _____ 19____

Physician: _____Phone:_____

Date: Time:	Comments: Init.
Date: Time:	Comments: Init.
Date: Time:	Comments: Init.
Date: Time:	Comments: Init.
Date: Time:	Comments: Init.
Date: Time:	Comments: Init.
Date: Time:	Comments: Init.
Date: Time:	Comments: Init.
Date: Time:	Comments: Init.
Date: Time:	Comments: Init.
Date: Time:	Comments: Init.
Date: Time:	Comments: Init.

Signature	Init.	Title	Date

Continuation of comments can be entered on back of this sheet.

Daily Log of Treatment Given by School Personnel
Continuation of Comments

Date & Time	Comments continued:
	Init.

Date & Time	Comments continued:
	Init.

Date & Time	Comments continued:
	Init.

Date & Time	Comments continued:
	Init.

Reprinted, with permission, from Colorado Department of Health, Colorado Department of Education. *Procedure Guidelines for Health Care of Special Needs Students in the School Setting.* Denver, 1988.

39 | IHP: Scabies

Wanda R. Miller

INTRODUCTION

Scabies is caused by *Sarcoptes scabiei var hominis,* also known as the human itch mite. It is a common, widespread, contagious disease that is transmitted from one person to another when they sleep together or share clothing and is frequently associated with sexually transmitted diseases. It may appear as a mild rash, but often causes serious skin irritations that lead to sleeplessness and secondary bacterial infections. Although the mite that causes scabies was described and drawn in 1687 by Giovanni Bonomo, it was not identified as the cause of the skin disease until the late Nineteenth Century.[1, 2] There are several varieties of mites, some of which are carriers of arthropod-borne diseases, but the scabies mite has not been shown to transmit infections among human beings.

Until recently, scabies epidemics were believed to occur in thirty-year cycles and to last for fifteen years. Researchers now believe the cyclical phases of scabies epidemics are less predictable than previously believed and that a wide variety of factors influence the development of a scabies epidemic. Some of those factors include overcrowding and close living conditions, poverty, wars, sexual promiscuity, immunosuppression, and resistance to medication treatments. With the increased number of adolescents engaging in sexual activities and homeless adolescents living on the streets, school nurses will need to know how to identify scabies and how to effectively treat the disease.

Pathophysiology

Scabies is a translucent, oval shaped, dorsoventrally flattened mite. The adult female is approximately 0.4 by 0.3 mm in size; the male is slightly smaller. The head is not evident, although the mouth parts may be mistaken for the head. The mite has four pairs of short, stocky legs that assist it in crawling along the skin.

The female mates once in her lifetime and within an hour burrows into the dead stratum corneum of the skin and remains there for the rest of her life. She lives for about thirty days, laying two to three eggs each day.[1, 3] The eggs are half the size of the female and take three to four days to hatch. The larva from the egg leaves the burrow about one day later, crawls across the skin to make a new burrow and after three molt stages as a nymph emerges as an adult mite.[1, 4] The nymph stage takes from nine to eleven days for the male and from fourteen to seventeen days for the female.[1, 5] In the most optimum conditions, high humidity and low temperatures, the mites will live from thirty to sixty days.[1]

The initial signs of scabies are erythematous, papular lesions which frequently go undetected. The primary clinical manifestation is itching, particularly at night. The itching may be intense enough to cause scratching that results in bleeding. Blood-stained underwear is a sign that should alert the nurse to the possibility of scabies. There is no specific onset of symptoms and itching begins slowly.

The distribution pattern of scabies on the body is usually symmetrical. The hands are frequently involved first. Lesions appear on the finger webs and the sides of the fingers. Additional common sites are: flexor aspects of the wrists; extensor surface of the elbows; anterior axillary folds; lateral borders of the feet, ankles, toes; the nipple area of the breasts in women; buttocks; abdomen; and in men, the penis and scrotum. Contrary to most practitioners' belief, in temperate climates scabies mites can be found above the neck. It is not unusual to find scabies in the folds behind the ears of young children and infants particularly. Infestations of the eyebrows and lashes in infants should raise the question in the school nurse's mind about the risk of sexual abuse.

A definitive diagnosis is made when the mite, eggs, or fecal pellets (scybala) can be identified. Some researchers believe that burrows can be seen in 95 percent of the patients with this disease; however, detection is difficult and the burrows are frequently missed.[1, 3] They appear as a reddened, elevated, scaly linear eruption and are frequently found on the interdigital areas, wrists, elbows, feet, and ankles. The use of mineral oil scrapings to produce microscopic slide observations is a reliable diagnostic method. The burrow ink test (BIT), using a felt-tipped pen followed by alcohol swab removal to outline the burrow,[2, 3] has also been used by Estes to clearly define the burrow.

Secondary infections have resulted in the development of acute glomerulonephritis with beta-hemolytic streptococci frequently being cultured from the site of the lesions.

Scabies is most frequently transmitted between individuals living in shared sleeping conditions, through sexual partners, and by holding hands in the home from friends and relatives. Scabies is frequently transmitted to young children through hand-holding behavior. The greatest risk of individual infection continues to be for those who sleep with an infected person or share their clothes and linens. Transmission of the disease rarely occurs by fomites.[4]

Treatment of scabies must include all family members and sexual contacts, since the symptoms of allergic reaction to the mites' digestive juices may not be evident in newly infected persons for four to five weeks.

Lindane, 1% (Kwell) has been the drug of choice for the treatment of scabies. Lindane lotion or cream is applied from the neck down to the entire surface of the skin and left on overnight for at least 8 to 12 hours and then washed off. The cure rates reported between 1948 and 1978 for lindane treatment were 96 to 98 percent[3]; however, treatment failures with the use of lindane have been reported with increasing frequency recently,[6] and the controversy continues over whether the mite has developed a tolerance to lindane or the treatment procedure is inadequate. Lindane is contraindicated for infants, small children, and pregnant and nursing women.

Topical permethrin cream in a 5 percent strength has been reported to produce a 89 to 92 percent cure rate.[6] Permethrin 5 percent topical cream has no demonstrated toxicity. This product is marketed under the trade name of Elimite and was approved as a treatment for scabies in 1989. It should not be mistaken for 1 percent permethrin rinse (NIX), which is approved for head lice but not for scabies.

Crotamiton, 10% (Eurax) and Sulfur 5% in petrolatum have been used to treat infants and children as well as Sulfur 10% for those adults who have scalp and face involvement. The effectiveness of these produces has been shown to be questionable.[6, 7]

INDVIDUALIZED HEALTHCARE PLAN

History

Update the student's history with particular emphasis on family and friends living in the home and sexual partners of any students who are pubescent. Scabies is a frequent imitator of other skin conditions. The most important information in the determination of scabies is itching, without itching scabies is unlikely. In any skin infection that has the potential to be a secondary infection, consider the potential of scabies as the primary cause of infection.

- When and how did the itching begin?
- How severe is the itching and is it worse at night?
- Are there scratch marks on your body from itching?
- Where are the scratches located on your body?
- Do you know anyone who has had frequent itching recently?
- Do you have your own bed or do you sleep with another person?
- Are you sexually active? If so, does that person have the same symptoms?
- What have you done to alleviate the itching?
- How do you think and feel about scabies?
- Would be willing to inform your family and/or your sexual partner(s) of the condition?
- If not, can I help you inform your family and sexual partner(s) of the condition or do you want me to inform them for you?

Assessment

Physical assessment

Describe the lesions in terms of pattern, onset, and cutaneous eruption.

Note any burrows, papules, scales, vesicles, bullae, crusts, pustules, nodules, or excoriation.

Note the distribution of the lesions on the hands (including the interdigital areas and palms), flexor aspects of the wrists, elbows, knees, feet, ankles, and toes, breasts, genitals (particularly the penis and scrotum of males), buttocks, and abdomen (periumbilical area).

Nursing Diagnoses (N.D.)

N.D. 1   Alteration in knowledge: deficit. (NANDA 8.1.1)*
N.D. 2   Alterations in self-concept: disturbance in self-esteem due to the situation. (NANDA 7.1.2.2)

---

* (See chapter 2, page 38 for explanation of the NANDA approved numerical system.)

N.D. 3   Alteration in physical integrity through impairment of the skin integrity, which may be an actual or potential. (NANDA 1.6.2.1.2.2, 1.6.2.1.2.1)

N.D. 4   Alterations in coping of the family in ineffective and compromised behavior. (NANDA 5.1.2.1.2)

Goals

The student and his/her family will be able to identify, prevent, and treat scabies. (N.D. 1)

The student will assume the responsibility for informing friends who have slept over or sexual partners of the risk of scabies. (N.D. 2)

The student is referred for treatment. (N.D. 3)

The family has effective strategies in place to cope with the scabies condition. (N.D. 4)

Nursing Interventions

The nurse will provide information to the family and student in order to identify, prevent, and treat scabies. (N.D. 1)

Update the above history to provide foundation for nursing assessment and intervention. (N.D. 1)

Provide information to the student and/or parent(s) about methods for disinfecting bedding and towels including machine washing, machine drying. (N.D. 1)

Educate the parents regarding noneffective treatments, such as, fumigating rooms and using insecticidal sprays on furniture and carpets. (N.D. 1)

The nurse will provide counseling to assist the student in understanding the scabies condition and in assuming an appropriate level of responsibility for the prevention of its transmission to others. (N.D. 2)

Discuss scabies with the student so the student is aware of the prevalence of the condition. (N.D. 2)

The nurse will assess the condition to determine that scabies are involved and recommend appropriate referral for treatment. (N.D. 3)

Follow up with the student upon return to school after the treatment and to determine that the medication was properly applied to kill the scabies and that the student understands that the medication has been effective and does not need to be repeated and that the continuing pruritus is caused by the allergic reaction. (N.D. 3)

The nurse will provide support in obtaining behavioral change in the family to establish effective coping skills. (N.D. 4)

Explain medication available to the student and/or parent(s), their effectiveness in killing scabies, the application time required in order for the medication to be effective, and the precautions necessary for children under 2 years of age and for pregnant and nursing women. (N.D. 4)

As with any medication, the nurse will want to instruct the parents to restrict use of the medication to the applications prescribed for treatment of the condition. (N.D. 4)

Expected Student Outcomes

The student and/or parent(s) will describe the signs of scabies infestation and a responsible medicated regimen that is safe for the student and the person administering the medication. (N.D. 1)

The student or parent(s) will report future infestations to the nurse in order to enhance surveillance of students in the school. (N.D. 2)

The student will comply with a follow-up schedule as evidenced by keeping appointments with the nurse. (N.D. 3)

The student will comply with prescribed treatment as shown by the absence of scabies. (N.D. 4)

REFERENCES

1. Green MS. Epidemiology of scabies. *Epidemiol Rev* 1989; 11: 126–50.
2. Taplin D, Meinking TL. Scabies, lice, and fungal infections. *Prim Care* 1989; 16 (3): 551–76.
3. Estes SA. The Diagnosis and Management of Scabies. Reed and Carnick Monograph. Piscataway, NJ. 1981.
4. Mellanby K. Biology of the parasite. In: Orkin M, et al., eds. *Scabies and Pediculosis.* Philadelphia: JB Lippincott, 1977.
5. Pratt HD. Mites of Public Health Importance and Their Control. Atlanta: Centers for Disease Control, 1975 (DHEW publication No. [CDC] 76–8297).
6. Taplin D, Meinking TL, Chen JA. Comparison of crotamiton 10% cream (Eurax) and permethrin 5% cream (Elimite) for the treatment of scabies in children. *Pediatr Dermatol* 1990; 7 (1): 67–73.
7. Meinking TL, Taplin D. Advances in pediculosis, scabies, and other mite infestations. *Adv Dermatol* 1990; 5: 131–52.

40 | IHP: School Phobia

Cynthia K. Silkworth

INTRODUCTION

School phobia occurs in approximately 1 to 2 percent of the school-aged population.[1, 2] Although it can occur at any age, it is most common in the first through fifth grades. School phobia seems to be evenly distributed among boys and girls and there appears to be no relationship to socioeconomic status, birth order, or ethnic origin. Children with school phobia tend to be of average or higher than average intelligence and have relatively good academic performance. Families of school phobic children tend to have a higher incidence of generalized anxiety or neurosis and have difficulty with parental separation and acceptance of school demands. School phobia is a serious emotional problem that needs prompt attention and intervention to prevent severe interruption and difficulties in learning.[1-5]

Pathophysiology

School phobia is a maladaptive coping strategy that evolves from the inability to make the transition into school. The child with school phobia exhibits an irrational fear and anxiety about going to or being in school. The child resists or refuses to go to school because of the dread of stressors in the school situation, such as peer conflicts, problems with teachers, problems with assignments, and so on. The fear or anxiety, however, is usually caused by anxiety or fear of separation from the parent (usually the mother). The child is reluctant to leave the mother and the mother is equally reluctant to have the child leave her.[3, 5, 6] Depression and having an unrealistic self-image also play a major role in school phobia.[2, 4]

The child with school phobia may express his/her anxiety in a variety of ways.[1, 3, 5, 6]

- somatic complaints—high incidence, such as abdominal pain, nausea, vomiting, anorexia, headaches, dizziness, fatigue, weakness, sore throat, pallor, leg pains, pain and spasm of neck muscles, low-grade fever, and so on; in most cases no physical cause can be found, symptoms tend to decrease on weekends, holidays, and school vacations

- crying

- withdrawal from school and recreational activities with other children

- other fears, such as being alone or being with people he/she does not know

  - dependent behavior
  - passive-aggressive behavior

377

School Phobia Management

Because school phobia involves the child, the parent, the healthcare provider, and the school, all must be involved in planning and implementation of interventions.

A team of school personnel is needed to effectively assist the student, parents, and healthcare providers resolve this problem. The school team should involve the following members: the principal, the student's teacher(s), the school nurse, the student's counselor, and the school psychologist, as well as the student's parents. School interventions include:

- forced attendance—physically brought to school by parent or school personnel.

- behavior modification—reward paired with behavior of coming to and staying in school, and participating in school activities.

- contracting—with parent, child, and school to have the child earn a privilege for attending school.

- alteration of school and classroom environment to decrease anxiety or fear with gradual transition back into the regular school and classroom environment.

- limit student complaints—physical complaints are assessed by the school nurse, appropriate interventions are implemented and the student is sent back to class.

- NO HOMEBOUND INSTRUCTION.

Home interventions include [2, 3, 5, 6]:

- expectation and attitude by parents that the child will go to school *every day*.

- school avoidance behaviors elicit strictly aversive consequences—restriction of privileges, withdrawal of attention, and so on.

- mental health counseling for parents and child.

There are several mental health counseling/treatment approaches that are effective. The selection of the approach depends on the nature and severity of the problem.

INDIVIDUALIZED HEALTHCARE PLAN

History

- student's general health status
- last visit with healthcare provider(s)
- last complete physical examination
- past history of illnesses and injuries
- student's sleeping pattern
- student's eating pattern
- health status of other family members
- student's and family's past experiences with stress, their response to the stress, and the outcome
- past periods of separation from his/her parents—circumstances, child's reaction, parent's and child's method of coping with the separation
- recent family transitions—move, death in the family, parental illness or injury, parental loss of a job, sibling moving away from home, other
- past school attendance pattern

- current school attendance pattern—frequency of absences, reasons for absences, when the absences occur (days of the week, after holidays and vacations), excessive absence with parent knowledge
- school performance
- behavior at school
- onset of somatic complaints—symptoms, intensity, duration, frequency, precipitating and alleviating factors
- school avoidance behaviors
- onset of refusal to go to school
- what does the student do when he/she stays home from school

Assessment

- student's perception of his/her health status
- student's concerns about his/her health
- student's concerns about the health of other family members
- student's locus of control
- student's fears, anxieties, and concerns
- student's feelings about school
- student's perception of stressors in the school setting—peers, teachers, schedule, assignments, tests, grades, specific classroom activities, other
- student's reaction to going to school and being in school—anxiety, behavior, physical symptoms
- student's perception of academic performance
- parent's perception of academic performance
- teacher's perception of academic performance
- student's ability to separate from parents—mother and father
- parent's reaction to student's ability or inability to separate from them
- parent's reaction to somatic complaints
- parent's reaction to school avoidance behaviors
- parent's attitude toward school
- student's environment—home and school
- student's ability to problem solve

Nursing Diagnoses (N.D.)

N.D. 1 Anxiety (NANDA 9.3.1)* related to stressors in the school setting resulting in school avoidance behaviors.

N.D. 2 Unresolved fear (NANDA 9.3.2) of going to school related to:
- separation from parent(s)
- school environment
- new environment (new school, new people)

N.D. 3 (Potential for) alteration in comfort (NANDA 9.1.1) related to response to anxiety/fear.

---

* (See chapter 2, page 38 for explanation of the NANDA approved numerical system.)

N.D. 4 Alteration in student role (NANDA 3.2.1) related to inadequate or maladaptive coping skills resulting in school avoidance behaviors.

N.D. 5 Ineffective family coping (NANDA 5.1.2.1.1) related to:
- parent-child inability to separate
- unmet psychosocial needs of parent and child
- child's school avoidance behaviors resulting in poor school attendance

Goals

Identify the causes of anxiety. (N.D. 1)

Utilize positive adaptive coping methods to decrease anxiety. (N.D. 1)

Identify sources of fear. (N.D. 2)

Utilize adaptive coping methods to decrease fear. (N.D. 2)

Decrease maladaptive coping methods. (N.D. 1, 2)

Increase adaptive coping methods. (N.D. 1, 2)

Decrease in physical symptoms/discomfort/pain related to anxiety/fear. (N.D. 3)

Decrease school avoidance behaviors. (N.D. 1–5)

Improve school attendance pattern. (N.D. 4)

Identify family difficulty coping with school avoidance behaviors. (N.D. 5)

Utilize adaptive methods for decreasing school avoidance behaviors. (N.D. 5)

Seek assistance and utilize resources in coping with and resolving school avoidance behaviors. (N.D. 5)

Nursing Interventions

Assist the student to identify and verbalize if he/she is feeling stress and anxiety and what the source(s) of those feelings are: at home, at school, separating from his/her parents, others. (N.D. 1)

Discuss ways to remove stressors or modify them so they cause less anxiety. (N.D. 1)

Remove or modify as many stressors as possible. (N.D. 1)

Assist the student and his/her parents to recognize the maladaptive responses they have chosen to alleviate anxiety (the student's specific school avoidance behaviors). (N.D. 1)

Assist the student and his/her parents to identify adaptive methods of reducing feeling of anxiety. (N.D. 1)

Assist the student to identify and verbalize his/her fears: at home, at school, separating from parent(s), and others. (N.D. 2)

Discuss ways to decrease or remove the cause of the fear(s). (N.D. 2)

Assist the student and his/her parents to recognize the maladaptive responses they have chosen to decrease the fear(s). (N.D. 2)

Assist the student and his/her parents to identify adaptive methods of reducing their feelings of fear. (N.D. 2)

Provide educational opportunities (individual or group) that will help the student to develop adaptive coping methods, such as: thought stopping, relaxation techniques, positive self-talk, and so on. (N.D. 1, 2)

Assist the student to demonstrate and practice adaptive coping methods. (It may take many gradual steps toward the desired method, such as coming to school for one class and gradually increasing it to all classes.) (N.D. 1, 2)

Provide positive reinforcement for improvements in utilizing adaptive coping methods. (N.D. 1, 2, 5)

Utilize behavior modification and contracting with the student and parents as a means of assisting them to try and maintain adaptive coping methods. (N.D. 1, 2, 5)

Assist the student to identify the physical symptoms he/she is feeling. (N.D. 3)

Assist the parent(s) to obtain a current *complete* physical examination for their child. (N.D. 3)

- If a physical cause is found, develop and implement a school management plan that will ensure the health needs of the student are met, as well as ensuring and encouraging a good school attendance pattern.
- If no physical cause can be found, develop and implement a school management plan that addresses symptom management at school, as well as requiring school attendance.

Collaborate with the student's healthcare provider(s) and parent(s) in addressing the mental health, as well as the physical health of the student. (N.D. 3)

If a physical cause is ruled out and school avoidance behaviors continue, refer the student and his/her family back to their healthcare provider and/or to community mental health resources for further assessment, care, and support. (N.D. 3)

Collaborate with the student's teacher(s), counselor psychologist, and adminstrators in assisting the student to come to and remain at school. Need to address: (N.D. 1–4)
- modifications to reduce the student's stress and anxiety
- support services needed
- health office visits
- mandatory school/class attendance

Assist the parent(s) to identify that a school attendance problem does exist. (N.D. 4, 5)

Discuss (possible) causes for the attendance problem and the behaviors that are occurring. (N.D. 4, 5)

Discuss how the school avoidance behaviors are affecting: (N.D. 4, 5)
- the parent(s)
- the student
- siblings and other members of the family

Assist the parent(s) to verbalize their feelings about their child's behaviors. (N.D. 5)

Discuss the way they and other members of the family have coped with the problem. (N.D. 5)

- Methods they have tried and the effectiveness of each method.
- Alternative methods they have thought of but not chosen to implement.

- Assistance they have sought from others (such as school personnel, healthcare providers, community mental health resources, friends, extended family members, others).

Discuss adaptive methods of coping with school avoidance behaviors. (N.D. 1, 2, 4, 5)
- behavior modification
- contracting
- modifying the environment to decrease anxiety and/or fear
- expectation and attitude that the child will attend school
- forced attendance Assist the parent(s) to implement adaptive methods of coping with school avoidance behaviors. (ND 4, 5)

Assist the parent(s) to communicate with school personnel, such as setting up and facilitating school conferences, keeping school personnel informed on the status of the student (health, attendance, behaviors—positive and negative), and so on. (N.D. 4, 5)

Assist parent(s) to effectively cope with and resolve their child's school avoidance behaviors and their cause(s). (N.D. 1–5)
- Assist in getting the student to school and keeping him/her in school.
- Provide the services needed to ensure the student's health needs are met at school.
- Provide positive reinforcement to the student and his/her parent(s) for good school attendance behaviors.
- Provide feedback to the parent and student when school avoidance behaviors are being used.

Refer the parent(s) to their healthcare provider(s) and/or community mental health resources for assessment, care, and support. (N.D. 1–5)

Assist the parent to utilize mental health services from their healthcare provider and/or community mental health resources. (N.D. 1–5)

Expected Student Outcomes

The student will:
- Identify sources of anxiety: at home, at school separating from his/her parent(s), and others. (N.D. 1)

- List adaptive and maladaptive responses to anxiety. (N.D. 1)

- Demonstrate adaptive methods to reduce anxiety. (N.D. 1)

- Identify sources of fear: at home, at school separating from his/her parent(s), and others. (N.D. 2)

- List adaptive and maladaptive responses to fear(s). (N.D. 2)

- Demonstrate adaptive methods to reduce fear. (N.D. 2)

- Identify the physical symptoms he/she is feeling. (N.D. 3)

- Accurately describe his/her physical health status. (N.D. 3)

- State or demonstrate a decrease in physical symptoms/discomfort/pain related to anxiety and fear. (N.D. 3)

- Identify behaviors that are used to avoid school. (N.D. 1–4)

- Decrease use of school avoidance behaviors. (N.D. 1–4)

- Attend school regularly. (N.D. 4)

The parent(s) will:

- Identify that a school attendance problem exists. (N.D. 4, 5)

- Identify that school avoidance behaviors exist. (N.D. 4, 5)

- Describe how these behaviors affect them, their child, siblings, and other family members. (N.D. 5)

- Verbalize their feelings about their child's behaviors. (N.D. 5)

- Describe methods they have used to cope with their child's behaviors and the effectiveness of the methods. (N.D. 5)

- List adaptive and maladaptive methods for decreasing school avoidance behaviors. (N.D. 4, 5)

- Choose and implement adaptive methods of decreasing school avoidance behaviors. (N.D. 4, 5)

- Communicate effectively with school personnel. (N.D. 4, 5)

- Attend parent-school conferences. (N.D. 4, 5)

- Seek assistance from healthcare provider and/or community mental health resource(s) for their child and themselves to assist them to cope with and resolve their child's anxiety, fear(s), and behaviors. (N.D. 1–5)

- Utilize healthcare provider and/or community mental health resource(s) for assessment, care, and support for themselves and for their child. (N.D. 1–5)

REFERENCES

1. Brulle AR, McIntyre TC, Mills JS. School phobia: its educational implications. *Elementary School Guidance* 1985; 20 (Oct): 19–28.
2. Want J. School–based intervention strategies for school phobia: a ten–step common sense approach. *Pointer* 1983; 27 (3): 27–32.
3. Glanville CL, Marshall L, Conley JF, Kelly GL. Nursing care of the child with dysfunctional behavior. In: Mott SR. *Nursing Care of Children and Families* Menlo Park, CA: Addison–Wesley Publishing, 1985.
4. McAnaly E. School phobia: the importance of prompt intervention. *J School Health* 1986; 56 (10): 433–36.
5. Porter E. The school nurse's role in school phobia. *School Nurse* 1987; (Nov/Dec): 8–11.
6. Hanvik LJ. The Child Afraid of School. Unpublished paper. 1982.

BIBLIOGRAPHY

Berg I. School avoidance, school phobia and truancy. In: Lewis M, ed. *Child and Adolescent Psychiatry: A Comprehensive Textbook.* Baltimore: Williams & Watkins, 1991: Chap 103.

Bernstein GA, Garfinkel BD. School phobia: the overlap of affective and anxiety disorders. *J Am Acad Child Psychiatry* 1986; 25: 235–41.

Gingrich-Crass J. Stress and crisis: specific problems of adaptation. In Wold SJ. *School Nursing: A Framework for Practice.* North Branch, MN: Sunrise River Press, 1981.

Harris SR. School phobic children and adolescents: a challenge to counselors. *School Counselor* 1980; 27 (4): 263–68.

Hsia H. Structural and strategic approach to school phobia/school refusal. *Psychology in the Schools* 1984; 21 (Jul): 360–67.

Paccione–Dyszlewski MR, Contessa–Kislus MA. School phobia: identification of subtypes as a prerequisite to treatment intervention. *Adolescence* 1987; 22 (86): 377–84.

IHP: Seizures

Mary J. Villars Gerber

INTRODUCTION

The school nurse plays an important role in identification of seizures and providing education and support to students, teachers, and parents. Students who experience seizures that are not well controlled will need the help of a school nurse in documenting seizures and providing feedback to parents and healthcare providers.

Concerns and needs that school personnel and students have may include healthcare planning for the student who has seizures, educational programs for staff and students, providing emotional support for students and staff, and promoting a positive social and educational climate for the student who may have seizures.

Epilepsy is a chronic disorder of the brain characterized by the tendency to have recurrent seizures. Seizures are sudden, uncontrolled episodes of excessive electrical discharges in some nerve cells of the brain, with associated sensory, motor, and/or behavioral changes. There are over thirty different types of seizures, each with its own characteristic behavioral and electroencephalographic changes.

Not all seizures indicate that a person has epilepsy. Other causes of seizures include high fever, alcohol or drug withdrawal, or an imbalance of body fluids or chemicals.

Etiology, or causes, of epilepsy include certain inherited diseases, problems during fetal development, lack of oxygen or brain injury during birth, problems in infancy including jaundice and infections, head injuries, infections such as encephalitis and meningitis, toxicity of mercury or lead, tumors of the brain, and circulatory problems including stroke.

Signs and symptoms vary according to the type of seizure a person experiences. Certain parts of the brain control different body functions. The function of the body which is affected is related to the part of the brain involved in the seizure. The International Classification of Seizures identifies two major groupings of seizures: generalized and partial.[1]

Generalized seizures are subdivided into tonic-clonic and absence seizures. Tonic-clonic seizures, also known as grand mal, generally last one to five minutes, and involve the entire body. The body falls, stiffens, and jerks. The person may cry out, bite their tongue, and become bluish due to lack of oxygen. They may become incontinent. The person is generally tired afterwards and may sleep.

Another form of generalized seizures is the absence seizure, also known as petit mal. It generally lasts a few seconds, the person may have a staring spell or blink their eyes. This type of seizure is most commonly found in children. It is sometimes mistaken for daydreaming in school.

Other forms of generalized seizures are myoclonic, clonic, tonic, and atonic seizures.

Partial seizures are subdivided into complex partial (psychomotor/temporal lobe) and simple partial (jacksonian/focal motor) seizures. Psychomotor/temporal lobe seizures usually last one to two minutes and consist of purposeless activity. Impairment of consciousness occurs. The person may appear confused, drunk, drugged, or psychotic. They may fidget with their clothing or lip smack. If restrained they may struggle.

The second type of partial seizure is known as a simple partial seizure. It usually consists of jerking of one limb or side of the body. Consciousness is maintained during the seizure.

A prolonged seizure, known as generalized convulsive status epilepticus, and severe recurrent seizures, represent a medical emergency. During a prolonged convulsive seizure, depletion of oxygen, blood flow, and nutrients to the brain occurs. Each child's physician will define what would represent a status seizure for a particular child. Generally a tonic-clonic seizure lasting longer than ten or fifteen minutes can be considered a medical emergency. Some children may have medications such as rectal valium to treat such a condition.

Medications/Treatments

The classic treatment for seizures are anticonvulsant medications. On occasion a ketogenic diet or surgery is indicated. Valium, administered rectally, may be ordered in the case of a status seizure.

Medication dosage is based on individual differences in body weight, rate of absorption, and other medications the person may be taking. Blood tests are periodically conducted to determine concentration of medications in the blood. Unacceptable side effects of all the medications include hypersensitivity or allergic reactions. Each medication is used to treat a specific type of seizure. One person may experience more than one type of seizure and therefore a combination of medications may be used.

Common medications used with children include: Clonopin, Depakene, Depakote, Dilantin, phenobarbital, Mysoline, Tegretol, and Zarontin.

Valium (diazepam) may be used to treat status epilepticus and severe recurrent seizures. Because of the central nervous system action of this medication, great care must be taken in administration of this medication in a school setting. Administered rectally, this medication is very fast-acting. The school nurse must be prepared to observe for side affects affecting the cardiovascular system and respiratory depression. Blood pressure and respirations must be monitored for signs of depression and the nurse must be prepared to act should they occur. The physician may order the use of oxygen during a status seizure as well. Preparation of the school nurse to manage this condition cannot be overemphasized.

The ketogenic diet includes foods high in fats and low in carbohydrates and protein. The reason for its effectiveness is not well known. Is is used in small numbers of children to treat specific types of seizures.

Surgical intervention is utilized in only a few select individuals and only after intensive evaluation. Extensive treatment with medication has been ineffective. The goal of surgery is to reduce the numbers or severity of seizures.

INDIVIDUALIZED HEALTHCARE PLAN

History

Health history; prenatal, perinatal, neonatal
History of seizures
- At what age did seizure activity begin?
- What kinds of behaviors were observed during a seizure?
- How often did seizures occur?
- How long did seizures last?
- What events might precipitate a seizure?
- Was there any aura (visual, auditory, olfactory) present before a seizure?
- Has the student experienced a seizure lasting longer than five minutes? If so, what intervention was needed?

What medications have been used in the past to control seizure activity?

Assessment

- Current status of seizure activity is needed to determine baseline:
   Frequency
   Date, time, and duration
   Specific behavior observed
   Activity that might precipitate seizure
   Aura
   Incidence of status epilepticus
   Changes in level of consciousness

- Observe seizure activity if possible to determine baseline.

- Emergency medical care information, including physician and phone number, hospital, parents' names and phone numbers, emergency phone numbers, and insurance coverage.

- Safety precautions that are routinely utilized and determination of those appropriate for school setting. Certain activities may be restricted. Some children are required to wear a helmet for head protection.

- Current medications at home/school and side effects. Side effects that will interfere with learning will be of particular importance. Medications may need to be administered at school.

- Social adjustment. Problems with self-esteem, self-image, and social relationships are frequently observed in children with chronic illness and may affect their overall school adjustment.

- Education/self-care needs including chronicity, healthcare needs and medications. Individuals may experience difficulties or lack of compliance with treatment regimen due to lack of knowledge or to fear.

- Classroom needs and modifications that are necessary due to seizure activity.

- Activity restrictions. Depending on type of seizures the student experiences, he/she may need to avoid contact sports or other situations that would pose risk if seizure occurred such as climbing on trees or certain play apparatus. Student should be accompanied during other activities such as bicycling or swimming.

Nursing Diagnoses (N.D.)

N.D. 1   Potential for injury (NANDA 1.6.1)* related to uncontrolled movements of seizure activity.

N.D. 2   Potential for aspiration (NANDA 1.6.1.4) related to seizure activity.

N.D. 3   Potential impaired social interactions (NANDA 3.1.1) related to chronic illness.

N.D. 4   Impaired social interactions (NANDA 3.1.1) related to (specify) secondary to chronic illness.

N.D. 5   Potential body-image disturbance (NANDA 7.1.1) related to chronic illness.

N.D. 6   Body-image disturbance (NANDA 7.1.1) related to (specify).

N.D. 7   Potential self-esteem disturbance (NANDA 7.1.2) related to chronic illness.

N.D. 8   Self-esteem disturbance (NANDA 7.1.2) related to (specify).

N.D. 9   Fear (NANDA 9.3.2) related to (specify).

N.D. 10   Potential altered health maintenance (NANDA 6.4.2) related to insufficient knowledge (specify).

Goals

Prevent injury during seizure. (N.D. 1)

Prevent aspiration during seizure. (N.D. 2)

Support and encouragement related to social interactions. (N.D. 3, 4)

Promote positive body image. (N.D. 5, 6)

Promote positive self-esteem. (N.D. 7, 8)

Identify source of fear and assist to reduce or eliminate. (N.D. 9)

Teach importance and benefits of treatment regimen. (N.D. 10)

Nursing Interventions

Protect child during seizure and educate staff in same measures. All staff need to know appropriate response to a child having a seizure to prevent injury. Protective head equipment and body straps used on wheelchairs may be necessary to prevent injury. (N.D. 1)

Establish appropriate activity restrictions in cooperation with parents/physician, based on real rather than perceived risk. Certain activity restrictions may need to be imposed to prevent injury during a seizure. Restrictions should be reassessed periodically to determine appropriateness. (N.D. 1)

Obtain current medical orders. (N.D. 1)

Provide for documentation of seizure activity during school and communication to parents/healthcare providers as appropriate. Include date, time, duration, objective facts about seizure behavior, and observer's name. (See examples of charts used to document seizure activity at the end of this chapter.) (N.D. 1)

---

* (See chapter 2, page 38 for explanation of the NANDA approved numerical system.)

Case management: Refer and follow up for medical care if needed, coordinate service providers. (N.D. 1–10)

First aid and emergency care as needed. Procedures for first aid should be established and known by school personnel. Emergency procedures in the case of status epilepticus need to be established and understood by staff. (N.D. 1)

Emotional support for students and staff. (N.D. 1–9)

Position child on his/her side if possible to prevent aspiration. Clear secretions from mouth if necessary. Provide instruction for staff in same interventions. (N.D. 2)

Update health history at least annually. (N.D. 2)

Support for development and maintenance of social skills. Health teaching and referral if indicated. (N.D. 3, 4)

Establish trusting relationship that will provide foundation for student to talk about issues related to body image. Provide support for social interraction. Specific interventions should occur depending on source of body image disturbance. (N.D. 5, 6)

Enhance sense of self-esteem. Provide opportunities for positive socialization. Make referral as indicated. (N.D. 7, 8)

Assess contributing factors to fear, reduce or eliminate contributing factors, provide health teaching or refer as indicated. (N.D. 9)

Reduce or eliminate barriers to learning. Provide instruction related to specific area where lack of knowledge is present. (N.D. 10)

Educational support for students and staff. (N.D. 10)

Self-care education for the student. (N.D. 10)

Expected Student Outcomes

Student will not experience injury during seizure. (N.D. 1)

Student will not aspirate during a seizure. (N.D. 2)

Identify problematic behavior and substitute constructive behavior for disruptive social behavior. (N.D. 3, 4)

Will share feelings about how s/he views self. Will begin to assume role-related responsibilities. Demonstrates confidence in ability to succeed at what is desired. (N.D. 5, 6)

Describe positive changes in feelings regarding self. (N.D. 7, 8)

Will discuss and identify source of fear and report increased sense of comfort. (N.D. 9)

Relates less anxiety, related to fear of unknown, fear of loss of control, misconceptions, or previously given misinformation. (N.D. 9)

Describes condition, causes, and factors contributing to symptoms, and procedures for disease or symptom control . (N.D. 10)

Understands condition and complies with medication and treatment regimen. (N.D. 10)

Actively participates in health behaviors prescribed or desired. (N.D. 10)

Collaborative Problems

Potential complication: Seizures

Potential complication: Respiratory arrest

Potential complication: Hypoxia

Developmental Issues

Very young children may tend to have less well-controlled seizures than older children. Changes in the type of seizure a child experiences may occur periodically and will need evaluation. Adolescents will often experience a change in seizure patterns due to maturation and hormonal changes.

REFERENCES

1. Santilli N, Dodson WE, Walton AV. *Students With Seizures: A Manual for School Nurses.* Cedar Grove, NJ: Health Scan, 1991.

BIBLIOGRAPHY

Arnold F, Casady L, Hadady B, Wilkes D, Williams S, Williamson M. *Individualized and Prescriptive School Nursing Services For Physically Handicapped Students.* 2nd ed. 1984. School Nurse Advocates for Children, P.O. Drawer 1538, Garden Grove, CA 92640.

Batshaw ML, Perret YM. *Children With Handicaps A Medical Primer* Baltimore: Paul H. Brookes Publishing, 1981.

Carpenito LJ. *Handbook of Nursing Diagnosis.* Philadelphia: JB Lippincott, 1989.

Carpenito LJ. *Nursing Diagnosis, Application to Clinical Practice.* Philadelphia: JB Lippincott, 1989.

Epilepsy Foundation of America, 4351 Garden City Dr, Landover, MD 20785. Publish numerous pamphlets, books, school alerts, posters, films/cassettes, and transcultural materials. Some titles are listed here:

> Questions and Answers About Epilepsy, 1989
> The Teachers Role, 1987
> Medicines for Epilepsy, 1990
> Seizure Recognition and First Aid, 1989
> Epilepsy School Alert, 1985
> A Child's Guide to Seizure Disorders, 1987
> Epilepsy and the School Age Child
> Epilepsy, Medical Aspects
> How to Recognize and Classify Seizures
> Because You Are My Friend
> Students With Seizures: A Manual For School Nurses, 1991

Larson G, ed. *Managing the School Age Child With a Chronic Health Condition: A Practical Guide For School, Families, and Organizations.* Wayzata, MN: DCI Publishing, 1988 (available from Sunrise River Press, 11481 Kost Dam Rd, North Branch, MN 55056, 612-583-3239).

Miller SL. Epilepsy and the School-Age Child. *Topics In Pediatrics* 1989; 8 (2): 17–22.

National Information Center for Children and Youth with Handicaps. General Information About Epilepsy. Fact Sheet Number 6, 1990. PO Box 1492, Washington, DC 20013.

Nichter C. Seizures: a developmental perspective. *Topics in Early Childhood Education* 1987; 6 (4) (Winter): 75–91.

Scheuer ML, Pedley TA. Current concepts: the evaluation and treatment of seizures. *N Engl J Med* 1990; 323 (21): 1468–73.

Walton A. Teaching children about epilepsy. *Education Unlimited* 1979; 1 (3): 16–19.

Whaley LF, Wong DL. *Nursing Care of Infants and Children.* St. Louis: CV Mosby, 1987.

Wong DL, Whaley LF. *Clinical Manual of Pediatric Nursing.* St. Louis: CV Mosby, 1990.

SUPPLEMENT

Log On Seizure Activity

Student Name _____

Date	Time	Duration	Description

This is a weekly log. Please complete and return to School Nurse at end of week.

Seizure Report
Flow Chart

Pupil Name _____ Grade _____ Class _____ D.O.B._____

	Date of Each Seizure							
	Time of Onset							
	Total Time Involved							
A.	Observations before seizure							
	cries out							
	other							
B.	Observations during seizure							
	Extremity involvement:							
	both upper & lower							
	arms affected right							
	left							
	legs affected right							
	left							
	straight							
	bent							
	stiff							
	limp							
	Verbal sounds before							
	during							
	Face twitching							
	Mouth open							
	closed							
	grimacing							
	Drooling							
	Vomited							
	Eye movement staring							
	open							
	closed							
	fluttering							
	rolled back							
	Head turned right							
	turned left							
	turned down							

Continued on next page

Date of Each Seizure	/	/	/	/	/	/	/
Hyperextended back							
Nodding							
Body-trunk							
rigid							
limp							
sitting							
laying							
trembling							
jerking							
standing							
Skin color							
pale							
grey							
blue							
red (flushed)							
Breathing							
difficulty during							
difficulty after							
15 seconds							
1 minute							
longer (amount?)							
Incontinent urine							
bowels							
C. **Observation after seizure**							
drowsy							
confused							
sleep (length of time)							
Other							
injury (elaborate)							
school nurse called							
health clerk called							
parent called							
child taken home (by whom)							
doctor called							
911 called							
Responder Initials							

Continued on next page

Responder's Signature

_____

_____

_____

Responder's Initials

_____

_____

_____

42 | IHP: Spina Bifida

Susan I. Simandl Will

INTRODUCTION

Spina bifida (split spine) is the result of embryonic maldevelopment of the spine. The spine fails to close, producing a cleft or split with one or more vertebrae remaining open over the spinal cord. This happens within the first twenty-five days of pregnancy and etiology is unknown. Spina bifida occurs worldwide yet incidence varies considerably throughout countries and cultures. Spina bifida with myelomeningocele, the most severe manifestation of the condition, occurs in a range of 0.67 to 2.50 per 1,000 births.[1]

Pathophysiology

Spina Bifida Occulta

One or more vertebrae fail to close in embryonic development leaving a cleft or split in the spinal column. This is a benign condition and frequently unknown. A tuft of hair or dimpling along the spine may mark a spina bifida occulta. There is no spinal cord pathology and there are no neurological deficits.

Spina Bifida Meningocele

The spinal cord meninges protrude through the spina bifida producing a sacklike mass. The mass can be skin-covered or be simply exposed meninges at birth. Neurologic deficits are unusual fol-

lowing rapid surgical repair of the meningocele. However, hydrocephalus can result following the repair because of resultant cerebrospinal fluid flow impairment.

Spina Bifida Myelomeningocele

This is the most severe manifestation of spina bifida because the meningeal sack protruding through the spina bifida contains neurofibers of the spinal column. Surgical repair of this condition may need to be accomplished in several procedures, however, initial closure of the defect is seen as an emergency requirement to prevent complications of meningitis. From 60 to 75 percent of the children with myelomeningocele will develop hydrocephalus, producing need for additional surgeries to shunt the cerebrospinal fluid to the peritoneum or vascular system and reestablish normal intracranial pressure.[2]

The amount of neurologic damage and subsequent pathology and lifestyle handicapping will depend on the level of the vertebral lesion. If the myelomeningocele is at or above the lumbosacral area, urine and bowel control will be compromised.

In the school setting a child with spina bifida may require assistance in managing a bladder or bowel program. The amount of lower limb paralysis will depend on the vertebral level of the myelomeningocele. A thorough nursing assessment will determine the amount of mobility and sensory functioning available to the child. Frequently orthotics such as braces or splints are used to stabilize the child. Range of motion exercises (active and passive) will be required to prevent contractures. Mobility aids (wheelchairs, wheelboards, crutches, walkers,etc.) will be used to facilitate locomotion.

The child with spina bifida may also experience learning disabilities or retardation. Involvement of the total educational team, including special education resources, will be necessary to facilitate a successful experience for the child at school.

INDIVIDUAL HEALTHCARE PLAN

Assessment

History

- What vertebral level was spinal lesion?
- What previous surgical procedures were performed and at what age?
  - closure of meningocele? age?
  - bladder and/or bowel reconstruction or diversion? Age?
  - reconstructive orthopedic surgery on hips, legs, feet? Age?
  - hydrocephalic shunt? Drainage site (peritoneal, atrial)?
- What previous physical therapy, occupational therapy, ostomy therapy has student received?
- What orthotics (splints, braces, stabilizers) have been used?
- What is family history in management of cares, stresses, finances, and demands of a physically disabled child?

Current Status

- Physical status:
    presence of visible myelomeningeal sac and its status or repair site status
    sensory disturbances: level
    motor disturbances: level
    contractures
    joint deformities (alkylosis, scoliosis, kyphosis, hip dislocations)
    hydrocephalus
    continence
- Student's description and definition of spina bifida
- Student's understanding of spina bifida
- What orthotics (splints, braces, stabilizers) does student use? When?
- What mobility equipment does student use (walker, wheelchair, wheelboard, etc.)?
- Transportation needs (car, van, equipment, assistance)?
- Urine and bowel management plan and frequency: What is needed at school?
    Urine: ostomy?
              catheterization (indwelling or intermittent)?
              diapering?
              artificial urinary sphincter (AUS)?
              abdominal pressure?

Bowel: laxative?
               diet?
               enema?
               ostomy?

- Family's current status in caring for child with disability:
  - finances
  - dynamics and interfamilial relationships
  - support sources
  - socialization
  - caregivers' skills
  - home physical environment
  - sources of assistance with cares, financial demands, emotional and family members personal needs
  - other stressors on family

- Activities of daily living strengths and limits:
  - mobility (transportation, getting on and off bus, stairs, elevators, hallways, class rooms)
  - feeding (cafeteria tray and table management)
  - dressing
  - elimination
  - recreation/leisure/diversion
  - classroom and learning activities

- School accessibility for handicapped youth (bathrooms, hallways, classrooms, doorways, cafeteria, peer and staff attitudes)
  - Students desire to be involved in self-care
  - Student's skill in management of cares

Psychosocial

- Age and developmental level
- Student's feelings about having spina bifida
- Student's perception of what family members think and feel about his/her having spina bifida
- Student's perception of what friends think and feel about his/her having spina bifida
- School club or athletic activities past and present
- Community and church activities past and present
- Depression or despondency
- Student's support systems: family, friends, other
- Student ability to appropriately accept dependence and appropriately maintain independence

Academic

- Review of academic or cumulative school record for patterns of academic performance
- Assessment of teachers' perception of student's performance and classroom adjustment
- Comparison of student's behavior, social skills, academic performance to peer norms

- School absence pattern
- Need for special education (P.L. 94–142) services to adequately educate the student (transportation, classroom adaptations, tutoring, occupational therapy, physical therapy, vocational guidance)
- Intellectual abilities: presence of learning disability or retardation?

Self Care

- Activities student states are limited by spina bifida
- What does student find useful to manage successfully in school?
- Need for learning support systems (special education, computer aids, tutors, adaptive physical education)
- What treatments, medications, activities of daily living, or cares can student manage on own?
- What treatments, medication, activities of daily living, or cares does student need assistance with?

Nursing Diagnoses (N.D.)

N.D. 1   Alteration in activities of daily living—personal, recreational, educational: hygiene, toileting, eating, writing, running, walking, stair climbing related to limits imposed by physical disability.

N.D. 2   Impaired physical mobility (NANDA 6.1.1.1)* related to impairment, orthotics, and/or mobility equipment.

N.D. 3   Alterations in self-care (NANDA 6.5.1, 2, 3, or 4 and 8.1.1) due to mobility limitations, developmental level, knowledge deficit, and/or skill deficit.

N.D. 4   Alteration in urine elimination (NANDA 1.3.2) (impairment or incontinence) related to spinal impairment, diversionary ostomy, presence of AUS (artificial urinary sphincter), or catheterization needs.

N.D. 5   Potential for urinary tract or kidney infection (NANDA 1.2.1.1) related to altered urine elimination.

N.D. 6   Urinary elimination knowledge (NANDA 8.1.1) or skill deficit related to altered elimination or presence of urinary drainage appliances.

N.D. 7   Alteration in socialization (NANDA 3.1.1, 3.1.2) related to mobility limits, dysfunctional grieving, embarrassment, stigma of chronic illness, lifestyle adaptations, feelings of differentness, sexuality or intimacy concerns.

N.D. 8   Independence-dependence conflict related to limits, lifestyle adaptations, perceptions of disability.

N.D. 9   Alteration in self-esteem (NANDA 7.1.2) and/or body image (NANDA 7.1.1) related to limitations, grieving, embarrassment, stigma perceptions, feelings of differentness, sexuality or intimacy concerns.

N.D. 10   Potential for infection (NANDA 1.2.1.1), or increased intracranial pressure related to presence of cerebrospinal fluid shunt or malfunction of shunt.

N.D. 11   Potential for skin injury (NANDA 1.6.2.1.2.1) related to presence of orthotics and/or decreased sensory perception in limbs.

* (See Chapter 2, page 38 for explanation of the NANDA approved numerical system.)

Goals

Student will acquire adaptations necessary to experience activities commensurate with capabilities in the school setting. (N.D. 1–3, 8, 10)

Student will be able to perform activities of daily living within his/her physical limits without excessive fatigue or development of pain. (N.D. 1–3)

Student will be involved in management of condition and improve self-management skills. (N.D. 1–3, 8, 9)

Student will have successful bladder elimination program. (N.D. 4–6)

Student will (acquire, progress in, maintain) effective and appropriate social involvement. (N.D. 7–9)

Student will demonstrate increased adaptation to and psychological comfort with bodily limits. (N.D. 7–9)

Student will be successful in activities which foster self-respect and scholastic progress. (N.D. 7–9)

Student will accept dependence when necessary for management of his/her condition. (N.D. 8, 9)

Student will not experience secondary infections or intracranial infections due to shunt. (N.D. 10)

Student will have skin maintained in good condition. (N.D. 11)

Nursing Interventions

School/Teacher Interventions

Assist teachers in development of alternative educational activities compatible with mobility abilities. (N.D. 1, 2)

Arrange for assistance as necessary for daily school activities: (N.D. 1,2,3)

- book carrying
- opening doors
- getting on and off bus
- extra time for passing between class
- toileting
- carrying food tray

Arrange for appropriate physical education activities and instruct physical education teachers in motor expectations appropriate to level of disability. (N.D. 1, 2)

Referral for special education (P.L. 94–142) evaluation for occupational therapy, physical therapy, tutoring, learning aids, transportation, vocational counseling. (N.D. 1–3)

Provide access to physically handicapped bathrooms, entrances, elevators as appropriate. (N.D. 1–3, 4, 8)

Arrange for special transportation as needed (van, wheelchair lift, other). (N.D. 1–3)

Provide appropriate nursing supervision to all personnel assisting the student with any cares. (N.D 4, 5)

Arrange for space and time for student to perform urinary care activities. (N.D 4–6)

See also Chapters 5 and 6 for additional mental health and psychosocial nursing diagnoses relevant to students with chronic impairment.

Student Interventions: Physical

Assist student with wheelchair, wheelboard, walkers, braces, splints, and other orthotics or mobility aids as needed. (N.D. 1–3)

Monitor limbs with braces, splints for fit, rubbing, or circulation impairment. (N.D. 11, 12)

Perform or assist student in performance of passive or active range of motion exercises. (N.D. 11)

Identify type of urinary elimination program student requires: diapering, manual abdominal expression, clean intermittent catheterization (CIC), indwelling catheter. (N.D.4)

Obtain physician orders for urine elimination procedures at school as required by school policy. (N.D. 4)

Identify student's ability to self-provide manual expression, diapering, CIC, or ostomy care. (N.D. 4–6, 8, 9)

Wound care of shunt if recent replacement or as appropriate or prescribed. (N.D. 10)

Monitor for signs of shunt infection (fever, malaise). (N.D. 10)

Monitor for signs of increased intracranial pressure (lethargy, irritation, transient confusion, eating poorly, vomiting, altered alertness or mental state, agitation, pupils changed or unequal, decreasing pulse, vertigo, seizures). (N.D. 10)

Instruct student in self-management of skin care. (N.D.11)

Instruct student in signs of early skin breakdown, early management techniques, and what signs and symptoms require physician evaluation. (N.D.11)

Observe pressure points for early signs of tissue breakdown. (N.D. 11)

Instruct student in safety precautions necessary because of sensory decrease: (N.D. 11)

- hot or cold injury prevention
- avoiding prolonged pressure, frequent position modification
- foot care

Monitor for signs of urinary tract infection (abdominal pain, strong or foul smelling urine, dark, cloudy or hazy character to urine, hematuria, vomiting, flank pain). (N.D. 5)

Instruct student in early signs of urinary tract infection. (N.D. 6)

Student Interventions: Psychosocial

Develop and maintain open, trusting communication with student. (N.D. 7–9)

Convey and model acceptance and appropriate cognitive interaction. (N.D. 7–9)

Provide for student and family referral to support groups. (N.D. 7–9)

Provide for student and family referral to supportive counseling. (N.D. 7–9)

Encourage student to share feelings and acknowledge these, encouraging additional appropriate sharing with family, friends, other involved healthcare providers. (N.D. 7–9)

Develop and maintain continuous communication with parents for planning and adjusting student's school care and activity. (N.D. 7–9)

Encourage and facilitate involvement in school extracurricular activities. (N.D. 7–9)

Encourage and provide opportunities for student's expression of feelings about condition, its management requirements, and limits it imposes. (N.D. 7–9)

Encourage student to identify own strengths and positive attributes. (N.D. 7–9)

Involve student in planning care routines and structuring adaptive helps. (N.D. 7–9)

Assist student in developing strategies to handle teasing and discrimination. (N.D. 7–9)

Assist student in realistic goal planning. (N.D. 7–9)

Assist adolescent student in verbalizing sexuality concerns and assist in developing healthy sexuality and intimacy goals. (N.D. 7–9)

Expected Student Outcomes

Student will be able to manage mobility around school and perform as many activities in the educational setting as possible. (N.D. 1–4, 8, 9)

Student will receive assistance for those activities with which s/he requires assistance. (N.D. 1–4)

Student will be able to physically attend all classes. (N.D. 1–3, 7–9)

Student will not be excessively fatigued from the activities of school attendance. (N.D. 1, 2)

Student will begin (progress in) self-care urinary program skills. (N.D. 4, 5, 6)

Student will demonstrate involvement in cares appropriate to age and developmental level. (N.D 4, 5, 6)

Student will not experience bladder or kidney infections due to distension, retrograde urine flow, or introduction of pathogenic organisms. (N.D. 4–6)

Student will verbalize positive feelings about self. (N.D. 7–9)

Student will identify several individual strengths. (N.D. 7–9)

Student will identify activities which are possible within mobility limits. (N.D. 7–9)

Student will be involved in one (or more) school or community activity. (N.D. 7–9)

Student will maintain (increase) peer contacts. (N.D. 7–9)

Student will begin to make realistic life goal plans. (N.D. 7–9)

Student (adolescent) will develop comfort with sexual or intimacy identity and abilities. (N.D. 7–9)

Student will not experience infection or malfunction of shunt. (N.D. 10)

Student will identify early signs of difficulty with shunt and they will be reported to physician. (N.D. 10)

Student will begin (progress in) self-skin-care management. (N.D. 11)

Student will not experience skin breakdown due to pressure points. (N.D. 11)

Student will identify early manifestations of skin irritation and identify how to manage early intervention. (N.D. 11)

REFERENCES

1. Murch R, Cohen L. Relationships among life stress, perceived family environment, and the psychological distress of spina bifida adolescents. *J Pediatr Psychol* 1989; 14 (2): 193–214.
2. Waechter E, Philips J, Holaday B. *Nursing Care of Children.* 10th ed. Philadelphia: JB Lippincott, 1985.

BIBLIOGRAPHY

Cleve L. Parental coping in response to their child's spina bifida. *J Pediatr Nursing* 1989; 4 (3): 172–76.

Faller N. Spina bifida: a team reviews the last 20 years. *J Enterostomal Ther* 1989; 16 (1): 42–43.

National Information Center for Children and Youth with Handicaps. General information about spina bifida. Number 12, 1990 (P.O. Box 1492, Washington, DC 20001).

Hafeman C. Teaching the younger patient. *J Enterostomal Ther* 1989; 16 (2): 52–57.

Willis C. Urinary incontinence in children with spina bifida. *Nursing Times* 1989; 35 (44): 48–51.

Wong D, Whaley L. *Clinical Manual of Pediatric Nursing.* 2nd ed. St. Louis: CV Mosby, 1990.

43 | IHP: Sports Injury

Susan I. Simandl Will

INTRODUCTION

Exercise and sports are a vital and valuable contribution to the school experience at all levels of education. Schools are offering a greater variety of physical education activities and increasing competitive sports options for both males and females. For the young athlete this means increasing the level of proficiency involved in these activities along with an improvement in muscular strength, flexibility, cardiorespiratory development, and self-esteem.

Along with increasing sports proficiency and greater numbers of student athletes, added to the regular physical education program, come the realities of periodic injury. Students often come to the attention of the school nurse for assessment and management of sports or physical education injuries.

Sports with the highest risk continue to be the contact sports of football, wrestling and gymnastics. The frequency and severity of injuries can be reduced with competent coaching, adequate time for conditioning and skill development, along with good safety equipment, safe playing surfaces, and limiting activities to those appropriate for age and size. The greater number of injuries occur in the older athlete who is competing rather than in those who are in physical education or recreational sports.[1] In addition, the risk is greatest both for injury and increased severity of injury for these older athletes during the Tanner Stage III of growth and development (maximum height velocity).[2] During this stage of peaking growth, coordination, strength, flexibility, and endurance may not be comparable to size. And at this time of growth the epiphyses are extremely vulnerable to permanent injury due to the decreased strength and maximum activity in the area. Often the epiphysis will fracture before tendon or ligament damage occurs.

Fortunately the majority of injuries are minimal in severity and do not produce prolonged impairment. Most injuries (over 50 percent) are soft tissue injuries; that is, sprains, strains, and contusions which frequently heal without complications and minimal effort.[3] More than 50 percent of these are never evaluated by a physician.[1] Many students have a small amount of physical damage and recuperate without complication in several days. Often a child will present to the school nurse to evaluate just these soft tissue injuries.

Some children's injuries will require lengthy recuperation and extensive school modifications. Other children will require minimal modifications to facilitate healing and reduce reinjury. A history, assessment, and individual school health plan are valuable in managing the entire range of disabilities a child experiences in school.

Pathophsiology

Contusions

Contusions are bruised muscle tissues. They are usually caused by external force directly to the muscle. A contusion does not eliminate function of the muscle as would a muscle rupture. The lower limbs are most frequently involved, especially the quadriceps, although contusions can happen to any muscle. Treatment will depend on the amount of damage to the muscle. R.I.C.E. (**Rest, Ice, Compression, and Elevation**) is the main principle of treatment for the first 48 hours to stop intramuscle bleeding. Any limit of motion should be evaluated by a physician as should an increasing hematoma which may represent difficulty in stopping the bleeding.

Strains

Strains are pulls in the musculotendon junction. These occur most frequently in the ankle but are possible in the hip (hamstring), groin, knee, shoulder, elbow, as well as in other joints. In a simple strain, tenderness is evident but there is no loss of joint flexibility. In more severe strains, disruption of the muscle-tendon function can be evident along with spasm and pain. R.I.C.E is the required first aid with physician exam to evaluate the more severe injuries.

Sprains

Sprains represent damage to the ligament which can involve only a few tissue tears to more complete tissue disturbance resulting in joint instability. The ankle is the most frequent joint involved in sprains and because of the epiphyseal weakness, avulsions of the ligament are possible. R.I.C.E is the required first aid with referral for physician exam to evaluate the more severe injuries.

Overuse Injuries

Overuse injuries represent microtrauma, or a repetitive activity stressing the muscle-tendon. A runner may experience this repetitive trauma as shin splints (multiple tears in the tibial tendons); a thrower or tennis player may experience this in the elbow; and the young softball pitcher may experience this as "Little League shoulder." Medical evaluation is always recommended to identify the type and severity of injury. Often the medical treatment is antiinflammatory medication along with cessation of the activity and occasionally limited immobilization. Return to the activity without evaluation and modification in the style, training, equipment, or playing surface will inevitably result in continued reinjury.

Fractures

Fractures are a traumatic disruption of bone mass. These can be of several types which include partial breaks, complete breaks, greenstick, and spiral breaks. Any injuries that produce swelling and severe pain, especially localized, should be suspected to be a break. Splinting, and referral for physician evaluation are necessary. Radiologic evaluation is the only sure way to identify the presence or absence of a fracture.

INDIVIDUALIZED HEALTHCARE PLAN

Assessment

History

- Other previous injuries of any type?
- Any other health condition or problem?
- How did this injury happen?
    - Where did injury happen? (gym, field, home, auto, school area, other)
    - How did injury happen? (fall, collision, twisting, other)
    - What body parts hurt at time of injury?
    - Did other body parts hurt at later time?

Evaluate at Time of Injury

- Emergency evaluation for Airway, Breathing, and Circulation
- Evaluate for consciousness and orientation to time, place, and person.
- History of injury
- Bone involvement
- Soft tissue involvement
- Range of motion in injured area
- Swelling, discoloration, circulation distal to injury
- Amount and severity of pain

Evaluate for Follow-up Care

- History of injury
- Soft tissue involvement
- Bone involvement
- Was student evaluated by a physician and what is the medical treatment plan?
- Presence of brace, sling, or cast
- Range of motion of affected limb
- Circulation and sensation distal to affected area
- Activity restrictions imposed by brace, cast, treatment plan, or pain
- Self-care activities which are limited:
    - bathing
    - dressing
    - toileting
    - eating, cafeteria management
    - writing
    - walking, negotiating school hallways, classroom accessibility
    - stair ability, competence, and safety
    - carrying belongings
- Sports the student is involved in currently and expects to play in next season
- Physical education classes in which the student is currently enrolled
- Degree and severity of pain

Nursing Diagnoses (N.D.)

N.D. 1 Alterations in activities on daily living—personal and educational: toileting, hygiene, writing, eating, walking, carrying, negotiating hallways, classrooms, and so on.

N.D. 2 Altered mobility and activity tolerance (NANDA 6.1.1.1, 6.1.1.2)* due to presence of pain, cast, brace, crutches, or sling.

N.D. 3 Potential for reinjury or additional injury (NANDA 1.6.1) due to limited mobility, inappropriate compensatory activities, crutches, cast, brace, or pain.

N.D. 4 Alteration in comfort, pain. (NANDA 9.1.1)

N.D. 5 Knowledge deficit (NANDA 8.1.1) relative to tissue healing needs and recuperation requirements.

Goals

Student will acquire adaptations necessary to continue as normal a lifestyle as possible in the school setting. (N.D. 1, 2)

The student will be able to perform activities of daily living within the limits of the physical impairment without excessive fatigue or exertion. (N.D. 1, 2)

The student will not experience reinjury, additional injury, or compensatory injury. (N.D. 2)

Student's pain will be successfully managed. (N.D.4)

Student will demonstrate ability to appropriately care for self and injury as much as developmentally possible. (N.D. 5)

Nursing Interventions

School/Teacher Interventions

Provide access to physically handicapped bathrooms, entrances, elevators as appropriate. (Crutch walking is especially dangerous in crowded hallways and on stairs. The students' limits may be easier managed in a handicapped-equipped bathroom for toileting.) (N.D. 1–3)

Provide for safe ambulation in hallways and classrooms: (N.D. 1–3)
Remove obstacles.
Arrange for extra passing time between classes or alternate passing time.
Arrange for use of elevator if necessary.
Arrange for monitored stair use if elevator unavailable for leg-impaired student.

Assist teachers in development of alternative educational activities if writing impaired: (N.D. 1–3)
Verbal reporting.
Computer or typewriter use with unaffected hand.
Student or teacher tutors.

---

* (See Chapter 2, page 38 for explanation of the NANDA approved numerical system.)

Arrange for pain medication at school as appropriate and in accordance with school district policy and procedure. (N.D. 4)

Arrange for elevation of limb in classroom (chair, padded wastebasket, extra desk). Inform teachers of need for this action as necessary. (N.D. 3, 4)

Arrange for partial day attendance, if full day inappropriate, increasing attendance as tolerated. (N.D. 1, 4)

Provide plan for cafeteria access and tray management during meal times. (N.D. 1–3)

Arrange for special transportation through school or community resources. (A three block walk on an affected limb to a bus stop may be impossible, especially in inclement weather conditions). (N.D. 1–3)

Alter physical education program as appropriate. (N.D. 1–3)

Student Interventions

Monitor activity tolerance, and observe for signs of inability to manage the demands of school activity. (N.D. 1–3)

Recommend physician evaluation for swelling, continued pain, limited motion, or obvious limb deformity. (N.D. 3)

Obtain physician recommendations for activity limitations and program for rehabilitation. (N.D. 3)

Encourage ambulation as much as reasonably tolerated and as permitted by medical treatment plan (decreases additional muscle atrophy and increases independence). (N.D. 2, 3)

Instruct student to limit activity and notify nurse of activity which causes pain or extreme fatigue. (N.D. 1–5)

Instruct student in injury care for first forty-eight hours: Rest, Ice, Compression, Elevation (R.I.C.E). (N.D. 3, 5)

Instruct student in appropriate crutch walking technique and to avoid hanging axilla on crutch handles (avoid inappropriate use and use which may result in neurologic or circulatory damage). (N.D. 1–3, 5)

Instruct student in signs which require follow-up physician attention: recurrent or increasing pain, swelling, discoloration, mobility decline. (N.D. 3, 5)

Instruct student to respond to pain (notify school nurse and/or teacher) early in onset to avoid excessive pain development. (N.D. 4, 5)

Instruct student in healing process. (N.D. 3, 5)

Instruct student in ways to care for injury which will promote healing: allow time, avoid reinjury, maintain good fluid and nutritional intake, obtain sufficient rest. (N.D. 3, 5)

Instruct student in cast or brace or sling care to prevent skin excoriation. (N.D. 3, 5)

Identify pressure points on affected limb.
Keep cast, brace, or sling dry.
Petal tape cast edges to prevent rubbing.
Tape or cork pin ends to prevent catching and displacement.

Instruct or arrange for instruction in muscle rebuilding after limb immobilization. (N.D. 3, 5)

- isolated muscle group isometrics
- active range of motion
- active muscle contractions and counter muscle group contractions for relaxation
- full activity
- full activity with weight bearing
- full activity for sports and or physical education class

Instruct student in use of pain medication as appropriate for school. (N.D. 4, 5)

Expected Student Outcomes

Student will apply appropriate first aid measures to an injury and seek medical evaluation. (N.D. 3)

Student will be able to perform as many activities in the educational setting as possible. (N.D. 1, 2)

Student will receive assistance for those activities which s/he requires assistance. (N.D. 1, 2)

Student will be successful in managing mobility to and around school. (N.D. 1, 2)

Student will be able to physically attend all classes. (N.D. 1, 2)

Student will not be excessively fatigued or compensated in healing program by activities in school attendance. (N.D. 1–3)

Student will not experience falls or reinjury in school. (N.D. 3)

Student will not develop circulatory complications. (N.D. 3)

Student will experience diminished or manageable pain at school. (N.D. 4)

Student will be able to accomplish progressively more activities as pain subsides. (N.D. 4)

Student will understand how to care for affected limb or injured site. (N.D. 5)

Student will follow medical limits on activity at school. (N.D. 2, 3, 5)

Student will prevent skin breakdown related to cast, brace, or sling immobilization. (N.D. 3, 5)

Student will understand how to recondition limb or injured site prior to return to sports activities. (N.D. 3, 5)

REFERENCES

1. Backx FJ, Erich WB, Kemper A, Verbeek A. Sports injuries in school-aged children: an epidemiologic study. *Am J Sports Med* 1989; 17 (2): 234–40.
2. Stanitski C. Management of sports injuries in children and adolescents. *Orthop Clin North Am* 1988; 19 (4): 689–98.
3. Webber A. Acute soft-tissue injuries in the young athlete. *Clin Sports Med* 1988; 7 (3): 611–24.

BIBLIOGRAPHY

Coady C, Stanish W. Emergencies in sports: the young athlete. *Clin Sports Med* 1988; 7 (3): 625–40.

Hergenroeder A. Diagnosis and treatment of ankle sprains. *Am J Disabled Child* 1990; 144 (7): 809–14.

McAuely E, Hudash G, Shields K, Albright J, Garrick RR, Wallace R. Injuries in women's gymnastics: the state of the art. *Am J Sports Med* 1987; 15 (6): 124–131S.

O'Neill D, Micheli L. Overuse injuries in the young athlete. *Clin Sports Med* 1988; 7 (3): 591–611.

Puderbaugh S, Canale S, Wendell S. *Nursing Care Planning Guides, A Nursing Diagnosis Approach.* Philadelphia: WB Saunders, 1986.

Roy S, Irvin R. Sports Medicine: *Prevention, Evaluation, Management, and Rehabilitation.* New Jersey: Prentice–Hall, 1983.

Spalj N, Buckwalter K, Oppliger R, Albright J, Stolley J. The school nurse's role in managing athletic injuries. *J School Health* 1989; 59 (6): 271–73.

Steiner M, Grana W. The young athlete's knee: recent advances. *Clin Sports Med* 1988; 7 (3): 527–47.

Wong D, Whaley L. *Clinical Manual of Pediatric Nursing.* 2nd ed. St. Louis: CV Mosby, 1990.

44 | IHP: Substance Abuse

Kathleen M. Kalb

INTRODUCTION

Substance abuse is a growing problem among adolescents.[1-3] By their senior year in high school, 64 percent of adolescents have tried illegal drugs[4] and 6 percent use those substances on a regular basis.[1] The school nurse has the opportunity to assess students in the initial stages of chemical use and help them avoid some of the negative consequences. There is sometimes a reluctance on the part of health professionals to recognize the potential for drug abuse in adolescence, especially in middle-class suburban youth.[4] By being aware of the prevalence of this problem, the nurse can begin to assess which students would benefit from particular types of interventions. Early detection becomes even more imperative in light of evidence that the severity of dependence is related to the age at which experimentation begins, with the youngest drug users at most risk for serious negative consequences.[5]

Process of the Disease

Chemical dependency is subtle and insidious in its early stages. Adolescence is the stage when many drug users begin the process that leads to hard-core substance abuse. Because the more dramatic negative consequences do not become apparent until later in the disease, it is common for

the adolescent to appear relatively symptom-free, thus making detection of the problem even more difficult.

"Dependence" is a term variously defined. Most sources agree that it has several universal characteristics. There is the initial exposure to the substance, which creates a physiologic response and a desire for continued use. With continued use the individual begins to feel increased physical and psychological need for the substance and eventually develops a tolerance to its effects.[1, 2, 5] These steps to dependence are not predictable in their time frames, since much depends on the individual's susceptibility to the substance and on the substance involved.

There is substantial cultural support for the use of drugs, and it is not surprising that 80 to 90 percent of all adolescents age eighteen and under have used alcohol.[1, 5] So called "licit" drugs such as nicotine and alcohol, although technically illegal for use by adolescents, are readily available to them. Developmentally, adolescents are seeking to form an adult identity out of which to function. With media and adult role models encouraging the use of these drugs,[1, 5] it becomes part of normal role rehearsal to try these substances. Ironically, drug-involved youth tend to become prematurely involved in adult life

411

situations (marriage, sexual relationships, employment) and fail to develop positive, internalized adult identities—the very thing they thought they were achieving by imitating the "grown-up" behavior of drug use.[2, 3] It is a very difficult task to pinpoint which adolescents are able to "try on" chemical use and abandon it as they mature, while others are pulled into a cycle of increasing use and eventual dependency.[4, 6]

The distinction between experimental use of chemicals and chronic or abusive use of a chemical is an important one and at times difficult to make.[2, 5] The first may be normal adolescent behavior and the latter represents a pathological response.[4] The nurse should not fall into the trap of seeing drug use as normal behavior, since this makes it less likely that a diagnosis will be sought.[4] At the same time it should be recognized that it is possible for an adolescent to engage in an "abnormal" behavior temporarily as (s)he tries to find a stable identity with which to transition into adulthood.

Use of alcohol rises steeply between the tenth and twelfth grades.[5] This makes it critical that adults who work with youth in the school setting are aware of the problem and are prepared to deal with it. Alcohol use seems to be more likely in white adolescents than in blacks, in higher socioeconomic groups, and highest of all among American Indian youth.[5] Chemical use tends to follow a general progression from legally available substances (such as alcohol and tobacco) to "harder," illegal substances.[5-8] The nurse should not inadvertently give students the impression that some drugs are less serious than others. (For example, parents have been known to express relief when learning that their adolescent is using alcohol instead of "hard" drugs.) Understanding this progression, as well as other behaviors associated with drug use, gives the nurse an awareness of which adolescents are most at risk. For

example, marijuana use is positively associated with use of alcohol and tobacco, with family use of chemicals, and with dating at an early age.[2, 5, 8] Youngsters who have eating disorders are more likely to be substance users.[8] In families with high levels of anxiety, tension between parents, rejection by parents, and/or little maternal control the adolescents are much more likely to begin drug involvement.[5, 7] However, it should be noted that: *the greatest single variable for predicting an adolescent's substance use is use by friends.*[2, 9] When evaluating an adolescent for chemical abuse, context is all-important.

The negative consequences of drug involvement are numerous and serious. Alcohol-related auto accidents are the leading cause of death among 16- to 24-year-olds.[5] Up to half of teen suicides and accidental deaths may be related to chemical use.[5] Learning impairment, as well as brain and organ damage have been seen in users of marijuana and/or alcohol.[5]

Beyond alcohol, tobacco, and marijuana are a host of other, "harder" drugs. Different categories of drugs have different effects on the individual, and varying addictive potential. See Table 1 for common classes of drugs and their effects.[1, 10]

Of the categories of drugs in the table, depressants and opiates lead to strong physical and psychological dependence; stimulants, hallucinogens, and volatile solvents lead to strong psychological dependence. Stimulants, hallucinogens, opiates, and volatile solvents produce tolerance as well.[1]

Treatment Options

Opinions vary on what constitutes appropriate treatment for chemically dependent children and adolescents. There are several options for treatment, depending on the stage of chemical dependency, availability of treatment alternatives, and the family's resources.

Table 1. Common Classes of Drugs and Their Effects

Class of Drug	Psychophysiologic Effect	Common Symptoms
Stimulants (Amphetamine, nicotine, caffeine, cocaine)	Increased alertness and activity, increased central nervous system activity	Restlessness, agitation sweating, dilated pupils dry mouth, diarrhea, increases in pulse, and temperature
Depressants Barbiturates (phenobarbital, pentathal sodium, amobarbital, butabarbital, secobarbital)	Decreased central nervous system activity, anxiety reduction, sleep induction	Respiratory depression, pupil constriction and/or lateral nystagmus, lethargy, drowsiness
Nonbarbiturate Sedatives (methaqualone, flurazepam, glutethimide, methypryllon)	Same as Barbiturates	Dilated pupils, hypotension fluctuating levels of consciousness
Narcotics/opiates (morphine, heroin, meperidine, methadone, others)	Pain Reduction	Similar to barbiturates, evidence of injection
Minor tranquilizers (diazepam, chlordiazepoxide)	Reduction of anxiety, muscle relaxation	Drowsiness, poor muscle coordination, confusion, skin rash, nausea
Major tranquilizers (mostly phenothiazines)	Reduction of psychosis	Pupil constriction, hypotension, tremors, extrapyramidal movements, cardiac arrythmias
Hallucinogens ("LSD," D-lysergic acid; Mescaline; "DMT," Dimethyltryptamine; "STP," dimetnoxy-4-methylamphetamine; "PCP," phencyclidine hydrochloride)	Alterations in sensation, emotional status, and awareness	Hallucinations, perceptual changes, psychosis
Tricyclics (Doxepin, imipramine, amitriptyline, desiprimine, nortriptyline)	Relief of depression	Hypotension, arrythmias, choreoathetoid movements, dry mouth, urinary retention
Volatile Solvents (glue, cement, various sprays, gasoline, some cleaning solutions)	CNS depressants	Similar to barbiturates

Adolescents are in a stage of identity formation. Since this identity almost invariably includes role-taking within a peer group, the peer influence on chemical use must be considered when referring a student for chemical dependency evaluation or treatment. It is important that referral sources be aware of the issues which differentiate adolescent chemical dependency treatment from adult chemical dependency treatment.[2, 4, 6, 7]

The context within which the student has become chemically involved must be considered in order to achieve successful treatment. Approaches which include group counseling (in a group of *adolescent* substance users), and family counseling stand the greatest chance of impacting the student's environmental factors.[1, 4, 5, 7, 11–13] (Individual therapy does not seem to be very effective in this age group, except in cases where there is serious underlying mental pathology.[5]) Family involvement may be resisted by both the adolescent and by individual family members.[5, 7, 11] When making a referral, it is best if the agency is one where the counselors are skilled at engaging families in the treatment process, and who can teach the families to respond in positive ways to the adolescent's problem.[7, 11, 12]

Once it has been determined that the student's chemical use is problematic, treatment is usually indicated on an outpatient basis. Only those whose chemical use has progressed to strong physiologic dependence are appropriate for inpatient therapy.[5] This may raise a number of ethical issues in cases where parents opt for inpatient therapy, and whose insurance covers such care, but whose child does not seem sufficiently compromised by chemical use to indicate such serious measures. Parents should be made aware of the danger in labeling their child chemically dependent if he or she is not yet at the stage of true dependence, as well as the danger involved in placing a relatively naive ado-

lescent in a peer structure of serious, chronic drug users.[2]

Evaluation of local resources is a difficult task. There are many factors to sort out in determining which programs might be appropriate for the students in a nurse's caseload. Following are some areas to consider when investigating treatment programs, and will provide answers to questions frequently posed by the student and his/her family.[4, 5, 7, 14]

- How successful is the program?
  Questions to ask:
  - What is the rate of recidivism (return to drug use following treatment)?
  - How do people in the program feel about it? (Ask this directly of participants and former participants.)

- Whom does it serve?
  Questions to ask:
  - How many clients are in the program?
  - What are their ages?
  - What is the process for admission? Referral process?

- What does the program include?
  Questions to ask:
  - What types of therapy or treatment are available? (Individual, family, group.)
  - What type of peer component is offered?
  - How long is the average course of treatment?
  - What provisions are made for aftercare? (Posttreatment success is influenced positively by participation in aftercare programs.[14]) Is the family involved in aftercare planning? Can the school be included in the aftercare planning?

- Is the program drug-free? (Programs that do not include total abstinence from psychoactive drugs seem to be less successful for adolescents than those which insist on a drug-free client.[4])

- What does the program cost? Is this cost covered by insurance? What provisions are made for those who can't afford the program?

- What are the credentials of the staff? (A combination of mature professionals and well-trained former users is desirable.[4])

- What are the program's connections with community and other resources? Listen for close relationships with medicine, psychiatry, educational resources, and job training programs.

- What sort of self-evaluation does the program do to foster improvement of services?

- What is the general attitude of the staff and personnel? As you explore the program, notice whether there seems to be a genuine concern for the clients. Do you notice an atmosphere of optimism, enthusiasm and respect? Note whether the program seems most oriented toward positive outcome or financial remuneration. How do you feel after talking to them on the phone or visiting the setting? Don't disregard subjective impressions, but don't make final judgments about a program after one phone call or interaction with the staff.

After gathering information on a given program or therapist, it is important to make a list of the most appropriate resources to which you might refer.[5, 7] Include on this list local physicians who are aware of the issues in chemical abuse and who would be willing to consult on cases from the school setting.

INDIVIDUALIZED HEALTHCARE PLAN

History*

An accurate history is of utmost importance in determining the student's current and projected substance use. Since this is a sensitive topic, with moral and legal implications, it is common for the student to be wary or defensive during any interview regarding chemical use.[4, 9] The nurse who is nonthreatening, honest, and nonjudging has a better chance of gaining the student's trust, and therefore of getting an accurate history.[1, 4, 8, 15] It is important to provide adequate time and privacy so the student may be as relaxed as possible.

It may be helpful to approach chemical use as part of the general history.[4, 7, 9] The school nurse could begin with a diet history, moving to use of prescription drugs, over-the-counter remedies, and finally illicit substances. This progression from least to most threatening questions will give the adolescent a chance to become comfortable with the nurse and with the process of giving information. Questions about tobacco products are an appropriate lead-in and can be followed by questions regarding alcohol use and finally by questions referring to use of street drugs. Confidentiality is a major factor in whether the adolescent feels safe answering questions honestly. The nurse should know what state law allows for protection of adolescent confidentiality and take this into account when gathering sensitive information.

---

*For a detailed and helpful description of the assessment process and interview, see: Anglin T. Interviewing Guidelines for the Clinical Evaluation of Adolescent Substance Abuse. *Pediatr Clin North Am* 1987; 34 (2): 381-398.

The adolescent's perception of peer activity is an indirect way to get information on his or her own drug use. Here are some questions that will give an idea of how the student perceives "typical" chemical use by others.[1, 8]

- Do most of the kids in your school drink or get into drugs?
- Do any of your friends use drugs? What kinds? How hard are they to get for someone your age? Is it easy for kids to get alcohol?
- Do most of the parties for high school kids include drugs or drinking? Have you been to any of these parties? What are they like?

If the teenager discusses the school as a place where the majority of his/her peers are using alcohol and other chemicals, this use is more likely seen as acceptable or even normative, which increases the chance that the student will be using chemicals on weekdays and jeopardizing school performance.

To get at the question of usage patterns, the adolescent may be more comfortable discussing this in a historical framework.[9] Note during the interview whether the adolescent seems particularly animated or positive when describing what it's like to get high. Here are some questions which might be useful.[5, 8]

- How old were you when you first tried alcohol (marijuana, tobacco, speed, other chemicals that the student has previously described using)?
- What was the experience like?
- When was the first time you ever got really high (drunk)?
- What was that experience like?

History of the usage pattern is also indicative of whether the chemical involvement is deepening or staying at an experimental level.

- When you get high, what do you usually use?
- How much does it take for you to get high? How does this compare to six months ago? A year ago?
- Where are you when you use? (home, school, friend's home, other)
- Do you use during the week, or on weekends only?
- Why do you usually use? Are you usually with friends or alone?
- How often do you use in a month?
- Have you noticed any problems that seem to be related to using?
- Do you ever have periods of time that you don't remember after you have been drunk or high? Are you ever ill or depressed the day after you have used?

Since family use of chemicals increases the risk that an adolescent will use,[1, 3, 5, 6, 8, 13] a few questions on family history are appropriate.[3, 4, 8]

- Does anyone in your family use alcohol or other chemicals?
  How often do they use?
- Do you think anyone in your family drinks too much or does drugs too often? What do you do when this is bothering you? What kinds of problems has this caused for you?
- Has anyone in your family been in treatment for alcohol or drug use? How did that go for them? How was it for you? Did it seem to change your family in any way?
- Has anyone in your family been ill or died from any illness related to drinking or drug use? Who was it and what was the illness?
- How are things going at home generally? Do you get along with your parents? If not, how do you and your parents usually solve conflicts?

Assessment

Note: Assessment of the adolescent chemical user is not solely the job of the school nurse. The questions and quidelines presented here are intended to give the nurse a baseline of information which can then be used to work with chemical health personnel, physicians, school social workers, family members, and the student to determine the best course of action in each particular case.

Current Status

Assessing current status for a student who is using chemicals includes some measure of where the student is functioning academically and socially as well as the usual physical and psychological assessments. Separating the experimental or one-time user from the chronic user can be a trying task, but the interview may provide clues. One place to start is in getting a sense of the adolescent's general development. Following are some questions the nurse can ask to determine whether the student is paying a developmental price for his/her chemical involvement.[4]

- Is school difficult for you? How are you doing in school this semester? Do you seem to be passing all your subjects? How does that compare to last year?
- Are you getting along with your friends? Do you have about the same friends as last year? How many of them do you consider really close friends?
- How old are most of your friends? Have any of them ever been in treatment for alcohol or drug use? Have any of them been in trouble with the law when they were drinking or getting high?

Falling grades, drastic changes in friendships, and friends either much younger or much older (greater than 2 years) are all indications that something in this student's life may be compromising development. Friends who have been in treatment or who have had involvement with the law increase the likelihood that this student is involved similarly.

Physical Assessment

The dramatic and serious medical complications resulting from chemical use are not evident until later in the disease and adolescents commonly have few or no medical conditions related to their drug use. More often there are subtle symptoms such as long-running upper respiratory symptoms, reddened eyes, or signs of trauma—either from needles or from violence. The nasal septum may show signs of irritation or perforation from cocaine use. Note any change in level of consciousness, alertness, and coordination.

There may be tachycardia with use of amphetamines, and changes in level of consciousness or abnormal vital signs may indicate acute drug use. For other typical responses to acute drug use, see the "Common Symptoms" column of Table 1.

Note the student's affect, appropriateness of eye contact, and physical appearance.[4] Although unconventional dress may be a normal manifestation of adolescence, note whether there is identification with drug culture through dress or jewelry.[4]

Psychological/Emotional Assessment

Psychological assessment is never clear-cut for an adolescent and this is doubly true in the adolescent who complicates the picture with drug abuse. Some questions to determine general psychological status are important.

- On a scale of 1 to 10 in which one is the worst and 10 is the very best, how would you rate your life right now? What are you good at? What plans do you have for when you finish high school?
- Have you felt down or depressed lately? How long did it last? What did you do about it?
- Do you feel sad or depressed now?
- Do your feelings change when you use chemicals? How do you usually feel when the drug wears off? Is this ever a problem for you?
- Have you ever felt like hurting yourself or anyone else? Was this when you were using any drug? What happened when you felt that way?
- Have you ever tried to hurt or kill yourself? Do you feel that way now?
- How are things going with your family? Friends? Teachers?
- Who do you talk to when things are going badly? Does that usually help?
- If you could change one thing about your life, what would it be?

Listen for the student's general attitude, self-esteem, hints of depression or suicidality. Note whether the student makes any connection between drug use and negative consequences. Follow up on hints of physical or sexual abuse, since children of substance abusers are more likely to be abused by their parents.[16] It is common for students at risk for substance abuse to show evidence of low self-esteem and depression.[1, 4, 9]

Nursing Diagnoses (N.D.)

N.D. 1 Ineffective individual coping (NANDA 5.1.1.1)* secondary to chemical use.
N.D. 2 Ineffective family coping (NANDA 5.1.2.1.2 and/or 1) secondary to chemical use.
N.D. 3 Self-concept: disturbance in self-esteem. (NANDA 7.1.2)
N.D. 4 Potential for injury (NANDA 1.6.1) secondary to drug use or overdose.
N.D. 5 Knowledge deficit (NANDA 8.1.1) regarding consequences of chemical use.
N.D. 6 Impaired social interaction (NANDA 3.1.1) secondary to chemical use.

Goals

The school nurse will:

- Assess student's current drug use.
- Work with other disciplines to form an optimal treatment plan for the particular student.
- Monitor student's progress in dealing with chemical involvement.

Nursing Interventions

Update history as above to provide foundation for nursing assessment and information for referral. (N.D. 1–6)

Determine whether student seems to be using chemicals regularly. (N.D. 3–5)

Determine what are the student's support systems are and whether they would support him/her through counseling for chemical use. (N.D. 1, 2)

---

* (See Chapter 2, page 38 for explanation of the NANDA approved numerical system.)

Communicate with other professionals within the school system as appropriate to form an effective treatment plan for the student. (N.D. 1–6)

Refer for further evaluation and treatment if the student is chemically involved. (N.D. 4, 5)

Refer for mental health counseling immediately if signs of depression or suicidality are noted during assessment. (N.D. 1)

Indicate genuine concern and inform student of nurse's availability for further support. (N.D. 1, 3, 5)

Work with other disciplines to encourage family involvement in assessment and treatment process. (N.D. 2)

Follow up with student on a weekly or biweekly basis to determine effectiveness of treatment and student's emotional status. (N.D. 1–6)

Expected Student Outcomes

- The student will cooperate with assessment process and counseling appointments as shown by attendance at same.

- The student will decrease chemical use as evidenced by self-report and improvements in areas compromised by chemical use (e.g., school performance, social interactions, family relationships, involvement with law enforcement agencies, other).

- The student will show increased ability to handle stress without chemical use as indicated by self-report and objective observation.

- The student will cooperate with involving family in assessment and treatment as indicated.

- The student will experience increased self-esteem as demonstrated by:
    Ability to take part comfortably in group activities.
    Ability to take social risks.
    Appropriate eye contact when interacting verbally.
    Affect reflecting comfort or positive emotional status.
    Ability to express positive opinion of self.

- The student will avoid injury both by avoiding intravenous use of chemicals and by avoiding violent situations which have potential for injury.

- The student will demonstrate awareness of the consequences of chemical use by both direct statement and behavior change to avoid negative consequences.

- The student will demonstrate appropriate social behavior as indicated by:
    Peer group which supports student's self-esteem.
    Self-reported comfort in social situations.
    Observed interactions with peers.

REFERENCES

*1. Neinstein LS. *Adolescent Healthcare, A Practical Guide.* Baltimore: Urban and Schwarzenberg, 1984.

2. Newcomb MD, Bentler PM. Substance use and abuse among children and teenagers. *Am Psychologist* 1989; 44 (2): 242–48.

*3. Robertson JF. A tool for assessing alcohol misuse in adolescence. *Social Work* 1989; (Jan): 39–44.

*4. Macdonald DI. Diagnosis and treatment of adolescent substance abuse. *Curr Probl Peadiatr* 1989; 19 (8): 389–444.

5. Henderson D, Anderson S. Adolescents and chemical dependency. *Social Work in Healthcare* 1989; 14 (1): 87–105.

*6. Bailey GW. Current perspectives on substance abuse in youth. *J Am Acad Adolesc Psychiatry* 1988; 28 (2): 151–62.

*7. Farrow JA, Deisher R. A practical guide to the office assessment of adolescent substance abuse. *Pediatr Ann* 1986; 15 (10): 675–84.

8. Riggs S, Alrio AJ. Adolescent substance use and the role of the primary care provider. *Rhode Island Med J* 1990; 73 (6): 253–57.

*9. Anglin T. Interviewing guidelines for the clinical evaluation of adolescent substance abuse. *Pediatr Clin North Am* 1987; 34 (2): 381–98.

10. Boston Women's Health Book Collective. *The New Our Bodies, Ourselves.* New York: Simon and Schuster, 1984.

11. Kurtines WM. Engaging adolescent drug abusers and their families in treatment: a strategic structural systems approach. *J Consult Clin Psychol* 1988; 56 (4): 552–57.

12. Szapocznik J, et al. Family effectiveness training: an intervention to prevent drug abuse and problem behaviors in hispanic adolescents. *Hispanic J Behav Sciences* 1989; 11 (1): 4–27.

13. Weis DM, et al. Family therapy and group counseling: therapeutic factors and the chemically dependent adolescent. *J Specialists Group Work* 1988; 13 (4): 218–23.

14. Fertman C, Toca O. A Drug and Alcohol Aftercare Service: Linking Adolescents, Families, and Schools. Pittsburgh: University of Pittsburgh, School of Education, *J Alcohol and Drug Ed* 1988; 34 (2): 46–33.

15. American Academy of Pediatrics, Center for Advanced Health Studies. *Substance Abuse: A Guide for Health Professionals.* American Academy of Pediatrics/Pacific Institute for Research and Evaluation, 141 NW Point Blvd, Box 927, Elk Grove Village, IL 60009-0927, 1988.

16. Bays J. Substance abuse and child abuse: impact of addiction of the child. *Pediatr Clin North Am* 1990; 37 (4): 881–904.

---

* These references contain guidelines, checklists, and/or tools which may be helpful in an assessment interview.

IHP: Tourette's Syndrome

Mary J. Villars Gerber

INTRODUCTION

Gilles de la Tourette syndrome (Tourette's syndrome) is a tic condition that may begin from the time of early childhood through adolescence, ages two through fifteen. Genetic studies suggest a familial incidence of tics. It is a disorder of the central nervous system. Criteria for diagnosis[1] include:

- Age of onset
- Rapid, recurrent, repetitive, purposeless, involuntary motor movements, affecting multiple groups of muscles
- Multiple vocal tics
- Ability to suppress movements voluntarily for minutes to hours
- Variations in the intensity of symptoms over weeks or months
- Duration of more than one year

Other behavioral difficulties may include attentional problems and compulsions and obsessions. Estimates indicate that up to 50 percent of people with Tourette's syndrome have attention deficit disorder.

Treatment with medication is indicated for tics only if symptoms are severe enough to cause psychosocial difficulties with family, teachers, or peers, or if they adversely affect the child's development or school functioning. Medications utilized include haloperidol (Haldol), pimozide (Orap), and clonidine (Catapres). Side effects of these medications can be significant. Side effects of haloperidol include depression, phobias, sedation, cognitive blunting, weight gain, acute dystonic reactions, parkinsonian symptoms, and akisthesia. Extra pyramidal side effects may be treated with Cogentin. Side effects of pimozide are similar to those of haloperidol. Clonidine is an antihypertensive medication that is sometimes used to treat Tourette's syndrome. Side effects may include sedation.

Other forms of treatment may include diet restrictions of sugar, chocolate, caffeine, and red/yellow food coloring.

INDIVIDUALIZED HEALTHCARE PLAN

History

At what age were tics first observed?
What type of tics (motor/vocal) have been observed?
Have there been changes in tics over time?
How long have symptoms been present?
What types of medical intervention have been used?

Assessment

- Family understanding of the condition and ability to provide support to the student. It is important for the child's family to understand the condition and be offered support as needed.

- Utilize "Teacher's Checklist on Tourette's syndrome: Range of Symptoms,"[2] to determine current symptoms observed.

- Assessment of student's level of development. The student may demonstrate delays in some areas due to nature and chronicity of the condition.

- Medications. The student may need medications in school. Side effects of the medication should be well known to the staff working with the student. Program accommodations may need to be established.

- Suppression of symptoms. Some individuals may have the ability to suppress symptoms for short periods of time. It will be important to know if the student is able to do this.

- Adjustment and coping. Assessment of social adjustment, peer relationships, and self-esteem will influence the student's educational performance.

- Stressful situations that will precipitate or exacerbate tic frequency. These situations will need to be determined and will influence the special program needs the student may have.

Nursing Diagnoses (N.D.)

N.D. 1 Altered growth and development (NANDA 6.6)* related to (specify).

N.D. 2 Alterations in family processes (NANDA 3.2.2) related to difficulty adjusting to family member with Tourette's syndrome.

N.D. 3 Impaired social interractions (NANDA 3.1.1) related to (specify) secondary to chronic condition.

N.D. 4 Self-esteem disturbance. (NANDA 7.1.2)

N.D. 5 Ineffective individual coping (NANDA 5.1.1.1) related to stress in response to presence of uncontrollable tics.

N.D. 6 Ineffective individual coping (NANDA 5.1.1.1) related to depression in response to uncontrollable tics.

N.D. 7 Noncompliance (NANDA 5.2.1.1) related to poor concentration or inability to suppress symptoms.

---

* (See Chapter 2, page 38 for explanation of the NANDA approved numerical system.)

Goals

Goals related to growth and development specific to student attainment of specified developmentally appropriate skills or behaviors. (N.D. 1)

Support positive family adjustment and growth. (N.D. 2)

Support positive social relationships. (N.D. 3)

Promote increased self-esteem. (N.D. 4)

Reduce stressful situations. (N.D. 5, 6)

Provide alternative methods to task completion. (N.D. 7)

Nursing Interventions

Provide opportunities for the student to meet age-related developmental tasks. (Specify) Based on assessment data, program modifications may be necessary for the student to have the opportunity to accomplish developmental tasks. (N.D.1)

Administer medications as appropriate. Observe for side effects. Maintain current medical orders and documentation of medications administered during school hours. (N.D. 1)

Assessment of family processes: family members' response to condition, behavior toward student, family communication and roles, access and use of healthcare, use of community resources. Family functioning and support for the child will influence student's adjustment at home and at school. (N.D. 2)

Be supportive to family. (N.D. 2)

Facilitate family strengths. (N.D. 2)

Facilitate understanding among family members. Clarification of misunderstanding can facilitate positive family responses. (N.D. 2)

Provide anticipatory guidance to family. (N.D. 2)

Initiate health teaching and referrals to family as necessary. Refer family to local Tourette's syndrome association. (N.D. 2)

Provide classmates with age-appropriate information to encourage understanding and empathy. Encourage parent participation as appropriate. (N.D. 3)

Provide opportunity for positive peer interraction and development of social skills. (N.D. 3)

Provide positive feedback to student. Give immediate feedback to student regarding social situations to foster appropriate interpretation. Regular counseling may be needed to promote positive self-esteem. Refer to appropriate professional for counseling as appropriate. (N.D. 4–6)

In-service staff on Tourette's syndrome. Provide support to staff. (N.D. 1–7)

Reduce or eliminate causative or contributing factors that result in increased stress and noncompliance. Provide alternative methods for task completion. Eliminate time limits if possible. Utilize oral methods of task completion if the student has difficulty with handwriting. Classmates can share copies of notes taken in class. Provide tape-recorded information or information to the student who has difficulty with blocking or "getting stuck" on printed material. Provide moderately structured classroom setting. Allow the student private space to discharge obsessive-compulsive urges until the urge has passed. Provide a safe "time-out" space for students whose symptoms become overwhelming. (N.D. 7)

Expected Student Outcomes

The student will demonstrate an increase in behaviors in personal/social, language, cognition, motor activities appropriate to age group (specify the behaviors). (N.D. 1)

The student will give/receive support within the family system. (N.D. 2)

The student/family will seek appropriate resources when needed. (N.D. 2)

The student will establish and maintain supportive relationships/friendships. (N.D. 3)

The student will identify positive aspects about self, interract appropriately with others, and participate in activities. (N.D. 4)

The student will demonstrate appropriate responses in situations geared to minimize stress. (N.D. 5)

The student verbalizes feelings related to emotional state. Accepts support from trusted individuals. Is able to make decisions and take appropriate action based on abilities. (N.D. 6)

The student will complete expected tasks given alternative methods for task completion. (N.D. 7)

REFERENCES

1. Ort S. Tourette's Syndrome and the School Nurse. Bayside, NY: Tourette's Syndrome Asssociation, 1984.
2. Colligan N. Recognizing Tourette's syndrome in the classroom. *School Nurse* 1989; (Dec): 8–12.

BIBLIOGRAPHY

Carpenito LJ. *Nursing Diagnosis, Application To Clinical Practice.* Philadelphia: JB Lippincott, 1989.
Hagin RA, Beecher R, Kreeger H, Pagano G. *Guidelines for the Education of Children With Tourette's Syndrome.* Bayside, NY: Tourette's Syndrome Association, 1980.
Parker K. Helping school-age children cope with Tourette's syndrome. *J School Health* 1985; 55 (Jan): 30–2.
Shapiro E. The role of the school nurse in tic and Tourette's syndromes. *School Nurse* 1982; (Fall).
Tourette's Syndrome Association. 42-40 Bell Blvd, Bayside, NY 11361. Resources for education of families, children, and professionals; legal aids; scientific and research materials.

46 | IHP: Ventriculo-Peritoneal Shunts

Mary J. Villars Gerber

INTRODUCTION

If the flow of cerebrospinal fluid (CSF) is obstructed from the fourth ventricle of the brain to the meninges surrounding the spinal cord, a condition called hydrocephalus occurs. This condition also occurs when there is an imbalance in the production and absorption of the CSF. Cerebrospinal fluid accumulates within the ventricular system causing the ventricles to become dilated and the brain tissue to be compressed against the surrounding bony tissue. If this condition develops before the cranial sutures fuse, there is an enlargement in size of the skull and dilation of the ventricles. This condition typically is evidenced in early infancy, but may occur into late childhood or early adulthood. Causes include tumors, infections such as meningitis, intraventricular hemorrhage, and trauma. Developmental abnormalities where this condition is evidenced account for most of the cases of hydrocephalus from birth to age two. They include Arnold-Chiari malformations, aqueduct stenosis, aqueduct gliosis, and myelomeningocele.[1]

Treatment includes relief of the hydrocephalus, treatment of complications, and management of problems related to the effects of the disorder on psychomotor development. Direct removal of an obstruction is sometimes possible. However, in most cases, children require the placement of a shunt that provides drainage from the ventricles usually to the peritoneum. This procedure requires fewer revisions than the ventriculoatrial shunt because there is more space for the placement of extra tubing to accommodate for the child's growth. Major complications include infection and shunt malfunction. Of those children treated for the condition, approximately one third are intellectually and neurologically in normal limits. About one half have neurologic disabilities with deficits in nonverbal processing skills. Children who are untreated and survive have significant physical and neurologic handicaps including ataxia, spastic diplegia, perceptual deficits, and poor fine motor coordination.

INDIVIDUALIZED HEALTHCARE PLAN

History

What is the medical diagnosis related to etiology of hydrocephalus?
What age was the diagnosis made?
What treatment has been provided?
At what age was shunt placement done and what type of shunt was placed?
What is the date of the last revision?

Assessment

- Emergency medical care information including physician name and phone number, hospital, parents' names and phone numbers, emergency phone numbers, and insurance coverage. This information will be necessary in the event a shunt malfunction is suspected.

- Observation of typical behavior in school setting. Irritability and changes in the child's interraction with their environment can be a sign of increased intracranial pressure.

- Physical exam. Observe site of shunt placement. Redness along the tract site can be a sign of a nonfunctioning shunt.

Nursing Diagnoses (N.D.)

N.D. 1 Potential for injury (NANDA 1.6.1)* related to inability to support large head and strain on neck.

N.D. 2 Potential for injury (NANDA 1.6.1) related to increased intracranial pressure.

N.D. 3 Potential for infection (NANDA 1.2.1.1) related to presence of mechanical drainage system.

N.D. 4 Potential impaired skin integrity (NANDA 1.6.2.1.2.2) related to impaired ability to move head secondary to size

N.D. 5 Potential altered health maintenance (NANDA 6.4.2) related to insufficient knowledge of (specify) signs and symptoms of infection, increased intracranial pressure, emergency treatment of shunt malfunction.

Goals

Prevent injury related to inability to support head. (N.D. 1)
Prevent injury related to increased intracranial pressure. (N.D. 2)
Prevent infection and/or assess for early signs of infection. (N.D. 3)
Prevent impaired skin integrity. (N.D. 4)
Health teaching for student/family as appropriate. (N.D. 5)

Nursing Interventions

Support student's head during transfers and change of position. Position to provide head support. Some students with very large head size will need assistance with all movement and positioning. (N.D. 1)

---

* (See Chapter 2, page 38 for explanation of the NANDA approved numerical system.)

Observe and teach others to observe for signs of increased intracranial pressure. These can be signs of a nonfunctioning shunt and will need immediate attention. (N.D. 2)

Infants

Bulging fontanelle
Vomiting
Irritability
Change in appetite
Lethargy
Sunsetting eyes
Seizures
Swelling along shunt tract
Redness along shunt tract

Toddlers

Vomiting
Lethargy
Irritability
Seizures
Headaches
Swelling along shunt tract
Redness along shunt tract

School Age

Headaches
Vomiting
Lethargy
Seizures
Irritability
Swelling along shunt tract
Decreased school performance

Establish plan of action should a shunt malfunction be suspected, or if trauma to the head has occurred. (N.D. 1, 2)

Establish activity restrictions. Generally all activities are allowed with the exception of contact sports which could pose risk of injury. (N.D. 1, 2)

Refer for speech and language assessment, occupational therapy, physical therapy, psychological assessment as appropriate. (N.D. 1, 2)

Observe for signs of infection along shunt tract. Shunt infection can occur at any time, but the period of greatest risk is one to two months following placement. (N.D. 3)

Inspect skin for signs of irritation, redness, or pressure points. Change position frequently. Use sheepskin, egg-crate foam or other resilient surfaces to protect pressure points when positioning. Observe for cleanliness of scalp. When a student is unable to assume normal mobility due to head size, these interventions are necessary to prevent skin breakdown. (N.D. 4)

Promote student/family learning and provide health teaching related to knowledge needed. (N.D. 5)

Expected Student Outcomes

Experiences no evidence of injury related to movement of head. (N.D. 1)
Experiences no evidence of increased intracranial pressure. (N.D. 2)
Receives immediate access to medical care should signs of increased intracranial pressure occur. (N.D. 2)

Exhibits no evidence of infection. Receives prompt medical care should signs of infection be evident. (N.D. 3)

Exhibits no evidence of skin breakdown. (N.D. 4)

Student/family is able to describe symptoms of infection, skin breakdown, shunt malfunction, emergency treatment needed for malfunction. (N.D. 5)

Collaborative Problems

Potential complication: increased intracranial pressure

Potential complication: sepsis

REFERENCES

1. Wong DL, Whaley LF. *Clinical Manual of Pediatric Nursing.* St. Louis: CV Mosby, 1990.

BIBLIOGRAPHY

Batshaw ML, Perret YM. *Children with Handicaps A Medical Primer.* Baltimore: Paul H. Brookes Publishing, 1981.

Carpenito LJ. *Handbook of Nursing Diagnosis.* Philadelphia: JB Lippincott, 1989.

Carpenito LJ. *Nursing Diagnosis, Application to Clinical Practice.* Philadelphia: JB Lippincott, 1989.

Whaley LF, Wong DL. *Nursing Care of Infants and Children.* St. Louis: CV Mosby, 1987.

Appendices

INDIVIDUAL HEALTH PLAN

ASSESSMENT	NURSING DIAGNOSES	GOALS	INTERVENTIONS	STUDENT OUTCOMES

EMERGENCY CARE PLAN

Date plan written _____ ID # _____

Student name _____ Birthdate _____ Grade _____

Parent _____ Emergency phone numbers _____

Doctor _____ Phone number _____

Hospital _____ Phone number (911) or _____

Medical insurance (optional) _____

****

Medical condition: _____

Usual treatment: _____

_____

Signs of emergency: _____

_____

_____

Actions for teacher to take: _____

_____

_____

_____

_____

_____

****

Date of event: _____

Student's response to emergency measures: _____

_____

Principal notified _____ Time _____ School Nurse Notified _____ Time _____

Doctor notified _____ Time _____ Parent notified _____ Time _____

ACADEMIC ASSESSMENT GUIDE
Susan I. Simandl Will

In planning an IHP for students, the school nurse's unique skill is integrating a plan to meet health needs with a plan to meet academic needs. This assessment guideline may be used to supplement the assessment in chapters for particular health problems. With assessment data from this tool, school nurses can develop nursing diagnoses, goals, interventions, and expectations for students which address their developmental, social, and academic needs.

DEVELOPMENTAL/ACADEMIC/SOCIAL ASSESSMENT	DATA SUMMARY
What is the student's age and developmental level?	
Is physical development appropriate to student's age?	
Do fine motor, gross motor, language and social skills seem age appropriate?	
How does the student get along with peers: Cooperative? Isolated? Conflictive?	
What are the student's support systems: family, friends, church, school groups, other?	
What is the student's knowledge level on issues of sexuality? Is this appropriate for age?	
Are sexual activities and interests age appropriate and developmentally appropriate? Safe?	
What are the student's developmental and social strengths? Weaknesses?	

	DATA SUMMARY
What are the student's patterns of academic performance as indicated by review of academic or cumulative school record? Grades? GPA? Failures? Retentions? Changes in academic performance?	
What are teachers' perceptions of student's performance and classroom behavior?	
How does the student compare in behavior, social skills, and academic performance to peer norms? (standardized tests, general perceptions)	
What is the student's school absence pattern? Current? Previous?	
Is there a potential need for special education services to adequately educate the student (P.L. 94-142)? (For example, transportation, classroom adaptation, tutoring, occupational or physical therapy, vocational guidance)	
What are the student's intellectual abilities? Presence of learning disability or developmental delay?	
What are the student's academic strengths?	
What are the student's academic weaknesses?	
How does the student feel about school? Likes? Dislikes?	
What are the student's perceptions of own school related strengths?	
What are the student's perceptions of personal areas for school related improvement?	

STUDENTS WITH SPECIAL HEALTH CARE NEEDS

EMERGENCY PLAN

Student: _____   Date: _____

Birthdate: _____

Preferred hospital in case of emergency: _____

Physician: _____   Phone #: _____

STUDENT-SPECIFIC EMERGENCIES

If You See This	*Do This*

IF AN EMERGENCY OCCURS:

1. If the emergency is life-threatening, immediately call 9-1-1.

2. Stay with student or designate another adult to do so.

3. Call or designate someone to call the principal and/or school nurse.

    a. State who you are.

    b. State where you are.

    c. State problem.

4. The following staff members are trained to deal with an emergency, and to initiate the appropriate procedures:

    _____

    _____

Adapted From: *Guidelines for Serving Students with Special Healthcare Needs*, Utah State Office of Education, August 1992

STUDENTS WITH SPECIAL HEALTH CARE NEEDS

TRANSPORTATION PLAN

Bus Number: _____   ☐ a.m.   ☐ p.m.

Bus Driver: _____

Student's Name: _____

Address: _____

_____

Home Phone: _____

Father's Work Phone: _____

Mother's Work Phone: _____

Student's
Photo

Babysitter's Name: _____   Phone: _____

Address: _____

School: _____   Teacher: _____

Disability / Diagnosis: _____

Medications: _____

Side Effects: _____

1. Mode of transportation on bus. (check one)

    ☐ wheelchair   ☐ car seat   ☐ seat belt   ☐ chest harness

2. Walks up bus stairs independently:

    ☐ Yes   ☐ No

3. Student's method of communication: _____

4. Behavioral difficulties student displays: _____

5. Equipment that must be transported on bus (including oxygen, life-sustaining equipment, wheelchair equipment, climate control, etc.)

    _____

    _____

Source: *Guidelines for Serving Students with Special Healthcare Needs,*
Utah State Office of Education, August 1992

6. Procedures for failure of life-sustaining equipment (if any): _____

    _____

7. Wheelchair restraint checklist: (check all that apply)

seat belt	❏ on	❏ off	❏	headrest up
chest harness	❏ on	❏ off	❏	abductor in place
wheelchair brakes	❏ on	❏ off	❏	other _____
tray	❏ on	❏ off		_____

8. Positioning and handling requirements: _____

    _____

    _____

9. Substitute bus drivers.

    Name: _____   Phone: _____

    Name: _____   Phone: _____

10. The bus driver and substitute(s) received training regarding the student's special needs.

    ❏ yes   ❏ no   Date of Training: _____

STUDENT-SPECIFIC EMERGENCIES:

If you see this...	Do this...

Source: *Guidelines for Serving Students with Special Healthcare Needs,*
Utah State Office of Education, August 1992

STUDENTS WITH SPECIAL HEALTH CARE NEEDS

TRAINING PLAN

_____   _____   _____
Date   Instructor   Person Trained

TYPE OF TRAINING _____

_____

_____

_____

Recommendations for follow-up and further training: _____

_____

Recheck Recommended: _____

_____   _____   _____
Date   Instructor   Person Trained

TYPE OF TRAINING _____

_____

_____

_____

Recommendations for follow-up and further training: _____

_____

Recheck Recommended: _____

_____   _____   _____
Date   Instructor   Person Trained

TYPE OF TRAINING _____

_____

_____

_____

Recommendations for follow-up and further training: _____

_____

Recheck Recommended: _____

Source: _Guidelines for Serving Students with Special Healthcare Needs,_
Utah State Office of Education, August 1992

STUDENTS WITH SPECIAL HEALTH CARE NEEDS

REFERRAL CHECKLIST   SCHOOL_____

STUDENT'S NAME_____   DOB_____

Person Completing Form_____   DATE_____

Does the Student:	YES	NO	COMMENTS
1. Have a medical diagnosis of a chronic health problem (such as: diabetes, tuberculosis, seizures, cystic fibrosis, asthma, muscular dystrophy, liver disease digestive disorders, respiratory disorder, hemophilia, etc.)? Condition_____			
2. Receive medical treatments during or outside the school day (such as: oxygen, gastrostomy care, special diet, tracheostomy care, suctioning, injections, etc.)? Condition_____			
3. Experience frequent absences due to illness?			
4. Experience frequent hospitalizations?			
5. Receive ongoing medication for physical or emotional problems (such as: seizure, heart, allergy, asthma, cancer, depression, etc.)? Medications_____			
6. Require adjustments of the school environment or schedule due to a health condition (such as: rest following a seizure, limitation in physical activity, periodic break for endurance, part-time schedule, building modifications for access, etc.)?			
7. Require environmental adjustments to classroom or school facilities (such as: temperature control, refrigeration/medication storage, availability of running water, etc.)?			
8. Require major safety considerations (such as: special precautions in lifting, special transportation, emergency plan, special safety equipment, special techniques for positioning, feeding, etc.)?			

Nurse _____   Date _____   Phone_____

Source: *Guidelines for Serving Students with Special Healthcare Needs,*
Utah State Office of Education, August 1992

STUDENTS WITH SPECIAL HEALTH CARE NEEDS

STUDENT INFORMATION   DATE_____

Personal

Student Name _____   Date of Birth _____

School _____   Age _____

Grade in School _____   Male / Female   Height_____   Weight_____

Contacts

Mother's Name_____

Mother's Address _____

Mother's Home Telephone _____   Work Telephone _____   Emerg. Telephone No._____

Father's Name_____

Father's Address_____

Father's Home Telephone _____   Work Telephone _____   Emerg. Telephone No._____

Guardian's Name_____

Guardian's Address_____

Guardian's Home Telephone_____   Work Telephone _____   Emerg. Telephone No._____

Physician   _____   Telephone No._____

Physician Address_____

Hospital Emergency Room_____   Telephone No._____

Hospital Address_____

Ambulance Service_____   Telephone No._____

School Nurse_____   Telephone No._____

School Liaison _____   Extension _____

Direct Care Staff_____   Extension _____

Medical

Diagnosis _____

Medications_____

Side Effects_____

Necessary Health Care Procedures at School_____

_____

_____

Health Care Plan for Period _____   to _____

Other Important Information ☐ *(check box if additional information is on back)*

Source: *Guidelines for Serving Students with Special Healthcare Needs,*
Utah State Office of Education, August 1992

STUDENTS WITH SPECIAL HEALTH CARE NEEDS

PHYSICIAN'S ORDER
FOR SPECIALIZED HEALTH CARE PROCEDURES

Student: _____

THE PHYSICIAN'S ORDER SHOULD BE UPDATED AT LEAST ANNUALLY.

HEALTH CARE PROCEDURES

Condition for which procedure is required: _____

_____

_____

Description of standardized procedure(s): _____

_____

_____

Precautions and possible adverse reactions and interventions: _____

_____

_____

Time schedule and suggested environment procedure(s): _____

_____

_____

The procedure is to be continued as above until (date): _____

_____

_____

Dietary recommendations: _____

_____

_____

Activity limitations: _____

_____

_____

Source: *Guidelines for Serving Students with Special Healthcare Needs,*
Utah State Office of Education, August 1992

MEDICATION PROCEDURES

Medications _____

Dose _____

Time _____

Procedure _____

Expected effects on learning _____

_____

Medications _____

Dose _____

Time _____

Procedure _____

Expected effects on learning _____

_____

PARENT AUTHORIZATION

I, _____, request the above health care procedures and/or medication treatment be administered to my child at school. I understand that qualified, designated person(s) will be performing these health care services. I will notify the school immediately if my child's health status changes, or there is a change or cancellation of the procedure/medication(s).

_____   _____
Parent/Guardian Signature   Date

PHYSICIAN AUTHORIZATION

❏   I have reviewed the Health Care Plan and approve of it as written.

❏   I have reviewed the Health Care Plan and approve of it with the attached amendments.

❏   I do not approve of the Health Care Plan. A substitute plan is attached.

_____   _____
Physician Signature   Date

Source: *Guidelines for Serving Students with Special Healthcare Needs,*
Utah State Office of Education, August 1992

STUDENTS WITH SPECIAL HEALTH CARE NEEDS

MEDICATION / TREATMENT / ADMINISTRATION RECORD

Student:_____   School:_____

Physician:_____   Grade:_____ DOB:_____

Date:_____

☐ Employee designated and trained to administer medication

Employee Name(s):_____

MEDICATIONS

Medication	Time / Frequency	Dosage	How Given	Possible Effects on Learning and Physical Functioning
1)				
2)				
3)				
4)				
5)				

Medication / Treatment Administration / Supervision		Medication / Treatment Administration / Supervision By Signature	Medication / Treatment Administration / Supervision		Medication / Treatment Administration / Supervision By Signature
Date	Time	Signature	Date	Time	Signature

Source: *Guidelines for Serving Students with Special Healthcare Needs,*
Utah State Office of Education, August 1992

Medication / Treatment Administration / Supervision		Medication / Treatment Administration / Supervision By Signature	Medication / Treatment Administration / Supervision		Medication / Treatment Administration / Supervision By Signature
Date	Time	Signature	Date	Time	Signature

Source: *Guidelines for Serving Students with Special Healthcare Needs,*
Utah State Office of Education, August 1992

STUDENTS WITH SPECIAL HEALTH CARE NEEDS

ADMINISTRATION OF MEDICATION CHECKLIST

The following checklist is to help school districts determine if they are consistent with state law regarding the administration of medication.

YES	NO	*The School District:*
_____	_____	1. Has designated employees who may administer medication.
_____	_____	2. Has a policy for proper identification and safekeeping of medication.
_____	_____	3. Has provided training for designated employees.
_____	_____	4. Has a procedure for the maintenance of records for administration.
_____	_____	5. Has current parent or guardian written and signed permission for medication to be administered at school.
_____	_____	6. Has a copy of the student's health care provider's signed statement describing the method, amount, and time schedule for administration.
_____	_____	7. Has a copy of the student's health care provider's statement that administration for medication by school employees during the school day is necessary.

Source: *Guidelines for Serving Students with Special Healthcare Needs,*
Utah State Office of Education, August 1992

Index